Veterinary Controversies and Ethical Dilemmas

This book identifies increasing concerns with the veterinary profession and confronts them provocatively, with a view to stimulating positive change. A central theme is the emergence of the profitable 'fur baby', which is being propagated through encouraged anthropomorphism, a limited evidence base, overdiagnosis, overtreatment, and practice corporatisation. Richly accompanied with thoughts on veterinary celebrity, the misrepresentation of veterinary 'success', research using client-owned animals, unregulated treatments and end-of-life decision-making, the book represents a small room full of large elephants. With experienced contributors from around the world, each chapter combines personal stories with evidence-based reflections.

While many of the subjects presented will have undergone some degree of ethical analysis, the book itself does not intend to teach veterinary ethics; instead, its role is to identify key concerns with the profession's current trajectory and to present them with candour, from the perspective of concerned veterinary professionals.

Ideal for use within the veterinary curriculum to stimulate undergraduate thought and discussion, this book will also be a valuable reference for practitioners as the veterinary profession comes to terms with life in a post-truth era.

CRC One Health One Welfare

Learning from Disease in Pets: A 'One Health' Model for Discovery
Edited by Rebecca A. Krimins

Animals, Health and Society: Health Promotion, Harm Reduction and Equity in a One Health World
Edited by Craig Stephen

One Welfare in Practice: The Role of the Veterinarian
Edited by Tanya Stephens

Climate Change and Animal Health
Edited By Craig Stephen and Colleen Duncan

Animal Welfare in a Pandemic: What Does COVID-19 Tell us for the Future?
By John T. Hancock, Ros C. Rouse and Tim J. Craig

Global One Health and Infectious Diseases: An Interdisciplinary Practitioner's Guide
Edited By William E. Sander

One Health: Veterinary, Ethical, and Environmental Perspectives
By Michael W. Fox

Veterinary Controversies and Ethical Dilemmas: Provocative Reflections on Clinical Practice
Edited By Tanya Stephens, R. Eddie Clutton, Polly Taylor and Kathy L. Murphy

For more information about this series, please visit https://www.routledge.com/CRC-One-Health-One-Welfare/book-series/CRCOHOW

Veterinary Controversies and Ethical Dilemmas
Provocative Reflections on Clinical Practice

Edited by Tanya Stephens, R. Eddie Clutton,
Polly Taylor and Kathy L. Murphy

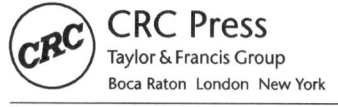

CRC Press
Taylor & Francis Group
Boca Raton London New York

CRC Press is an imprint of the
Taylor & Francis Group, an **informa** business

Designed Cover Image: Harry Stephens

First edition published 2026
by CRC Press
2385 NW Executive Center Drive, Suite 320, Boca Raton FL 33431

and by CRC Press
4 Park Square, Milton Park, Abingdon, Oxon, OX14 4RN

CRC Press is an imprint of Taylor & Francis Group, LLC

© 2026 selection and editorial matter, Tanya Stephens, R. Eddie Clutton, Polly Taylor, and Kathy L. Murphy; individual chapters, the contributors

Reasonable efforts have been made to publish reliable data and information, but the author and publisher cannot assume responsibility for the validity of all materials or the consequences of their use. The authors and publishers have attempted to trace the copyright holders of all material reproduced in this publication and apologize to copyright holders if permission to publish in this form has not been obtained. If any copyright material has not been acknowledged please write and let us know so we may rectify in any future reprint.

Except as permitted under U.S. Copyright Law, no part of this book may be reprinted, reproduced, transmitted, or utilized in any form by any electronic, mechanical, or other means, now known or hereafter invented, including photocopying, microfilming, and recording, or in any information storage or retrieval system, without written permission from the publishers.

For permission to photocopy or use material electronically from this work, access www.copyright.com or contact the Copyright Clearance Center, Inc. (CCC), 222 Rosewood Drive, Danvers, MA 01923, 978-750-8400. For works that are not available on CCC please contact mpkbookspermissions@tandf.co.uk

Trademark notice: Product or corporate names may be trademarks or registered trademarks and are used only for identification and explanation without intent to infringe.

ISBN: 978-1-032-58260-3 (hbk)
ISBN: 978-1-032-57986-3 (pbk)
ISBN: 978-1-003-44930-0 (cbk)

DOI: 10.1201/9781003449300

Typeset in Times
by Apex CoVantage, LLC

Contents

Foreword xix
Preface xxiii
Acknowledgements xxvii
About the Editors xxix
List of Contributors xxxiii

PART I Introduction

Chapter 1 Veterinary Controversies and Ethical Dilemmas:
An Introduction 3

R. Eddie Clutton

1.1 Changes in the Veterinary Profession 3
1.2 Ambivalent Beneficence 4
1.3 The Elephant in the Room 4
1.4 The Origin of the Book 5
1.5 Veterinary Overtreatment 5
1.6 Pets as Experimental Animals 6
1.7 Australian Developments 7
1.8 Contributors 7
1.9 Veterinary Curmudgeons 8
1.10 Jodi Ware 8
1.11 Final Thoughts 9

Chapter 2 Veterinary Killing: History and Ethics 10

Andrew Gardiner

2.1 Introduction 10
2.2 Killing and Caring 10
2.3 Killing as 'Treatment' 11
2.4 Caring about Killing: Technology and Techniques 14
  2.4.1 Companion Animals: Ethics and Aesthetics 14
2.5 Conclusion/Provocation 16

v

Chapter 3	The Law, Animals, and Veterinarians 20
	Peter Fordyce

	3.1	The Veterinary Surgeons Act 1966 and the Social Contract with Society 20
	3.2	The Law, Suffering, Sentience, and Ethics 21
	3.3	Common Law Property Rights and the Tension Between Legislative Ethical Imperatives: Anthropocentricism and Animals as a Means to a Human End 24
	3.4	Unnecessary Suffering and the Unwritten Social Contract Implicit within the VSA 1996 25
	3.5	Potential Sources of Ethical Conflict 27
	3.6	Summary 28

Chapter 4	Sentient Beings: Our Duty of Care: Who Are our Patients? 29
	John Webster

	4.1	Rights and Responsibilities; Moral Agents and Moral Patients 29
	4.2	Justice: The Ethical Matrix 31
	4.3	Justice for Pets 33
	4.4	Coda 34

Chapter 5	Let's all March for (Veterinary) Science: Veterinary Science in a Post-Truth Society 36
	Tanya Stephens

	5.1	Marching for Science 36
	5.2	Evidence-Based Veterinary Medicine (EBVM) 37
	5.3	Can we Trust the Evidence? 38
	5.4	Caregiver Placebo Effects 40
	5.5	Living Longer and Better Lives 40
	5.6	Does the Public Trust Veterinarians? 41
	5.7	Science, Ethics, and Clinical Decision-Making 41
	5.8	Veterinary Science in a Post-Truth Era 42

Contents

PART II Some Ethical Challenges Facing the Veterinary Profession

PART IIA Too Much Veterinary Medicine

Chapter 6 Just Because We Can Doesn't Mean We Should 47

Polly Taylor

Chapter 7 Overdiagnosis 50

Brennen McKenzie

    7.1   What is Overdiagnosis? 50
    7.2   How Do We Know Overdiagnosis Exists? 51
    7.3   What is the Harm of Overdiagnosis? 55
    7.4   What Causes Overdiagnosis? 57
    7.5   How Do We Reduce Overdiagnosis and Overtreatment? 58

Chapter 8 Do You Want Bloods with That? 60

Tanya Stephens

    8.1   Background 60
    8.2   If All Else Fails, Look at the Animal 61
    8.3   A Hypothetical Scenario 63
    8.4   Have I Changed My Mind? 64
    8.5   Good Guidelines would be Useful 66

Chapter 9 Oncology and Ethics 69

Tanya Stephens

    9.1   Background 69
    9.2   Prognosis 70
    9.3   Oncology, Chemotherapy, and Ethics 71
    9.4   Is Palliative Care in the Best Interests of an Animal? 72
    9.5   Should We be Euthanising Cancer Patients? 74
    9.6   Summary 75

Chapter 10 Small-Animal Overtreatment: Intensive Care 77

Peter Fordyce

10.1 Intensive Care 77
10.2 The Problem of Recognising What Suffering is in
      Animals, and Quantifying it 80
10.3 Confounding Human Factors Potentially Obscuring
      The Patient's Best Interests... 82
10.4 What Might be Done to Help Avoid Overtreatment
      in the Vicu?... 85

PART IIB Research on Companion Animals

Chapter 11 Innovation versus Experimentation: Experiments on Pets? 89

Polly Taylor

11.1 Fido.. 89
11.2 Innovation Versus Experiment... 89
11.3 Experiments on Pets 90
11.4 Clinical Veterinary Research 92
11.5 Independent Ethical Review 94
11.6 Informed Owner Consent 94
11.7 Where Now?... 94

Chapter 12 Veterinary Ethical Review – A Multitude of Questions 97

Stephen N. Greenhalgh

12.1 Introduction 97
12.2 Why (Should Ethical Review be Undertaken)?................... 97
12.3 What (Should Undergo Ethical Review)? 98
    12.3.1 Retrospective, or Secondary, Use of
            (Clinical) Data 99
    12.3.2 Retrospective, or Secondary, Use of Tissue
            or Previously Collected Samples 99
    12.3.3 Observational Research 99
    12.3.4 Interventional Research 100
    12.3.5 Zoological or Wildlife Research......................... 100
    12.3.6 Conservation or Management Practices 100
    12.3.7 Obtaining Data About Animals from Humans.... 100
    12.3.8 Secondary Use of Tissue (or Data) from
            Experimental Animal Research 100
    12.3.9 Clinical Case Management 101

		12.3.10	Use of Animals in Teaching and Education 101
		12.3.11	Use of Animals for Food Production, Clothing, Sport, Work, and Service etc 101
		12.3.12	Setting the Bar for Ethical Review 101
	12.4	When (Should Ethical Review be Undertaken)? 102
	12.5	Who (Should Undertake the Ethical Review)? 103
	12.6	Where (Should the Ethical Review be Carried Out)? 105
	12.7	How (Should the Ethical Review be Carried Out)? 106
	12.8	Conclusion 106

Chapter 13 Can Considering Laboratory Animal Legislation Improve Animal Welfare in Innovative Veterinary Practice? 109

Ngaire Dennison

13.1	Background 109
13.2	The Legislation 109
13.3	Harm Benefit Analysis 110
13.4	ASPA; Other Legal Requirements 110
13.5	The 3Rs (Table 13.1) 111
13.6	AWERBs 112
13.7	Calculating Study of Harms of Under ASPA 112
13.8	Predicting Study Success and Subsequent Benefits Under ASPA 113
13.9	Harm–Benefit Analysis Under ASPA 114
13.10	How Similar Procedures are Restricted by the Veterinary Surgeons Act 114
13.11	Routine Veterinary Practice 114
13.12	Confusion Over Clinical Veterinary Research 116
13.13	Can ASPA Assist in Clinical Decision-Making? 116
13.14	Lack of Transparency in Ethical Decision-Making in Veterinary Practice 117
13.15	Lack of Independent Oversight of Decisions 117
13.16	Lack of a Robust System Evaluating the Animal's Overall Experience 118
13.17	Animal Advocacy 120
13.18	Mixed Messages: The Profession and the Public 120
13.19	Inadequacy of Current Systems 121
13.20	Lack of Clarity in Critical Terminology 121
13.21	What Can be Learned from Laboratory Animal Practice? 121
13.22	Summary 122

PART IIC Evidence-free Veterinary Medicine

Chapter 14 Why Believe in Magic? The use of Ineffective Therapies has Welfare and Ethical Implications 127

Tanya Stephens

- 14.1 Introduction 127
- 14.2 Complementary and Alternative Veterinary Medicine (CAVM): Where is the Evidence for Increasing Demand? 128
- 14.3 Where is the Evidence? What is the Point of Needless Needling? 130
- 14.4 CAVM and Animal Health and Welfare 132
- 14.5 Donkeys, Bears & Pangolins 132
- 14.6 The Pet Wellness Industry 133
- 14.7 Counteracting CAVM 134

Chapter 15 Should Complementary and Alternative Veterinary Medicine be Considered Malpractice? An Ethical–Legal Analysis 137

Manuel Magalhães Sant'Ana and Alexandre Azevedo

- 15.1 Background 137
- 15.2 Alternative Medicine – What's in a Name? 138
- 15.3 Regulatory Approaches to CAVM 139
- 15.4 CAVM and Professional Malpractice 141
- 15.5 Recommendations 143
- 15.6 Disclosure Statement 143

Chapter 16 Pointless Supplements and 'Therapeutic' Pet Foods 146

Andrea Tarr

- 16.1 What are Supplements? 146
- 16.2 Do Pets Need Supplements? 147
- 16.3 So Why do Pet Owners Buy Supplements? 147
- 16.4 Giving an Impression of Efficacy 148
- 16.5 Why is Evidence of Efficacy Needed for Supplements? 149
- 16.6 They Can't do Any Harm Can They? 150
- 16.7 Pet Owners Need Help to Make Better Choices 150

PART IID   Exotic Animal Medicine

Chapter 17 Zoo Vet Dilemmas – A Personal Perspective 155

Andrew Routh

    17.1   Introduction 155
    17.2   What is a Zoo? 155
    17.3   What is a Zoo Vet? 156
    17.4   Regulation, Legislation, and Zoo Ethics 157
    17.5   The Patients 159
    17.6   Detecting Illness 160
    17.7   How to Treat a Patient 160
    17.8   When Not to Treat a Patient 161
    17.9   Overall Welfare 162
    17.10 Husbandry and Managing the Captive Population 162
    17.11 The Goal 163
    17.12 Conclusion 164

Chapter 18 The Value of Mice 166

R. Eddie Clutton and Amanda Novak

    18.1   Introduction 166
    18.2   The Implicit and Explicit Values of Animals 166
    18.3   Wild Mice: History and Intrinsic Value 168
    18.4   Wild Mice: Extrinsic Value 169
    18.5   Wild Mice: Legal and Ethical Considerations 169
    18.6   Wild Mice and Veterinary Care 170
    18.7   Pet Mice: History and Intrinsic Value 170
    18.8   Pet Mice: Extrinsic Value 171
    18.9   Pet Mice: Legal and Ethical Considerations 172
    18.10 Pet Mice and Veterinary Care 172
    18.11 Laboratory Mice: History and Intrinsic Value 173
    18.12 Laboratory Mice: Extrinsic Value 174
    18.13 Laboratory Mice: Legal and Ethical Considerations 176
    18.14 Laboratory Mice and Veterinary Care 176
    18.15 Conclusion 177

PART III Why Are These Controversies Arising Through Changes at Numerous Levels of the Veterinary–Client–Patient Relationship?

PART IIIA The Animal Population

Chapter 19 Problems with Pedigrees: Righteous Rage and the Need for Nuance 183

Alison Skipper

    19.1   Introduction 183
    19.2   Background 183
    19.3   The Controversy 184
    19.4   Pathways to Progress? 185
    19.5   Bothersome Breeders 186
    19.6   Veterinary Re-Evaluation? 188
    19.7   Conclusion 189

Chapter 20 Ageing Pets and Physical Rehabilitation 192

Mary Ellen Goldberg, Sheilah Robertson, and Polly Taylor

    20.1   Introduction 192
    20.2   Physiology of Ageing 192
    20.3   Quality of Life 194
    20.4   Physical Rehabilitation for Ageing Animals 194
            20.4.1   Pain Management 195
            20.4.2   Physical Therapy 196
            20.4.3   Environmental Adjustments 197
    20.5   Life Cannot be Prolonged Forever 197
    20.6   Conclusion 198

PART IIIB The Veterinary Profession

Chapter 21 Veterinary Education and the Changing Profession 203

Sarah Wolfensohn

    21.1   Different Approaches to Treatment 203
    21.2   The Effect of Business Ownership and Pet Health Insurance 204
    21.3   Veterinary Specialisation 206

	21.4	Ensuring Good Animal Welfare 206
	21.5	The Bigger Picture – Influencing Policy and Legislation 208

Chapter 22 The Art of Veterinary Science 211

Kendal Shepherd

	22.1	Background 211
	22.2	What is 'The Art'? 212
	22.3	The Consultation 213
	22.4	Behaviour of the Patient 214
	22.5	Euthanasia 214
	22.6	Guilt – A Salutary Tale 215
	22.7	The 'Art' of Consulting 216
	22.8	Record-Keeping 216
	22.9	Student Selection 217
	22.10	Accepting Help without Losing Face 218
	22.11	'Having a Go' 218

Chapter 23 Veterinary Academia, Clinical Specialisation, and Animal Welfare 221

R. Eddie Clutton

	23.1	Introduction 221
	23.2	Veterinary School Curricula 222
	23.3	Clinical Specialisation 223
	23.4	Clinical Specialisation and Undergraduate Education 224
	23.5	Gold Standard Care 225
	23.6	Studies using Client-Owned Animals 226
	23.7	Clinical Ethical Review Committees 227
	23.8	The Moral Disassembly of Veterinary Graduates 229
	23.9	Conclusion 229

Chapter 24 What are General Practitioners Good for? 231

Brennen McKenzie

Chapter 25 Do Vets Need to Love Animals? 238

Kathy L. Murphy

	25.1	Introduction 238
	25.2	Is Love Necessary for Good Animal Welfare? 239
	25.3	Is Love Sufficient for Good Animal Welfare? 239
	25.4	The Dual Role of the Veterinarian 241

25.5	The Changing Landscape of the Veterinary Profession	241
25.6	The Complexity of Human-Animal Relationships	243
25.7	Governance, Pragmatism, and the Limits of Love	243
25.8	Conclusion: Love as a Potential Advantage but not a Necessity	245

Chapter 26 It is Time to Ditch the Gold Standard 247

Tanya Stephens

26.1	Background	247
26.2	The Mythical Gold Standard	248
26.3	What is the Gold Standard Anyway?	249
26.4	The Spectrum of Care and Evidence-Based Veterinary Medicine	250
26.5	Costs of Veterinary Services	251
26.6	Human Behaviour and EBVM	253
26.7	Best Evidence is Best!	253

Chapter 27 Informed Consent – In Whose Interests? 256

Carol A. Gray

27.1	Introduction – If Our Patients Could Give Consent	256
27.2	We Need to Talk About Money	257
27.3	We Need to Talk About Best Interests	258
27.4	We Need to Talk About Shared Decision-Making	259
27.5	We Need to Talk About Contextualised Care	260
27.6	We Need to Come Back to Informed Consent	262
27.7	We Need to Consider the Practical Aspects of the Consent Process	263

Chapter 28 The Death of Veterinary Euthanasia 265

R. Eddie Clutton

28.1	Introduction	265
28.2	Changing Attitudes to Animal Euthanasia	265
28.3	Reasons for Eschewing Animal Euthanasia	267
28.4	Palliation and Hospice	267
28.5	Client-Driven Treatment in Preference to Palliation, Hospice, or Euthanasia	267
28.6	Client-Driven Treatment with Veterinary Concurrence	268
28.7	Veterinarian-Driven Treatment with Owner Concerns	269

	28.8	Too Expensive to Die?.. 269
	28.9	Fewer Convenience Killings?... 270
	28.10	Concerns with Complex Ethical Questions Concerning Animal Euthanasia 270
	28.11	Over-Moralised Vets?... 270
	28.12	Genuine Advances in Veterinary Medicine 271
	28.13	Gold Standard Care 271
	28.14	Specialisation and Credentials.. 272
	28.15	A Taboo Subject?... 273
	28.16	Conclusion 273

Chapter 29 Moral Stress, Emotional Labour, and Mental Health in the Veterinary Profession 276

Vanessa Ashall

	29.1	Introduction 276
	29.2	Saturday Morning... 276

PART IIIC Veterinary Practice

Chapter 30 The Customer Isn't Always Right: Why Business Ethics is not Professional Ethics 287

Tanya Stephens

	30.1	Background.. 287
	30.2	What is a Profession?... 289
	30.3	Moral Reasoning 289
	30.4	Veterinary Professional Ethics... 289
	30.5	Ethical Issues Unique to the Veterinary Profession........ 290
	30.6	Business Ethics 291
	30.7	'The Customer is Always Right' 292
	30.8	Who is the Customer? 292
	30.9	Professional Ethics Vs Business Ethics........................... 292
	30.10	Veterinary Practice as a Business 293
	30.11	Ethical Issues Associated with the Costs of Veterinary Service 293
	30.12	Contemporary Factors that Can Have an Impact on Veterinary Professional Ethics.. 294
	30.13	Strengthening Ethical Practices 295
	30.14	Summary... 295

Chapter 31 Corporatisation: Do Shareholders Care about Animal Welfare? ... 297

John Innes

 31.1 Introduction 297
 31.2 Why do Consolidators Exist? 298
 31.3 How do Funding Models Influence Company Behaviour? 299
 31.4 Collateral Effects of Consolidation 300
 31.5 Benefits of Consolidation 301
 31.6 Future Perspectives 302

Chapter 32 Costs of Veterinary Services as an Animal Welfare Issue 304

Nigel R. Taylor

 32.1 Addendum 311

PART IIID *Veterinary Clients*

Chapter 33 Anthropomorphism in Veterinary Practice 315

R. Eddie Clutton

 33.1 Introduction 315
 33.2 History 315
 33.3 Science and Anthropomorphism 317
 33.4 Changes in the Human–Companion Animal Bond 318
 33.5 Anthropomorphism in Veterinary Practice 319
 33.6 Anthropomorphism and Public Health 319
 33.7 Anthropomorphism and Animal Benefits 319
 33.8 The Human Benefits of Anthropomorphism 320
 33.9 Anthropocentricism and Animal Harms 320
 33.10 Anthropomorphic Owners and Animal Harms 320
 33.11 Anthropomorphism and the Veterinarian-Client Relationship 321
 33.12 Anthropomorphic Owners 321
 33.13 Anthropomorphic Vets 322
 33.14 The Perfect (Anthropocentric) Storm 322
 33.15 Anthropomorphism, Anthropocentricism, and Death 322
 33.16 Conclusions 323

Contents   xvii

Chapter 34 Going to Extremes: High Financial Cost, Overtreatment
and Palliative Care 326

Polly Taylor

    34.1   Funding Advanced Veterinary Treatment 326
                34.1.1   Insurance 327
                34.1.2   Crowdfunding 328
                34.1.3   Lines of Credit 328
    34.2   Overtreatment 328
                34.2.1   Gold Standard Treatment 329
    34.3   End of Life and Palliative Care 330

Chapter 35 Give the Dog a Bone 333

Tanya Stephens

    35.1   Pets are Plentiful 333
    35.2   The Carbon Pawprint 335
    35.3   Should Dogs and Cats be Vegan? 336
    35.4   Robotic Pets 339
    35.5   Is it Time to 'Eat the Dog'? 340

PART IIIE   Vets in Society

Chapter 36 Is the Veterinary Profession Encouraging Exploitation of
Horses in Sport? 345

Sue Dyson

    36.1   A Personal Experience 345
    36.2   Conflicting Pressures 346
    36.3   Establishing Moral and Ethical Boundaries 346
    36.4   Appropriate Training to Deal with the Challenges 348
    36.5   Communication between Veterinarians and Clients;
the Conflicts that Fee Scales Generate and Managing
Clients' Expectations 348
    36.6   The Conflicts Generated by the Pressures of Horse
Sports 349
                36.6.1   Steeplechasing 350
                36.6.2   Flat Racing 350
                36.6.3   Eventing 351
                36.6.4   Dressage 352
                36.6.5   Showjumping 352
                36.6.6   Western Performance Horses 352

	36.6.7	Endurance 353
	36.6.8	Bull Fighting and Rodeos 353
	36.6.9	Showing 353
	36.6.10	Polo 354
	36.6.11	Lower-Level Sports and Leisure Horses 354
36.7	Conclusions 354

Chapter 37 Vets Speaking up for Animal Welfare 356

Sean Wensley

37.1	Veterinary Animal Welfare Responsibility 356
37.2	Veterinary Animal Welfare Strategies 357
37.3	Veterinary Animal Welfare Advocacy 359
37.4	Ongoing Challenges 361
37.5	A Two-Tier Veterinary Profession? 364
37.6	A Three-Stage Evolution 365

Chapter 38 An Approach to Ethical Conflicts in Clinical Practice 368

Brennen McKenzie

38.1	Introduction 368
38.2	General Principles of Medical Ethics 370
	38.2.1 Preserving Life Versus Relieving Suffering 372
38.3	An Approach to Clinical Ethics? 372
	38.3.1 What is Best for the Patient? 374
	38.3.2 What Does the Owner Want, Need, and Believe about their Pet's Needs? 376
	38.3.3 What Limitations are Imposed by the Context? 377
	38.3.4 What is the Best Approach to Meet the Needs of the Patient within the Limits Set by the Owner and General Context? 378
	38.3.5 It's a Circle, not a Point 379
38.4	Managing Conflict and Disagreements about Patient Care 380

Index 383

Foreword

I've often been asked what kept me awake at night in my days as a partner in a large-animal and mixed-animal practice. I've answered, 'Money worries, human resource issues, dissatisfied clients, not enough vets to carry out all the work that builds up after a bank holiday'. However, nobody ever asked what *haunted* me and, for that matter, no one still does.

Quite simply, it is when I got animal welfare wrong, whatever the species – dog, cat, cow, sheep, or horse. Whether it was due to my ignorance or whether, together with the owner, we embarked on a course of action which, in uncomfortable hindsight, was not in the animal's best interests. I signed up all those years ago to ensure animals' health and welfare came first. However, it took time to fully appreciate that there can be a difference between health and welfare, usually taken as synonymous. This realisation increased the migraine of ethical dilemmas. This book would have helped me to navigate through the complexities of owner attitudes, my perceptions of the profession's expectations, and all the wonderful diagnostics and treatments at my disposal, without losing sight of the most important factor – the patient's welfare. I was very struck by one of the contributor's insightful questions – 'What do you think your dog would prefer and why?' (see Kendal Shepherd, Chapter 22). This is also an insight into this intriguing book.

I became a trustee for the BVA's Animal Welfare Foundation selfishly to be surrounded by both experts in the welfare field and evidence-based studies, hoping that by osmosis the position could help me understand and calibrate my moral compass. One of the charity's key events is the discussion forum, where we hear from experts in their fields and together discuss contentious issues affecting animal welfare and our profession, including topics around overtreatment, all done in a comfortable space. In many cases, the issues discussed have resulted in further debate and action within the profession. Well, here is a similar discussion, but on steroids.

I know, and am in awe of, a number of the authors involved in this work, including two of the editors, Polly Taylor and R. Eddie Clutton, both highly regarded experts in their field who have spoken at various forums on overtreatment and overdiagnosis and are ardent in their views – with justification. Other contributors I've the pleasure of knowing and working with include a former AWF trustee Sean Wensley and Sarah Wolfensohn, both of whom have spoken frequently for AWF and are widely recognised leaders in animal welfare. So I forgave myself for being both apprehensive and honoured in equal measure to be asked to write this foreword, even more so after reading the absorbing contributions from all the authors.

I read this to the gentle accompaniment of the sound of Maud drinking, an abandoned cat we adopted some years ago. She was plagued by awful skin disease which no doubt led to her abandonment, and it took an enormous effort from both of us to eventually control. 'Why don't you put her to sleep?' was a question I was often asked. What was the motivation in asking? Was it because they thought she was suffering (indeed she was), or was it because of the endless pills being administered, entailing a daily fracas neither of us relished? Was it because of an understandable degree of revulsion at her appearance? Few people were willing to touch her. Was it because of the cost of all the diagnostics and treatment? I often wondered which of these, if not all, were the original reason for her abandonment. However, she and I persevered.

Now her kidneys are not what they used to be; she is rapidly becoming an old cat. 'What would you do if it was yours?' is now ringing in my ears, a familiar question from the consult room and one I have to admit I am struggling to answer.

Why do I mention this? This collaborative book is one I wish I had had to hand in my practice days, even better when I was a student with the prospect of qualifying soon; it has expertly recalibrated my sometimes-uncertain moral compass regarding what levels of diagnostics and treatment to impose on the cat, bringing with it a welcoming sense of comfort and assurance.

The book is a compelling read, enhanced by contributions from multiple authors. Each brings their own style and perspective to a captivatingly wide variety of topics, ranging from the history of our profession, ageing pets, zoo animals, the art of veterinary medicine to students' education. Some topics, such as laboratory mice, may seem initially unrelated to daily practice, but I found them to be surprisingly relevant and thought-provoking as they explore many themes, attitudes, and even relevant laws regarding animal treatment and consequent welfare. One of the joys of the discussion forums is hearing about other disciplines and species and finding there is a commonality, shared values, and relevance found among all veterinarians which all go towards fine-tuning that moral compass, as many tell me afterwards.

I relished the fact that the contents are both delightfully controversial and deliberately provocative. While you may not agree with all their stances or the conclusions, and I found myself bristling on occasion, it is important to be challenged in an authoritative way; it didn't half make me think as their papers are expertly laid out, backed with evidence. This is a unique book offering an intriguing mix of being an informative, educational, thought-provoking, and valuable reference resource; above all, animal welfare rings out.

One of the great joys of our profession is the ever-advancing knowledge, skills, and multitude of tools at our disposal, including the findings of proper scientific research on animal welfare. Having read this collection of expert opinions, I was left with that gratifying sense of satisfaction bestowed when you finally understand some complex pathophysiology and how the appropriate treatment works.

The authors are not trying to turn the clock back 30 years to rose-tinted halcyon days, a critique that could be thrown at the book without having truly read the contents first. Such expertise takes time to accumulate, along with arguments to

Foreword

become ordered. 'Been there, done it, and have the T-shirt' (covering the scars of practice?) is a useful attribute to have.

'Well, the stances here are going to stifle our profession's clinical advancement' is another critique some may aim at this book. It's a stance familiar to the medical profession in the past, where the pendulum of law swung between favouring the medics or the law. Some within the medical profession were arrogantly keen on performing their own experimental procedures, citing it was needed to advance medicine; now this is much less so a result of the use of evidence-based medicine, much to the benefit of patient's welfare. It is interesting to see how a similar conflict exists within our profession, as highlighted by many of the authors who do offer solutions and alternatives rather than just highlighting the problems (this book is far from naïve). A take-home message, whether for the medical or veterinary profession, is the giving and gaining of proper informed consent. Something we could learn from the medical profession?

An unexpected side effect of reading this book was to be filled with renewed pride in having been a GP vet, such that I almost wanted to get back into the clinic – luckily for the sake of animal welfare, I will abstain.

So as Maud (an Old German name meaning 'powerful battler') now totters off to insistently scratch at her litter tray – a teeth-grinding noise – I ponder again, what should I do? Am I falling into the trap of 'the cobbler's children are the worst shod'? Or should I be doing more? Have I done 'gold standard diagnostics and treatment' because she deserves it or because I am bowing to perceived peer or public pressure? No, I am going to take her welfare first because I know her better than anyone, and I follow a pragmatic approach or a 'contextualised care' approach – a much better terminology and an approach the BVA is keen to promote.

Although not the primary aim of this book, it has been a surprising help in shaping my own ethical understanding and stance – recalibration of the moral compass. Developing this critical faculty is essential for all of us when we deal with animals and their welfare. This work offers us valuable insights that can help us determine one's own stance between health and welfare.

Monty Python (referenced within the book) had a sketch where someone keen for an argument paid the argument clinic – well, buy this book and have a good one. We exist in polarised times – right or wrong. It is never binary, and whilst the contributors have a strong standpoint, eloquently and expertly presented, here is a chance to ruminate and, if necessary, agree disagreeably. Our profession is being uncomfortably buffeted at the moment as it faces question and scrutiny. We cannot be entirely innocent of this, and the views here question why and proffer some answers. Has that pendulum swung too far towards the mythical 'gold standard' and heroic treatments, expensive machines that go bleep (Monty Python again), and dazzling diagnostics?

Collectively, as a profession, we must be accessible to everyone, not just to those with deep pockets. Our focus should not be exclusively on the disease to the costs, literal and metaphorical, of the pet and their owner. Instead, we should focus our efforts more holistically so that we treat the individual client and their pet as well – a contextualised care approach – whilst constantly prioritising the pet's welfare, even when this, in all honesty, means euthanasia. Should we make a stand against this perplexity of 'fur babies', 'gold standard' treatments, and often misguided owner perceptions about what is best for their pet? Now that we have this book, perhaps that's one thing less to lose sleep about.

Julian Kupfer
Chair of the Board of Trustees
Animal Welfare Foundation

Preface

As a practitioner, with a particular interest in professional ethics, I have for some time expressed a concern regarding some aspects of contemporary veterinary practice. When Alice Oven (senior editor, *Veterinary Medicine*, Taylor and Francis/CRC Press) and I were chatting about this, Alice suggested the possibility of editing another book in their veterinary series. It became very clear to us that there were more than enough contemporary and controversial issues to fill a book. I have not been alone with these concerns, and I therefore reached out to R. Eddie Clutton, Polly Taylor, and Kathy L. Murphy, to join me as co-editors. When we sought expressions of interest from potential contributors, it quickly became obvious that one book might not be enough to cover the subject as the response was so enthusiastic. With our efforts hugely shored up by Jodi Ware, the project took off.

As a longstanding small-animal practitioner and practice owner I am at the coalface of the effects of societal changes on veterinary practice, as well as changes within the profession, such as the emergence of the term 'veterinary industry' (even though we don't work in factories) and veterinary practice as a 'business', and I am all too aware of the challenges associated with practice ownership. Nevertheless, I find practice most enjoyable and rewarding, even the parts which involve dealing with difficult two-legged animals, and I find it an enormously satisfying occupation. I can't imagine doing anything else. I am pleased to be able to enjoy the positive advancements which allow me to better care for animals and their owners, whilst at the same time I feel comfortable expressing concerns about some aspects of veterinary practice which I think are problematic.

The key role of professional ethics can be lost in today's world; however, it is important that veterinarians acknowledge that an essential aspect of being a professional is a need for self-reflection, which is particularly relevant for practitioners making clinical decisions. Any profession where the entrenched professional response to a problem is to reflect on it, seek to understand it, and link it to knowledge, beliefs, values, and practice will often respond more effectively to challenges.

This is what this book aims to do. Contributors were asked to write about contemporary and controversial issues from a personal and professional perspective, providing an opinion piece with few references rather than an academic paper. Whether you agree with them or not is less important than whether they make you think: the aim of the book is to give contributors a voice and engage in debate about the current state of the profession with the aim to stimulate positive changes in areas found wanting.

The book is certainly not a criticism of the profession. Clearly, there are some things that are not quite right in the profession. The high dropout rate of new graduates and falling trust (at least in Australia, where I am) and mental health concerns are just three examples, but there are many more which are dealt with in this book, alongside reflections on being a veterinarian. The book covers a wide range of views from a wide range of authors who have shared their thoughts and ideas.

Hopefully, these reflections and comments will inspire future generations of veterinarians to realise that they are in a great profession where critical examination is acceptable and will lead to better public awareness and appreciation of our role in society. All too often there is an emphasis on ethical dilemmas making life difficult for practitioners, whilst for me these dilemmas (which should be called challenges as they aren't between two choices) are what makes practice so interesting and intellectually stimulating.

Surveys have shown that the public wants veterinarians to demonstrate accountability and transparency, care about animal welfare, possess good clinical skills, be professional, have good client relationships, and not have money-making as their first priority.

It is therefore disturbing to read that, in Australia at least, trust in the profession is falling, and we are considered less trustworthy than teachers, pharmacists, nurses, and firefighters. At least we're above politicians and used-car salesmen, if that is any consolation. Unfortunately, if there is a loss of trust in the profession, it risks losing its social license to operate, and if the public no longer trusts the profession, there is a risk we will lose our special status. This isn't a case of defending our privileged place in society but ensuring that, as professionals bound by rules, regulations, and professional ethics, we rightly remain the primary source of information on animal health and welfare.

Veterinarians have had to deal with changes in the profession, from education, specialisation, new diagnostic tools, new therapies, and changes in society, with pet owners becoming more demanding. It is said that new diagnostic tools and treatments have allowed companion animals to lead longer, healthier lives. However, these longer lives could partly be attributed to better preventative healthcare, including avoidance of fast-moving vehicles. Moreover, longer lives may not necessarily be happier ones if the animal is riddled with old-age ailments and the owner and veterinarian are reluctant to say the last goodbye. Increasing specialisation and lack of recognition of generalists and their connection to local communities is an ongoing topic of conversation in the profession.

It doesn't help that we live in a post-truth era where feelings are more important than facts, science has been downgraded, and opinion holds more attention than evidence. Anyone can tweet any kind of nonsense, and scientists' voices are drowned out in a sea of misinformation. Pity the poor practitioner who has to deal with the pet owner who has already consulted 'Dr Google' on their way to the practice and is now an 'expert' in veterinary matters. All this is more than enough reason for the veterinarian to avoid abrogating their professional responsibility onto the owner at the expense of the animal's health and welfare.

We know that all may not be well in the profession on a number of fronts. For example, a Pet Industry Association of Australia 2022 survey cited widespread dissatisfaction, high stress, understaffing, long working hours, and abuse by pet owners. A 2023 State of New South Wales (NSW) parliamentary inquiry into veterinary workplace shortages in the State received over 200 submissions. Approximately 85% of veterinary services are in the companion animal sector, and the pandemic led to an increase in pet ownership, at the same time as a move towards part-time and casual work. This change in workplace culture where veterinarians are no longer willing or able to work long hours and undertake after-hours on-call marks a seismic change in the profession.

On the other side of the world in the UK, the Competition and Markets Authority is undertaking a review of companion animal practice based on nearly 45,000 client and over 11,000 veterinary professional responses to a call for information.

Who would want to be a veterinarian nowadays? In the past, being a veterinarian was a common career aspiration for young people, but in a recent poll of high school students in Australia, it doesn't rate a mention in the top 10 for boys and, at number 10 for girls, well behind other careers such as law, medicine, and motor mechanics.

In any case, should we be asking if pet ownership is a luxury we can't afford? Is the human-animal bond so special that it must be maintained at all costs, and society and veterinarians must subsidise those who cannot afford veterinary care? Or should we be keeping pets at all, given the environmental impact of pet keeping? Maybe we should all keep robots instead, and companion animal veterinarians turn their minds and hands to small-scale engineering!

When Claude Bourgelat established the first veterinary school in Lyon in 1761, it was with the aim for veterinarians to serve humanity. Of course, the profession is much more complex than it was in 1761, but surely the ideals should be unchanged, given the essential role of veterinarians in animal health and welfare and public health. What is surely unchanged is that veterinarians owe a special duty of care to those they serve; they have duties to other professionals and responsibilities to society in general.

The book is timely as there is a need to allay concerns from the public as well as from inside the profession which erode trust. It is essential that veterinarians do all they can to surgically dissect what could be a problem and fix it! The profession needs to be forward-looking and veterinarians need to be engaged in issues where they can be the trusted professionals. To regain and retain trust, veterinarians need to be constantly alert to and confront issues that affect the profession rather than turning a blind eye.

Tanya Stephens

Acknowledgements

This book would not have been possible without Alice Oven (senior editor, *Veterinary Medicine*, Taylor and Francis/CRC Press). It was Alice who encouraged Tanya Stephens to submit a proposal for this book after discussing controversial and contemporary topics in veterinary medicine. We are also very appreciative of the help and guidance from Shikha Garg, senior editorial assistant.

Our profound thanks to Jodi Ware for her devotion to this project and her patience with four prehistoric digital-agers.

Finally, our gratitude to our enthusiastic contributors for penning their own reflections on veterinary practice and helping bring this book to life.

Tanya Stephens, R. Eddie Clutton, Polly Taylor, and Kathy L. Murphy
October 2024

About the Editors

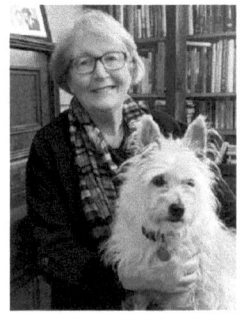

Tanya Stephens was born and raised in Somerset and then Derby before her family set sail for Australia when she was a teenager. She is a graduate of the University of Sydney in Veterinary Science and has a Masters in International Animal Welfare, Ethics and Law from the University of Edinburgh, is a Member of the Australian and New Zealand College of Veterinary Scientists in Animal Welfare and was made a Fellow of the Royal College of Veterinary Surgeons in 2020 for meritorious contribution to the profession. Tanya established her own small animal practice in Haberfield Sydney and very much enjoys practice. She is also a wildlife researcher with original research on galactosaemia in kangaroos. Her interests lie in professional ethics, animal welfare, research, evidence based medicine, wildlife, the environment and sustainable agriculture. She is a regular presenter and published author on these topics and is the editor of One Welfare in Practice: the Role of the Veterinarian. Tanya holds leadership positions in the Australian Veterinary Association and is the current President of the Conservation Biology Special Interest Group and Chair of the AVA's Animal Welfare Trust, member of a number of Animal Ethics Committees, honorary consulting veterinarian for the Children's Medical Research Institute, veterinary member of the NSW Civil and Administrative Tribunal, Chair of the NSW Kangaroo Management Advisory Panel and Chair of the NSW Greyhound Welfare Integrity Commission Animal Welfare Committee. She is a recipient of the Belle Bruce Reid Medal awarded by the University of Melbourne to Australia's 100 most notable women veterinary science graduates. Tanya is married to Harry, an architect, who designed this book cover, and they have four children and nine grandchildren.

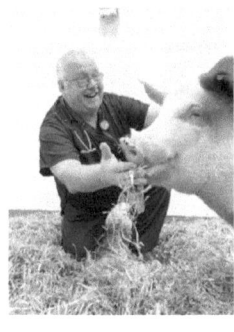

Eddie Clutton graduated (BVSC [hons]) from the University of Liverpool in 1981before beginning post-graduate training in the Department of Anaesthesia, The Royal Liverpool Hospital. He worked in the University of Virginia – Maryland, USA for 5 years as assistant professor in Veterinary Anesthesiology. He gained the RCVS Diploma in Veterinary Anaesthesia in 1985. He became Head of Veterinary Anaesthesia in the Royal (Dick) School of Veterinary Studies (Edinburgh) 1990–2015. He became a Diplomate of the European College of Veterinary Anaesthesia in 1996. He was editor-in-chief of *Veterinary Anaesthesia and Analgesia* (2000–2005). He was President of the Association of Veterinary Anaesthetists (2005–2008). He is a member of the Royal College of Anaesthetists, the Association of Veterinary Anaesthetists, the Animal Welfare Science, Ethics and Law Association, the Laboratory Animal Veterinary Association and the Laboratory Animal Science Association. His research interests include: pain management and depth of anaesthesia monitoring in pigs and sheep; and medical ethics. He was awarded a Chair of Veterinary Anaesthesiology (University of Edinburgh) August 2007. He was a co-founder of EthicsFirst (2016). He was awarded the Morpheus Award in 2019 for exceptional contributions to Veterinary anaesthesia, analgesia and intensive care, and to the European College of Veterinary Anaesthesia and Analgesia. He is currently the Clinical Director of the Wellcome Trust Critical Care Laboratory for Large Animals (Roslin Institute). He was awarded the Fellowship (RCVS) June 2019 for his meritorious contribution to knowledge. In 2024 he was awarded the British Veterinary Association's Dalrymple- Champneys Cup and Medal for the distinctive contributions he has made to the field of veterinary anaesthesia.

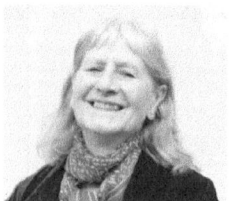

Polly Taylor graduated as VetMB from Cambridge University in 1976 and worked in general practice before moving to the Cambridge University Veterinary School where she obtained the RCVS DVA. She became chief of anaesthesia at the Animal Health Trust in 1983 and gained her PhD (Cambridge University) in 1987 for her thesis in equine anaesthesia. In 1994 she became University Lecturer and subsequently Reader at the Cambridge University Veterinary School where she was responsible for the clinical anaesthetic service, teaching undergraduates and post graduates and for research in anaesthesia. She became a Diplomate of the European College of Veterinary Anaesthesia in 1995 and was founding President of the College. She has been honoured with a number of awards for her work in anaesthesia and analgesia. In 2024 she was awarded an Honorary Doctorate from the University of Zurich for "contributions to veterinary anaesthesiology and analgesia research, education and animal welfare worldwide". Since 2002 she has worked as an independent consultant in anaesthesia, with work ranging from clinical anaesthesia of numerous species and teaching to drug registration, as well as research, particularly in analgesia. She has published numerous papers on anaesthesia and analgesia in many species, particularly horses and cats. Since its inception in 2008 she has been a director of Topcat Metrology Ltd, developing and supplying bespoke nociceptive threshold testing systems for a wide range of animal species. She was a member of the UK Advisory Council for the Misuse of Drugs (2002–2010) and has continued to be an advocate for the veterinary profession in matters concerning drug legislation. Her most recent activity putting her head above the parapet is to join a growing group showing the profession that overtreatment of animals "just because we can" is often not in their best interests.

About the Editors

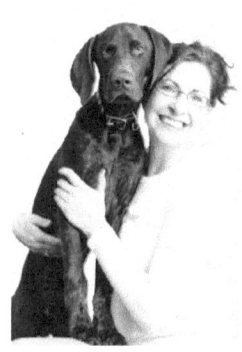

Kathy Murphy graduated from the Royal Veterinary College, London, in 1999. After spending several years in mixed general practice she moved to the University of Oxford where she completed Certificates in Veterinary Anaesthesia and Analgesia, and Laboratory Animal Science, whilst working as a clinical laboratory animal vet. Remaining at the University of Oxford she was awarded a Wellcome Trust Fellowship for her PhD in behavioral neuroscience and went on to the position of Assistant Professor of Neuroscience and Anesthesiology at the Icahn School of Medicine, Friedman Brain Institute, in New York City and returned to the University of Oxford in 2013 for the clinical academic position of Laboratory Animal Anaesthetist; and then to Newcastle University, UK, in 2016 for the position of Director of the Comparative Biology Centre. During this time she carried out a concurrent alternate track European College residency in Veterinary Anaesthesia and Analgesia, which provided the opportunity to return to companion animal work in a variety of settings, both first opinion and referral practice – private, academic, corporate and independent. She currently works as a consultant in change management, and holds non-exec board positions. She is founder and director of Barking Brains Ltd, a science communication platform; is co-founder of EthicsFirst; past Trustee and veterinary advisor for the Rottweiler Welfare Association and fills time on ethical review panels, working groups and with ad hoc reviewing, lecturing and MSc/PhD supervision.

Contributors

Vanessa Ashall
University of York

Alexandre Azevedo
Escola Universitária Vasco da Gama

R. Eddie Clutton
The University of Edinburgh

Ngaire Dennison
University of Dundee

Sue Dyson
Independent

Peter Fordyce
The University of Cambridge

Andrew Gardiner
Royal (Dick) School of Veterinary Studies
University of Edinburgh

Mary Ellen Goldberg
Independent veterinary technician

Carol A. Gray
Hartpury University

Stephen Greenhalgh
The University of Edinburgh

John Innes
Movement Referrals Independent Veterinary Specialists

Manuel Magalhães Sant'Ana
Faculty of Veterinary Medicine
University of Lisbon

Brennen McKenzie
Adobe Animal Hospital

Kathy L. Murphy
Barking Brains Ltd.

Amanda Novak
Merck KGaA

Sheilah Robertson
Lap of Love Veterinary Hospice

Andrew Routh
Independent conservation veterinarian

Kendal Shepherd
Veterinary Behaviourist

Alison Skipper
Royal Veterinary College

Tanya Stephens
Veterinary Practitioner Sydney
Australia

Andrea Tarr
Veterinary Prescriber

Nigel R. Taylor
Locum Veterinary Surgeon and Named Veterinary Surgeon

Polly Taylor
Taylor Monroe

John Webster
The University of Bristol

Sean Wensley
People's Dispensary for Sick Animals (PDSA)

Sarah Wolfensohn
The University of Surrey

Part I

Introduction

1 Veterinary Controversies and Ethical Dilemmas
An Introduction

R. Eddie Clutton

1.1 CHANGES IN THE VETERINARY PROFESSION

Perhaps the easiest way for anyone to appreciate the major changes that have occurred in the veterinary profession over the last 40-odd years, i.e. over most of the career spans of the current co-editors, is to watch and critically compare episodes of *All Creatures Great and Small* (BBC) and *The Supervet* (Channel 4). The former portrays a young, self-effacing, and inexperienced Glasgow veterinary graduate (James Alfred Wight) gingerly assimilating himself into an alien (Yorkshire) culture through, amongst other things, the exercise of veterinary professionalism. This he bases convincingly on an apparently genuine devotion to the preservation of the health and welfare of a wide range of (predominantly agricultural) animal subjects. And he does this whilst remaining constantly aware that many of his clients are not well-off. Importantly, much that Herriot does in *All Creatures Great and Small* serves to constantly remind viewers that vets are human beings and make mistakes, but as professionals, they can accept responsibility and 'make good'. In the course of time, the humble Herriot becomes a respected and valued member of the community, both as a person but importantly as a 'vitinry' – a veterinary surgeon – a member of the Royal College of Veterinary Surgeons, a fact signified by a simple post-nominal (MRCVS), which he proudly displayed on a small brass plaque on the wall of his principal's practice.

In contrast, the *Supervet* programme has, for the past decade, broadcast selected footage from a small-animal referral hospital in Surrey. Predominantly featured have been complicated, often 'first-ever', 'heroic' operations on dogs, cats, and tortoises being performed by Noel Fitzpatrick. This 'reality' show reveals the lengths to which some modern vets will go and portrays a fundamentally different form of veterinary surgeon. The curated, sensationalistic content has probably heightened public expectations (Lamb 2018) and encouraged other veterinary professionals around the world to push the limits in an animal population that cannot decline treatment in the first place, nor complain about painful complications later.

1.2 AMBIVALENT BENEFICENCE

To be clear, most of the changes that have occurred over the last 40 years have been of major benefit to the animals committed to veterinary care. Advances in imaging, diagnostics, and therapeutics have allowed major improvements in case management. As veterinary anaesthetists, two of the co-editors (PMT and REC) would propose that the management of animal pain has been the greatest of these benefits, not only in recognition of the technical and pharmacological advances that have made this possible, but because of an ideological shift amongst general veterinary practitioners that has seen the dismissive 'pain is natural – leave it alone' attitude become one in which effective pain management is a prioritised and promoted consideration in most spheres of veterinary influence – from laboratory fish to the traditional farmyard species. However, new ideas and innovations are seldom uniquely good or bad: improved animal pain management is likely to provide some veterinarians with a justification to conduct more invasive, noxious operations of questionable animal value. The same 'ambivalent beneficence' applies to other innovations and developments. For example, used correctly, advances in bench-top analytical technology and imaging, e.g. ultrasonography, CT, and MRI, have substantially improved veterinary diagnostic capabilities but, used thoughtlessly, result in overdiagnosis, which obfuscates appropriate treatment, contributes little to case management, and adds considerably to the client's bill – because innovation is not cheap and someone must pay. Similarly, new technologies now allow animals to undergo radiotherapy, open-heart surgery, kidney transplants, prolonged lung ventilation, and operations whereby their legs are replaced with expensive metal stumps. Some of these innovations are procedures that humans in many parts of the world are unable to receive, which makes them even more questionable: a human patient might at least appreciate the differences between medical overenthusiasm and torture, and the possibility that the former may be of some benefit. Consequently, the first part of this book dwells on the question 'Is there too much veterinary medicine?' and in answering this question, examines overdiagnosis and overtreatment, the dangers of research conducted on client-owned animals, quackery (or evidence-free veterinary medicine), and finally, veterinary medicine for uncommon species (attractions and reality).

1.3 THE ELEPHANT IN THE ROOM

The book then attempts to determine how these problems have arisen and does so by reviewing changes that have occurred within the animal population, the veterinary profession, veterinary practice, animal owners, and society in general. It finds that the principal driver (and the elephant in the room) of change is not difficult to identify: the veterinary profession is now commonly referred to as the veterinary *industry*, and those whom Herriot would have called owners or clients are now called *consumers*. Many practices have become clumped into conglomerates which, some 'consumers' believe, price-fix for the benefit of their shareholders. Sadly, one end-result of these collective changes is a breakdown in the relationship between veterinary surgeons and their clients (or consumers), and the reason is not bad service, overly long waiting times, incompetent practitioners, or limited specialist facilities – it's simply cost. Many clients believe the cost of animal treatment is far too high – but then some of these complainants will have spent several thousands of pounds buying a pet which cannot breathe, walk, or think properly – and then buy it Dracula suits to wear at Hallowe'en. Pet insurance, the corporatisation of practices and crowdfunding to cover the costs of veterinary specialist overtreatment all indicate the real nature of the *elephantis in locum*, and it is not a nice view of the profession nor the society it serves.

1.4   THE ORIGIN OF THE BOOK

This book represents a convergence of grumpiness originating some 10,500 miles apart. The UK component started about 10 years ago when anaesthesia residents at an unnamed UK veterinary college chose not to participate in a Home Office–licensed large-animal research project – not through any ethical objection to experimenting on animals but because more challenging, interesting, and 'heroic procedures' were being conducted on client-owned companion animals in the university clinic. This prompted three co-editors (PMT, REC, and KM) – all of whom were anaesthetising animals under A(SP)A (the Animal (Scientific Procedures) Act 1986) to question the residents' motives. The 'ranters' (as we then called ourselves) wondered why trainee veterinary specialists would prefer involvement in an ethically unevaluated, untested, potentially noxious, complicated, and expensive procedure with no guarantee of success and on a single client-owned animal, in preference to the experimental work. This, after all, was technically challenging (thoracotomy in sheep), so it had great educational and training value and would have benefitted from their participation. Furthermore, the experimental work aimed to benefit humans (and possibly animals) worldwide and involved animals which were protected by two ethical review and approval processes, the law, and pre-established humane endpoints which would have minimised any subsequent suffering related to the procedure.

1.5   VETERINARY OVERTREATMENT

This prompted an examination of veterinary overtreatment (or 'pet vivisection', as we described it) in general. The questions 'Are we going too far?' and 'Just because we can, should we?' had been circulating for some time, but disappointingly, neither question nor answer seemed to be of sufficient concern to prevent many veterinarians, including anaesthetists, from participating in it. This was all the more unexpected because veterinary anaesthesia had weathered an overdiagnosis storm in the 1990s. This began with the widespread uptake of bench-top clinical chemistry analysers, which was driven not by an acute clinical need but by technological advances and more benign financing options. Not surprisingly, blood sampling became popular because it helped pay for the device, though the reasons for sampling were seldom justified. For example, the more accurate assessment of anaesthetic risk was amongst the most popular justifications for the phlebotomy frenzy that ensued – despite evidence-based unanimity amongst medical anaesthetists in both the UK and the USA that pre-operative blood screening added nothing to anaesthetic risk assessment beyond a thorough medical history review and a physical examination – other than financial cost. Veterinary studies asking the same question came to the same conclusions. A debate held at the Association of Veterinary Anaesthetists' Conference in 1998 saw the motion 'Routine pre-anaesthetic blood sampling is expensive and unnecessary in animals' being carried with 119 in favour swamping a singular and forlorn 'nay'. But while overdiagnosis – by definition – is costly and not useful, overtreatment is costly and often harmful – except to those who inflict it and benefit reputationally and financially. Overtreatment is the core of the question 'Just because we can, should we?' and is defended in numerous ways by the reverse question 'We can, so why shouldn't we?' After all, 'It's what the client wants' or 'It's the animal's last and only chance' or 'How else are we going to improve veterinary surgery?' or even 'Why shouldn't animals get the same standard of care as humans?' At the bottom of the barrel the inexhaustible scraper will find 'This will help us advance medical science and help humans without the use of poor laboratory animals!' This book, it is hoped, will help the reader see the fragility of these excuses and recognise an urgent need for more veterinary ethicists.

1.6 PETS AS EXPERIMENTAL ANIMALS

An editorial published in *Nature* in December 2016 calling for the deregulation of the EU Directive 2010/63 in order to facilitate the use of client animals in clinical trials next caught our attention and prompted a letter of objection. *Nature*'s editorial board gave several reasons why they couldn't publish this letter, so it finally appeared in the (good old) *Veterinary Record* of the following year (Clutton et al. 2017). The basis of the objection was straightforward: the use of client-owned animals for research needs considerably more governance, ethical review, and regulatory oversight than animal-based research regulated under the EU Directive and/or A(SP)A – not less, which was *Nature*'s proposal. There were two important consequences to this published objection. First, an animal owner in the US – Jodi Ware – emailed to applaud us after discovering that her own dog, Lightning, had undergone experimental surgery without her knowledge or permission. This was revealed only after acute and severe complications necessitated radiographs which showed an unexpected and unexplainable implant. The case did not end well with Lightning's painful condition persisting until he was finally put to sleep. Jodi's efforts in the US to ensure some form of control over the use of pets in 'bad science' have not been successful, but she catalysed the formation of EthicsFirst in 2018 and has been its driving force ever since. The second consequence of the *Nature* editorial was the revelation that numerous elements of A(SP)A and the EU directive formulated to protect laboratory animals have much to offer clients' animals at risk of veterinary overtreatment. Consequently, two webinars sponsored by the European Society for the Laboratory Animal Veterinarians (ESLAV), the Laboratory Animal Veterinary Association (LAVA), the University Federation for Animal Welfare (UFAW), and EthicsFirst which focused on the question 'Can we work together to improve the process and transparency of ethical decision-making in veterinary medicine and surgery?' were held during the COVID-19 lockdown. The results of this are summarised by Ngaire Dennison in Chapter 13.

1.7 AUSTRALIAN DEVELOPMENTS

The Australian component of this book took root somewhat earlier. Tanya Stephens (TS), a veterinary practitioner with interests in animal welfare, research, evidence-based practice, professional ethics, and sustainability had been challenging dubious practices since at least 2009 when she raised concerns with vets using 'magic potions' in a letter published in the *Australian Veterinary Journal*. Challenging overdiagnosis with the question 'Do you want bloods with that?' asking that 'Hospice care needs rational debate', and presenting on land clearance at a One Welfare conference drew TS to the attention of Alice Oven, senior editor at Taylor and Francis, who consequently asked her to produce a book titled *One Welfare in Practice: The Role of the Veterinarian*. In 2019, both EthicsFirst and TS published independent concerns with veterinary oncology, which revealed a large area of common ground. Consequently, when Alice Oven asked TS to edit a book describing general grumbles with veterinary practice, the EthicsFirst group seemed an obvious choice as co-editors.

1.8 CONTRIBUTORS

Selecting contributing authors was not too difficult, as many had already written on the areas selected. Potential authors were told that we would not be looking (necessarily) for a heavily referenced evidence-based argument but more for a personal reflection/opinion on the subject of interest. As the book title suggests, we encouraged provocative writing. The intent was for the book to be read predominantly by veterinary undergraduates, but we hoped that it would be of interest to those who care about the profession, are interested in veterinary ethics, and are committed to improving the way vets meet their obligations to animals and the people who own them. In the final analysis, the ultimate objective was to give the whole profession and the laity 'food for thought'. We believe our selection of authors has achieved the book's intended objectives, and we hope the readers agree.

One consequence of inviting the views of numerous contributors for their personal reflections has been to reveal – if it wasn't already known – that considerable worldwide variation exists in writing styles, grammar, and spelling. Classical examples include 'euthanise' and 'euthanatize' (or is it 'euthanize'?) as well as 'anaesthesia' (the first American version) versus 'anesthesia', the more recent and less correct option. The minefield that was hyphenation ('post-operative' *versus* 'postoperative') has grown: is it 'overtreatment' or 'over-treatment'? Rather than let Microsoft or Channel 4 decide whether 'supervet' or 'super-vet' is the most appropriate term, the editors decided that, with very few exceptions, the contributing authors' versions will be accepted. We apologise for the resulting inconsistencies, but modern English, like a personal view, is difficult to prescribe.

1.9 VETERINARY CURMUDGEONS

Initially, it was very difficult to write this introduction (and other chapters in the book) without sounding like veterinary curmudgeons who hadn't kept pace with modern developments in veterinary practice. Given what social media were saying about some examples of veterinary overtreatment, we felt at times to be quite out of touch. What many appeared to be claiming were veterinary successes and breakthroughs seemed to us to be anything but; indeed, many seemed to be downright cruel. However, several events have since occurred that convinced us we were not entirely off course – at least in the eyes of the veterinary profession – rather than the emotionally incontinent who haunt social media. First were the overwhelmingly positive responses to PMT's and REC's contributions to the BVA's AWF forums held in 2019 and 2021. Second was the near-unanimous support received at the various webinars held during the COVID-19 lockdown, promoting the process and transparency of ethical decision-making in veterinary medicine and surgery. Then, in March 2024 came the 'Consultation on proposed market investigation reference' by the Competition and Markets Authority (CMA), which initiated and will likely sustain a useful professional self-analysis for some time to come. In the following April, an article published in the *Atlantic Monthly* titled 'Why Your Vet Bill Is So High' indicated that our ivory tower perceptions were not entirely unfounded, and that the basis of concerns was similar in both the USA and the UK. Finally, there was a steady publication of letters in the *Veterinary Record* from veterinary surgeons which echoed our thoughts and concerns on matters ranging from the profession-client relationship (Davies 2024) to 'contextualised care' (McGettigan 2024; Benyon 2024). These thankfully confirmed that there were a few other 'old grumblers' out there.

1.10 JODI WARE

This book owes incalculable gratitude to Jodi Ware (see previous section). Since co-founding EthicsFirst, setting up and maintaining the website, Jodi has capitalised on her insomnia to ensure that no item of interest to the group might possibly get away. Whilst continuing to seek redress for her own bitter experiences with non-consenting veterinary overtreatment in the US she has supplied energy, information, assistance, and guidance to EthicsFirst and to say we are extremely grateful to her would be an understatement. However, despite being the tireless director of operations for this book, she has, for good reasons of her own, elected not to be a co-editor. Instead, she took the sole and unenviable responsibility for bringing this project to its conclusion. Jodi Ware, we salute you!

1.11 FINAL THOUGHTS

For several years now, Channel 4 seems to have been unaware that the veterinary profession in the UK is awash with 'supervets'; indeed, they are the norm, and it is the default state. This majority serve their clients diligently, sincerely, honestly, and professionally, working hard and incessantly, often under difficult conditions, night and day, and for comparatively little financial reward, to help animals (and their owners) in trouble. Some supervets don't help individual animals directly, but through their research, policy creation, animal advocacy, regulatory function, charitable work, animal disease prevention, public health commitments, animal and habitat conservation, and educational activities, they quietly bring huge benefits to large numbers of animals and society in general. Usually, the normal supervet remains loyal to their profession, the RCVS, and the commitment they made when their careers began, i.e. to the health and welfare of animals committed to their care. In focusing on unpleasant areas which seldom – if ever – apply to these common-or-garden supervets, we hope this book at best offers some food for thought for everyone who reads it. More importantly, though, we hope it serves as a navigational aid to those who may have lost their bearings and as a very clear 'Here there be dragons' to those sixth-formers, veterinary undergraduates, and new veterinary graduates preparing to set sail on the adventure of their lives – as veterinary surgeons.

REFERENCES

Benyon P. The meaning of contextualised care. *Vet Rec.* 2024;195(1):34.
Clutton E, Bradbury G, Chennells D, et al. Pets in clinical trials. *Vet Rec.* 2017;181(8):209–210.
Davies T. Impact of the CMA review. *Vet Rec.* 2024;194(7):268.
Lamb H. Are TV vets good or bad for the profession? *Vet Rec.* 2018;183(2):73.
McGettigan S. The meaning of contextualised care. *Vet Rec.* 2024;195(2):75.

2 Veterinary Killing
History and Ethics

Andrew Gardiner

2.1 INTRODUCTION

Killing/euthanasia is a common procedure in veterinary medicine. While generally seen as unproblematic in terminal disease, and when carried out for welfare reasons, the process is complicated by advances in veterinary care which can prolong animals' lives to an extent that may be considered overtreatment. Veterinarians may experience moral distress if they feel they are keeping animals alive when they should be euthanised. At the same time, healthy animals are sometimes killed to prevent diseases from spreading or for spurious reasons. Such decisions do not operate solely across animal category lines (e.g. companion vs farmed) but reflect differing conceptions of animal value within species as well. This chapter takes a historical approach to the ethics of killing animals. It concludes that veterinarians may be helped in decision-making by trying to triangulate thinking across species lines, and focusing on sentience, not species, when considering the profession's broader ethical responsibilities towards all animals.

2.2 KILLING AND CARING

Unlike doctors, veterinarians routinely kill their patients. The oath of declaration that British veterinarians take on admission to their regulatory and licensing body, the Royal College of Veterinary Surgeons, states (emphasis retained):

> I PROMISE AND SOLEMNLY DECLARE that I will pursue the work of my profession with integrity and accept my responsibilities to the public, my clients, the profession and the Royal College of Veterinary Surgeons, and that, **ABOVE ALL**, my constant endeavour will be to ensure the health and welfare of animals committed to my care.
>
> **(RCVS 2024)**

Globally, not all veterinary professions use oaths. In those that do, animal welfare is not always mentioned, but there is often an obligation to relieve animal suffering (WSAVA 2024). The 'mercy killing', or euthanasia, of sick or suffering animals has generally been seen as unproblematic in veterinary medicine. Recently, an increasing interest in veterinary palliative care has begun to explore the timing, location, and normative use of euthanasia in veterinary patients (Goldberg 2016). Traditionally, many veterinarians have maintained that death is not an animal welfare issue, although the process of killing may be a welfare issue (Webster 1994, 15). In other words, an animal's welfare is not compromised by a painless death, which is the literal meaning of the term *euthanasia*.[1] Others, some veterinarians included, have argued that death is a welfare issue for animals, even when killing is painless (Višak 2013; Yeates 2009). One such argument, along the lines of preference utilitarianism, is that even a painless and 'perfect' death is a welfare issue because it deprives the animal of positive and enjoyable experiences that may have occurred had that life continued. That is a hypothetical proposition and, while true for some animals, it is also true that many animals live lives of suffering inflicted by humans, or due to challenges of living in the wild, and that under these circumstances death could be a release.

The euthanasia/welfare issue is of fundamental importance to the veterinary profession and there are many ways to explore it. This chapter uses a historical perspective to discuss some ethical aspects surrounding caring and killing. The term 'killing' is used to encompass all contexts in which animal death is brought about. Many (most) animal deaths cannot properly be termed euthanasia if we use this term to suggest that animals' interests are best served by dying. In keeping with the remit of the book, the chapter is written in the spirit of a 'provocation' to encourage discussion and debate.

2.3 KILLING AS 'TREATMENT'

Killing has been the mainstay of veterinary disease control policy since the 19th century. Most countries have legislation which demands the slaughter of animals in the presence of a number of notifiable diseases; these are mainly (but not exclusively) diseases affecting that category of animal known as 'livestock'. It is an arbitrary categorisation, with no basis in considerations of animal sentience: a pig is as sentient as a dog; a farmed llama is no different from a companion one except in terms of how humans construct situation and consequence (for the llama). This is an important point to bear in mind in a profession which is forced to be 'speciesist' because of the differing value attributed to different animal lives in human societies. Just as relevant as species are the differing contexts under which animals find themselves being cared for by humans.

The livestock policies and practices referred to derived from the success of a rigorous cull that took place during 1865–1866, and which eventually halted a devastating pan-European outbreak of cattle plague (rinderpest), a disease that had ravaged human civilisation since antiquity. The late 19th century outbreaks coincided with emerging ideas about the cause and nature of spreading disease, both animal and human, and consequent ideas about treatment.

Two broad theories of disease co-existed and to some extent overlapped in the 19th century. Contagionism held that disease was always around. It spread from infected individuals to healthy ones by contamination or close contact, causing periodic outbreaks. Prior exposure to disease might give immunity in surviving animals. A typical event causing an outbreak would be the accidental importation of disease into a new area by moving and mixing animals. Such movements became common from the 1840s as international livestock trade increased.

A rival set of theories, anticontagionism (sanitarianism), stated that disease could arise (or generate) spontaneously due to poisoned air, local climatic influences, or poor sanitation. Anticontagionists believed that once a disease had generated, individuals became infected if they were predisposed by their constitution and general health. According to anticontagionists, given the right unsanitary conditions, disease could generate simultaneously in multiple locations. This could give the impression of the disease 'spreading' in a population, whereas it was, in fact, multiple spontaneous appearances. The differences between the two theories could however be subtle, and by the 19th century, the possibility of a disease arising spontaneously and then propagating contagiously was recognised.

Treatment followed on from cause. Contagionists pursued quarantine and isolation to prevent disease *transmission*; anticontagionists emphasised environmental measures and sanitation to prevent disease *generation* and diffusion (Worboys 2000, 40). After two royal commissions on cattle plague in 1865 and 1866, a slaughter policy was introduced. It gained support from the farming industry in the face of a mounting national crisis. It was supported by most in the veterinary and medical professions, even as it was also criticised as barbaric, unscientific, and wasteful of animal life. However, it eventually brought the epizootic under control.

This use of killing as 'treatment' has shaped the veterinary profession ever since. Initially, it was seen as all that was needed for animal disease control. Towards the end of the 19th century, veterinarians were less interested in identifying and exploring the causes of animal diseases than in stopping outbreaks once they had occurred. Prevention and treatment at the level of the individual patient was not pursued. Experimental research directed towards those aims was even considered dangerous because of the risk of introducing diseases. Major livestock diseases like cattle plague became administrative and legislative issues rather than clinical or scientific ones. As Worboys (1992) notes, 'Veterinarians were not interested in the nature and action of germs, as their main approach to disease management and control worked at the level of whole animals and above, and [by] killing, nor curing'.

The 'stamping out' of cattle plague by slaughter contributed to the development of germ theory, 'probably the most important single concept in the history of modern medicine' (McGrew 1985, 25). Cattle plague and its control, therefore, helped to establish veterinary authority in relation to animal disease at a time when the profession was struggling to gain a foothold amongst the many individuals and groups claiming to be able to treat animals. Killing as 'treatment' was tied into the emergence of a more scientific and epidemiological veterinary medicine that sought to replace empiricism, even if there were clear limits as to how far the veterinary profession wished to pursue the *science* of spreading diseases because, in killing, they had the ultimate cure for any disease.

'Stamping out' approaches operated across all species groups, although large-scale culls are now rarely used for companion animal disease in Europe, North America, and Australia, as they were when rabies was prevalent (Pemberton & Worboys 2007). However, the destruction of large numbers of healthy companion animals in shelters throughout the world can be viewed as an ongoing companion animal cull, which, in ethical terms, complicates the nature of companion animal patient-hood in an era when the treatment of these animals in wealthy countries can look like 'human medicine for animals', with some individuals receiving advanced life support that would not be out of place in medical intensive care units. Routine culling, often in those same wealthy countries, stands in stark contrast to such 'gold standard treatment': one veterinary source estimates 355,000 healthy companion animals were euthanised in US animal shelters in 2021 (Special Reports Team 2024). Other sources cite much higher numbers: 'Taking a middle-of-the-road estimate, about three million animals are killed every year [in US shelters]. That's 342 every hour' (Pierce 2016).

Given that 99% of domestic animals are involved in global agriculture (Miele 2016), the use of killing as a livestock disease control policy has enormous implications for animal life, especially when, in the veterinary context of disease outbreaks, many of the animals killed may not be suffering from any disease but are killed in order to establish a *cordon sanitaire*. In the 2001 foot-and-mouth outbreak in Britain, when 6–10 million animals[2] were killed, most of them healthy, the contiguous cull to create 'fire breaks' amidst spreading disease was one of the most controversial aspects. It caused a crisis for the British government (Anderson 2002). More recently, the acrimonious row over the UK government policy of culling wild badgers to prevent the spread of tuberculosis to cattle has reached new heights when Brian May, astrophysicist and guitar legend of the rock band Queen, presented a BBC documentary questioning the science behind badger culling (Gibney 2024). New data appear to exonerate badgers in favour of cattle-to-cattle spread, with the government testing system apparently failing to detect a significant number of infected cattle. The debate is playing out as a classic case of disputed science for a modern day cattle plague (Cassidy 2012). The veterinary tendency to tackle spreading disease by 'stamping it out' (killing) is now focussed on an iconic wild mammal whose role in the propagation of the disease seems anything but clear. The result is a battle between various interest groups who claim to be advocating for animal welfare in one way or another, with 'science' currently unable to provide a definitive answer acceptable to all. The historical echoes over debates about germ theory are hard to ignore.

It should be remembered that killing also 'stamps out' disease in the individual animal body when treatment becomes ineffective. This aligns more to 'mercy killing' and the true meaning of euthanasia. Although the situation, context, and timing are different, the underlying rationale and response to disease is the same, but now killing is seen as a positive solution to intractable health or welfare problems. This contextual factor, operating as a cultural assumption within the veterinary profession, has been suggested as a possible contributory factor to the increased suicide rate amongst veterinarians (Bartram & Baldwin 2010; Dalum et al. 2024).

2.4 CARING ABOUT KILLING: TECHNOLOGY AND TECHNIQUES

Initially, the veterinary profession did not take a prominent role in shaping the technologies of animal killing, for example, in the promotion of reliable mechanical stunning prior to exsanguination of farm animals and horses at slaughter. Speaking at a meeting of the National Veterinary Medical Association (NVMA) in London, one leading veterinarian stated, 'We are not very much concerned with the slaughtering of animals, but in preserving animals. We are not out to kill; we are out to save life' (MacQueen 1922, 642). This is an interesting statement of veterinary professional ethics, especially given the (by then) well-established slaughter policy surrounding cattle plague and other diseases. It might be read in the context of the aftermath of the colossal slaughter of humans and animals that occurred during World War I, 'the horse war', which traumatised the nation. MacQueen's was not a view uniformly held throughout the profession. Others argued that veterinary expertise should be brought to bear on slaughter methods, but some distancing of veterinarians from what was going on in the slaughterhouse is shown in the relatively minor role the profession played in the humane slaughter debate, especially in the inter-war period. Medical practitioners and others, notably the Model Abattoir Society, were at least as active as veterinarians, mainly because of related interests in public health, slaughterhouse sanitation, and meat hygiene. The Council of Justice for Animals and its sister group, the Humane Slaughter Association, promoted a welfarist angle on slaughter, nationally and internationally, by advocating for captive bolt pistols and often supplying them to abattoirs (Hughes 2011). Veterinary reticence on large animal killing is in contrast to the more proactive role veterinarians took when considering methods of companion animal killing in the 1930s.

2.4.1 Companion Animals: Ethics and Aesthetics

In fact, the movement to promote humane slaughter included companion animals from the start, even if they were not the main focus. At its founding in 1911, the Council of Justice for Animals (CJA) set out to campaign for both food *and* pet animals, and methods of humanely killing the smaller companion animals were promoted. For example, in 1916, the Animal Rescue League judged electricity safe for killing cats; in 1919 the CJA was supplying 'lethal boxes' for companion animals; and from the 1920s, captive bolt pistols were used on companion animals, especially dogs, and became the standard method used by the police when dealing with strays.

Whereas a limited number of people associated with the meat trade killed livestock animals, many people took on the 'professional' killing of smaller companion animals. These included veterinary surgeons, farriers, non-qualified animal doctors, employees of welfare charities, the police, chemists (pharmacists), scientific researchers, kennel owners, breeders, and others. A much greater diversity of methods of killing existed, many of questionable humanity.

Veterinary Killing

The emergence of large-scale humane society 'destruction clinics' in the 1930s, as well as ongoing tension between some of these societies and the veterinary profession, caused the British veterinary profession to publish the result of an enquiry into companion animal killing methods in 1937 (NVMA 1937). The committee of enquiry consisted of eleven veterinarians drawn from Britain's five veterinary schools existing in 1937 (London, Edinburgh, Glasgow, Liverpool, and Dublin). The chair was G. W. Dunkin, who was the veterinary superintendent at the National Institute for Medical Research in London. The aim of the work was 'to explore in all its bearings the subject of small-animal euthanasia, i.e. of dogs, cats and birds, with a view to arriving at an authoritative opinion as to which is the most efficacious method of humanely destroying these animals' (NVMA 1937, 6).

The committee investigated existing methods of small-animal euthanasia (see Table 2.1); they did not set out to develop new techniques. The committee was keen to emphasise that their work was not experimental in the usual sense, i.e. a Home Office licence was not needed as the animals observed were already destined for euthanasia. In the introduction, the authors stated this clearly:

> From the outset it appeared to the Committee that any operation in the nature of an experiment, the result of which was doubtful or unknown, would be repulsive, and further it appeared to be quite unnecessary since, in the opinion of the Committee, known and tried methods were sufficiently numerous to allow of their arriving at a satisfactory conclusion without adopting this unacceptable line of attack.
>
> **(NVMA 1937, 7)**

TABLE 2.1
Common Dog- and Cat-Killing Methods Investigated by the NVMA Committee.

Chemicals	Lethal chambers
By injection or oral route	
Hydrocyanic acid	Carbon dioxide and chloroform
Prussic acid	Motor car exhaust
Hydrogen cyanide	Coal gas
Strychnine	
Magnesium sulphate*	**Shooting**
Chloral hydrate	Free bullet
Nembutal*	Captive bolt*
Evipan sodium*	
Avertin*	**Electricity**
Chloroform *(inhaled)*	Electrolethalers – probes
	Cabinet method

Note: Methods endorsed by the Committee, sometimes with conditions attached, are asterisked. The others were mostly judged unsuitable except in moribund, anaesthetised or heavily sedated animals.

This framing made the animal welfare agenda explicit. In this sense, it closely resembled the approach of the Humane Slaughter Association, which ran a wide-reaching programme of demonstrations at slaughterhouses and elsewhere. The NVMA authors accepted that views on what constituted humane killing of animals 'are very varied'. The investigations were supported by diverse organisations who provided expertise or materials. This included most of the humane societies, as well as equipment and drug manufacturers, chemical, gas and electrical companies, livestock organisations, and medical practitioners. The Committee even sought information from countries in which capital punishment was carried out.

Killing methods that were widely perceived as being humane, such as the lethal chambers popular with humane societies, were rejected because of apparent distress caused to the animals and because 'the patients were able to observe their companions undergoing similar discomforts' due to the fact that multiple animals were usually placed in the chamber together (NVMA 1937, 33). Such considerations had also been applied to slaughterhouse reform. Ideal slaughterhouse design prevented livestock witnessing the slaughter of those preceding them.

It was understood that, in the early stages of anaesthesia, animals tended to become excited or hyper-aroused. This was seen with several methods of killing animals also. Because of the difficulty of differentiating this from distress, the Committee erred on the side of caution. Methods which produced any form of heightened emotional state prior to loss of consciousness were mostly rejected. In this sense, the *intent* of the procedure was highly relevant, i.e. a 'side effect' that could be acceptable for routine anaesthesia became unacceptable for killing, even although the effect on the animal would be qualitatively similar and the recipient animal would not know the difference. This manifestation of 'care' around killing marked an important stance in relation to animal euthanasia that would inform developing notions of companion animal practice in the later 20th century (Gardiner 2009).

2.5 CONCLUSION/PROVOCATION

An ethical tension exists in veterinary medicine: veterinarians treat many (in effect all non-human) animals, but there is great variation in how different species of equivalent sentience are constructed as the subjects of veterinary care and consequently the type of treatment they receive. Veterinary medicine is highly speciesist in this way. This is especially apparent in the language used to describe animal killing (Jepson 2008).

It is, however, more than a matter of language and metaphor. The locations, circumstances, and technologies of veterinary killing vary greatly. Even in a single wealthy country such as Britain, it can be difficult to situate veterinary killing within any unified ethical framework. This makes it challenging to address the subject in general, all-species terms, even although the articulation of such an overarching ethic could be helpful to veterinarians, who may find themselves experiencing considerable moral distress when called upon to kill animals or when they are prevented from killing animals whose lives are being prolonged under poor welfare for anthropocentric reasons. Veterinary medicine is essentially a form of private medicine where finances dictate the extent of treatment. There is a danger that the veterinarian emerges as a kind of technician to service the needs, wants, or even whims of animal owners or a wider animal industry. Indeed, the emergence and now wide currency of the term 'veterinary industry', replacing 'veterinary profession', seems to signal this might already be happening.

What can we learn from this short historical survey of veterinary killing? Killing remains a fundamental veterinary intervention, one which is at the same time a privilege, a responsibility, a sometime legal requirement, and a technical matter, an ethical one, even an aesthetic one. Context is everything and while there may be no easy answers regarding veterinary killing, I believe the issue should be talked about more in veterinary schools and elsewhere and that this should, whenever possible, be done in a comparative way, focusing on sentience not species, and taking account of the many and varied contexts of veterinary care around the world. A form of ethical triangulation could be helpful which crosses species lines and encourages reflection about our nonverbal patients and their predicaments, including the predicament of how they are attributed value in human society. This avoids the danger of an ethical division along species lines, whereby a strand of companion animal medicine peels away as 'human medicine for animals' and other forms of veterinary medicine operate along entirely different lines. The risk is that at either extremity, the animal suffers: from overtreatment at one end to under or no treatment at the other, at times approaching denial of sentience.

Because of the risk of moral distress caused to veterinarians by both killing animals and being prevented from doing so, it is important to remember that the associated ethical issues cannot be the responsibility of the veterinary profession alone. To young vets caught up in difficult situations, it is not your fault! The question of animal value and the ambiguous moral status of animals in human society is one that requires broader debate, with veterinarians advocating for the animal wherever they (the animals) find themselves. It would be a mistake to enter a situation where, paraphrasing an earlier quotation, one species of veterinarian claims, along medical lines, 'We are not out to kill; we are out to save life' as the *defining* ethic of veterinary medicine. This ignores the many positives of compassionate and timely euthanasia – a topic now ever more prominent in human medicine, with assisted dying legislation consistently receiving high public support but remaining problematic for the medical profession.

Veterinarians are caught in the middle between animals and human culture and society. The latter continues to use and exploit animals in ever more inventive ways, but perhaps, as animal advocates, the middle is where veterinarians should be, as long as they can nurture and sustain an overarching ethic which encourages debate and guides actions, progress, and some developing degree of equity for animals wherever they find themselves. One that also supports veterinarians in their challenging role.

This chapter is based on a paper, 'Killing and Caring', delivered at the Association of Social Anthropologists of the UK conference, Durham, 2016, and is a condensed version of an article of the same name later published in *Veterinary History* (Gardiner 2019), with new material for this volume.

NOTES

1 Euthanasia: the act or practice of putting painlessly to death, especially in cases of incurable suffering; an easy mode of death. From the Greek *eu* well and *thanatos* death. *The Chambers Dictionary*, 10th ed., Edinburgh: Chambers Harrap, 2006.
2 Around 6 million adult animals were slaughtered, as well as approximately 4 million lambs and calves; the latter were not counted accurately.

REFERENCES

Anderson I. *Foot and mouth disease 2001: lessons to be learned inquiry*. London: The Stationery Office; 2002 Jul. Report No.: HC888.

Bartram DJ, Baldwin DS. Veterinary surgeons and suicide: a structural review of possible influences on increased risk. *Vet Rec*. 2010;166(13):388–397.

Cassidy A. Vermin, victims and disease: UK framings of badgers in and beyond the bovine TB controversy. *Sociol Rural*. 2012;52(2):192–214.

Dalum HS, Tyssen R, Moum T, et al. Euthanasia of animals – association with veterinarians' suicidal thoughts and attitudes towards assisted dying in humans: a nationwide cross-sectional survey (the NORVET study). *BMC Psychiatry*. 2024;24(1):2.

Gardiner A. The animal as surgical patient: a historical perspective in the 20th century. *Hist Philos Life Sci*. 2009;31(3–4):355–376.

Gardiner A. Killing and caring. *Vet Hist*. 2019;20(1):6–27.

Gibney E. Don't stop me now: Queen's Brian May on saving badgers and the scientific method. *Nature*. 2024 Aug 22. Online ahead of print.

Goldberg K. Veterinary hospice and palliative care: a comprehensive review of the literature. *Vet Rec*. 2016;178(15):369–374.

Hughes T. *Making a difference: 100 years of the Humane Slaughter Association*. Wheathampstead: Humane Slaughter Association; 2011.

Jepson J. 2008. A linguistic analysis of discourse on the killing of nonhuman animals. *Soc Anim*. 2008;16(2):127–148.

MacQueen J. Annual general meeting. *Vet Rec*. 1922;36(2):636–645.

McGrew R. *Encyclopedia of medical history*. New York: McGraw-Hill; 1985.

Miele M. Killing animals for food: how science, religion and technologies affect the public debate about religious slaughter. *Food Ethics*. 2016;1(1):47–60.

National Veterinary Medical Association (NVMA). *Report of the special committee appointed by the NVMA to study the subject of small animal euthanasia*. London: NVMA; 1937.

Pemberton N, Worboys M. *Mad dogs and Englishmen: rabies in Britain, 1830–2000*. Basingstoke: Palgrave Macmillan; 2007.

Pierce J. *Run, Spot, run. The ethics of keeping pets*. Chicago: University of Chicago Press; 2016.

Royal College of Veterinary Surgeons (RCVS). *Code of professional conduct for veterinary surgeons and supporting guidance* [Internet]. Undated [cited 2024 Jan 4]. Available from: https://www.rcvs.org.uk/setting-standards/advice-and-guidance/code-of-professional-conduct-for-veterinary-surgeons/pdf/.

Special Reports Team. Animal shelter statistics: state rankings and nationwide data. *Onevet.ai Animal Shelter Statistics* [Internet]. 2024 May 18. Available from: https://onevet.ai/animal-shelter-statistics/.

Višak T. *Killing happy animals: explorations in utilitarian ethics*. Basingstoke: Palgrave Macmillan; 2013.

Webster J. *Animal welfare: a cool eye towards Eden*. Oxford: Blackwell Publications; 1994.

Worboys M. Killing and curing: veterinarians, medicine and germs in Britain, 1860–1900. *Vet Hist*. 1992;7(2):53–71.

Worboys M. *Spreading germs: disease theories and medical practice in Britain, 1865–1900*. Cambridge: Cambridge University Press; 2000.

World Small Animal Veterinary Association (WSAVA). *WSAVA global oath* [Internet]. Undated [cited 2024 Jan 4]. Available from: https://wsava.org/resources/global-oath/.

Yeates JW. Death is a welfare issue. *J Agric Environ Ethics*. 2009;23(3):229–241.

3 The Law, Animals, and Veterinarians

Peter Fordyce

The law recognises that animals are both property, thus subject to the owner's 'property rights', and also sentient, hence capable of suffering. While legislation recognises that animals may suffer when used for human purposes, it seeks to limit this by curtailing some of the owner's property rights, and criminalising behaviour that causes 'unnecessary suffering'.

Implicit within society's social contract with the veterinary profession is that veterinary surgeons will act in the best interests of their patients, albeit within the constraints of other legislative strictures, and an owner's property rights.

Modern veterinary medicine can give rise to ethical dilemmas about what is genuinely in the patient's best interests. If members of the profession cannot demonstrate their actions were always 'those of a reasonably competent and humane person' in relation to 'best interests', it will undermine their social contract with society.

3.1 THE VETERINARY SURGEONS ACT 1966 AND THE SOCIAL CONTRACT WITH SOCIETY

The Veterinary Surgeons Act of 1966 regulates who can practice veterinary medicine and surgery in the UK. It gives power to the Royal College of Veterinary Surgeons to define what is and what is not an act of veterinary surgery and hold to account members of the college for their actions. To paraphrase a former registrar of the RCVS, the VSA 1966 is a legally enforceable social contract between society and the profession that gives a monopoly for members of the college to practise veterinary surgery, and in return for that monopoly, it protects society from 'the unqualified, the incompetent and the unethical' when it comes to the veterinary care of animals.

The act and the college provide for mechanisms requiring minimum standards of professional competence before membership can be obtained and, once obtained, allows ongoing monitoring of competence of veterinary surgeons (henceforth vets), as well as ensuring the minimum standards of care the public would expect for their animals. The act also provides mechanisms by which concerns about a member's competence and ethical behaviour can be challenged by the public; a complaint, if successful, given the monopoly that membership of the college confers, can lead to an individual losing their ability to practice.

The Law, Animals, and Veterinarians 21

On becoming a member of the RCVS, vets are required to swear an oath, where they 'promise and solemnly declare that they will pursue the work of my profession with integrity and accept their responsibilities to the public, my clients, the profession and the Royal College of Veterinary Surgeons, and that, above all, their constant endeavour will be to ensure the health and welfare of animals committed to their care'. One of the tenets inherent in the promise to 'accept their responsibilities to the public' is that vets should respect and obey their obligations to not only the legislative requirements of other laws that impinge on their working lives, but also the ethical underpinning behind them.

Where vets perceive their duty 'to ensure the health and welfare of animals committed to their care' conflicts with duties to other laws, ethical dilemmas may arise. These may include direct conflicts between obligations to the legal rights of others involved in the care of animals, such as the owner of the animal (who has 'property rights' and may have selfish interests), the organisation where the vet works (who may have selfish financial motivations for not prioritising the client's best financial interests or the animal's best welfare interests), and to society, where legislative provisions put the welfare of an individual animal subordinate to wider public policy imperatives (e.g. public health and safety legislation such as the Animal Health Act 1981 and the Dangerous Dogs Act 1991). Additionally, ethical dilemmas can occur where interpretation of what is in the best interests of an individual patient becomes a matter of debate as there is room for disagreement about whether an animal is suffering, and whether its suffering is unnecessary. The legal and ethical concepts regarding unnecessary suffering are a cornerstone principle for understanding the legislative landscape in which vets practice, and how wider society may view the profession's activities.

3.2 THE LAW, SUFFERING, SENTIENCE, AND ETHICS

The term 'unnecessary suffering' comes from the English Animal Welfare Act 2006, replicated in similar animal welfare protection legislation across the UK, including the Animal Health and Welfare Act (Scotland) 2006 and Welfare of Animals Act (Northern Ireland) 2011. While the precise legislative requirements imposed on humans relating to animal welfare varies in the different jurisdictions of the UK, the legal concept of 'unnecessary suffering' is universally applicable across the UK. These acts are particularly relevant to the duties imposed on vets practising veterinary medicine given the legal necessity and moral duty to abide by the requirements of these acts. The consequences of this are discussed subsequently, but understanding what the terms 'suffering' and 'unnecessary' might mean are helpful in understanding how society may interpret how the profession governs itself, particularly as there is room for interpretation of these terms.

The concept of animal suffering is not a new one, and whether animals can suffer has been a matter of philosophical debate for at least a millennium. From a legal perspective, statutory recognition that (some) animals can suffer first occurred in 1822, when Martin's Act (The Cruel Treatment of Cattle Act 1822) was passed to prevent cruel practices associated with the cattle trade. The evolution of animal welfare protection legislation over the last 200 years is beyond this chapter; however, in more recent years there are perhaps three key drivers that have resulted in current UK animal welfare protection legislation; these are the recognition of animal sentience, the development of animal welfare science, and how these have effected ethical debate surrounding human interaction and use of animals.

In 2022, the UK Parliament passed the Animal Welfare (Sentience) Act. This act had its roots in the EU Treaty of Amsterdam 1997, with the treaty's protocol establishing legal recognition of animals as 'sentient beings', and requiring legislators in the EU to take this into account when formulating policy. (A more detailed discussion of animal sentience occurs in the next chapter). Neither the treaty nor this act defines sentience. However, John Webster's statement that 'a sentient animal is one that has feelings, and its feelings matter to it' is particularly useful in understanding what sentience is. In this context, 'feelings' would be construed as mental states the animal is aware of, which may range from the spectrum of joyous or happy to egregiously miserable/suffering. While some would argue that animals don't have feelings, legislators and much of the population now accept that higher animals do have them and are therefore sentient. Much of the scientific rationale behind this assumption comes from Darwinian theory, and information from the recently developed academic field of animal welfare science.

In Darwinian terms, feelings are considered to have evolved in higher species as a way of motivating behaviour that promotes the success of the individual (and hence the species). They do this by causing the animal to seek situations that promote the animal's ability to reproduce and propagate its genes into the future, while trying to avoid situations that reduce its viability, and hence ability to reproduce. In simple terms, for example, finding nutritious food is good for your survival and makes you happy, things causing bodily damage are potentially detrimental to your survival, and pain is a mechanism to help you avoid such damage.

Attempting to establish what animals require to be evolutionarily successful, with their associated positive mental states, and what situations they need to avoid (hence avoiding unpleasant mental states), is the purpose of the academic subject of animal welfare science. It has its origins in the 1966 Brambell report, a report commissioned by Parliament to examine public concern arising from the increasing prevalence of factory farming in the UK – a concern pithily expressed by Ruth Harrison in her 1964 book Animal Machines, who contended; 'animals don't live before they die, they merely exist'.

The enquiry led to funding for and the foundation of the Farm Animal Welfare Council. This was established to advise government on improving animal welfare by scientific examination of what the needs and preferences of various species were, focusing on their physiological behavioural and health needs. Scientific rationale could then be used to support legislation to improve animal welfare.

The ethical justification behind the legislative imperative driving improvements in welfare were/are encapsulated in FAWC's Five Freedoms, published shortly after the Brambell report. The Five Freedoms are essentially ethical concerns about what egregiously unpleasant mental states (feelings) animals should be free from, i.e. not suffer from. These include the aspiration that they should be free from hunger and thirst, free from discomfort, free from fear and distress, free from pain, injury, and disease, and free to express normal behaviour.

While the Five Freedoms set out ethical imperatives to reduce suffering by setting legislative policy ambitions, they also set principles for how this might be achieved. These include requirements for ready access to water and a suitable diet that maintains health and vigour, provision of an appropriate environment for the animal to live in, ensuring the conditions and treatment of animals avoid causing mental suffering, and avoiding management procedures that cause pain and injury, along with preventing disease, or rapidly diagnosing and treating it if it occurs. Additionally, animals should be provided with sufficient space, proper facilities, and appropriate company of the animal's own kind so they can indulge in the natural behaviours that are normal for animals of that species.

While the practical imperatives behind FAWC's Five Freedoms are clear (e.g. 'provision of a suitable diet that maintains health and vigour'), exactly what an appropriate diet is for a species, what an appropriate environment might be, or what does or does not cause mental suffering became the focus of scientific investigation. Provision of such information by experts in the field of animal welfare science was (and continues to be) able to provide rational and creditable data to inform policy decisions by legislators, and to courts, about whether human actions involving animals will cause suffering, and the degree of suffering caused. Such data acts as a powerful counterbalance to arguments that animal welfare is mere anthropomorphic sentimentality.

The intervening years have provided a substantial peer-reviewed scientific literature supporting the fact that animals are sentient and can suffer, along with knowledge about what makes them suffer, and the physiological, behavioural, and pathological changes that occur in them when they are suffering. While legislators and courts have used this information to inform their decisions, information about the lives of animals, and how they may suffer has increasingly entered the public domain through the media in recent years, and this information has helped provide the political pressure for legislative change that further improves animal welfare.

Improvements in animal welfare protection legislation are driven by political pressure, and over the last 70 years, the public's increasing understanding of animal sentience, the nature of animal's lives, and ways in which animals may suffer have caused a shift in the public's approach to the ethics of animal use. As the academic lawyer Mike Radford (a strong proponent for improving animal welfare through legislation) put it, if law is the means (of improving animal welfare), animal welfare science and ethics are the justification'.

Concern in society about how humans use animals is not new (e.g. the Brambell report), and extensive discussion about the history of animal ethics is beyond this chapter. However, the modern study of animal ethics really started in the 1970s, when academic philosophers such as Peter Singer, Tom Regan, and Richard Ryder began investigating and questioning the morality of how animals were treated at that time, with books such as *Animal Liberation* and *The Case for Animal Rights* reaching relatively large public audiences. While philosophically and politically contentious at the time (and to some extent they still are), they opened a debate in wider society about the morality of how we use animals, and where the limit of good moral behaviour lies.

The debate about the ethics of human treatment of animals has moved forward since the 1970s, and major academic institutions across the world now provide courses in 'animal rights law'. While current debate about legal rights for animals is perhaps somewhat esoteric for many, the voting population, and legislators appear better informed about the ethical concerns surrounding the use of animals.

If one were to summarise where society's ethical perspective about where legislative protection for animal welfare was at present, the Banner Principles are a good starting point. These principles came from another parliamentary review into animal welfare and encapsulate the moral intent behind much current animal welfare protection legislation:

A. Harms of a certain degree and kind ought never to be inflicted on animals.
B. Any harm to an animal requires justification and must be outweighed by the good which is realistically sought in subjecting an animal to it.
C. The harm which is justified by the second principle ought to be minimised as far as possible.

While some proponents of animal rights legislation might argue that this is an anthropocentric utilitarian approach to protecting animal welfare, and therefore morally inappropriate, it is this legislative and ethical landscape in which vets must practice today, while also recognising their legal and ethical obligations to others, including owners, their employers, and wider society.

3.3 COMMON LAW PROPERTY RIGHTS AND THE TENSION BETWEEN LEGISLATIVE ETHICAL IMPERATIVES: ANTHROPOCENTRICISM AND ANIMALS AS A MEANS TO A HUMAN END

In virtually all jurisdictions across the world, animals have long been considered to fall into the legal category of 'property'. This contrasts with the category of 'legal persons' (such as humans and some 'non-human entities' such as corporations) who have legal rights and can bring legal actions in criminal and civil courts to protect those rights. This remains so in the UK today and was one of the major philosophical objections to Martin's law at the time, i.e. that the state should not interfere with the property rights that owners had over their animals.

Prior to Martin's Act, owners of animals had common law legal rights to do as they saw fit with their property, including rights to 'use' their property, to profit from the use of their property, to exclude others from using their property, to sell it, or to destroy it (in the case of animals, to kill the animal); these legal rights were (and some still are) enforceable by the owner (the 'legal person') in court.

Martin's Act was the first to set limits on the caprice of animal owners over their 'property' and reflected developing ethical views about animal use in society at the time. As discussed, ethical views about how animals should be treated have evolved massively in the last 200 years, not only restricting the property rights of animal owners, but also placing legal duties on them in relation to preventing certain harms. However, animals are still categorised as 'property' in law, with owners retaining (albeit curtailed) property rights over their animals.

The situation may place vets in a difficult ethical and legal dilemma, where respecting 'property rights' may conflict with their legal and ethical duties to prevent unnecessary suffering in their patient. This is likely to occur when there is a disagreement between the veterinary surgeon (or veterinary team) and the animal's owner about whether an animal is suffering, how much it is suffering, and what is the best way to deal with that suffering. While legislation can be used to override the owner's property rights surrounding consent about what happens to their property in certain circumstances where the animal is suffering unnecessarily, exactly where the levels of acceptable suffering and of necessity lie may be debatable in some cases. The selfish interests of the client, the vet, and the vet's employer may also cloud judgement over where the best interest of the patient lies. Brief examination of some of the ethical principles behind the AWA 2006 and the Animals (Scientific Procedures) Act 1986 (A(SP)A 1986) may assist the profession to see how society might interpret its action in this situation.

3.4 UNNECESSARY SUFFERING AND THE UNWRITTEN SOCIAL CONTRACT IMPLICIT WITHIN THE VSA 1996

As discussed, the Animal Welfare Act 2006 (as devolved) clearly accepts the principle that animals can suffer, hence the term 'unnecessary suffering'; the ethical and legal issues relating to suffering are ones of necessity, proportionality, and intent. Two major pieces of legislation that impact on the clinical work of vets illustrate how society might expect these ethical imperatives to be interpreted by the veterinary profession; these are the Animal Welfare Acts(s) and the Animals (Scientific Procedures) Act 1986 (A(SP)A 1986).

The A(SP)A 1986 regulates biomedical research in the UK, where animals undergo surgical, medical, and toxicological procedures that are of no benefit to the animal undergoing them; the argument that this is 'necessary suffering' is a utilitarian one, in so much as the suffering they endure is for the 'greater good' – predominantly human good. Societal unease at situations where animals may suffer for no benefit to themselves in biomedical research has resulted in an extremely rigorous legislative environment for this activity, not the least a requirement that statutory pre-emptive expert ethical analysis of any planned procedures on animals is required before it can happen. This analysis follows the ethical principles espoused by Banner. Clearly, where procedures that cause animals to suffer are not conducted for the animal's benefit, society wishes for rigorous ethical analysis of those actions. This may even apply if 'experimentation' might be for the benefit of the patient. The RCVS recognises this societal concern, setting parameters about what constitutes 'routine veterinary practice' and what might count as 'experimentation' in terms of A(SP)A 1986. However, as discussed in later chapters of this book, where the exact border lies may be indistinct.

The AWA 2006 additionally gives an indication regarding society's ethical approach to the importance of considering the best interests of an animal that might be suffering (albeit in an anthropocentrically caveated way). It provides guidance to courts into matters they may consider when determining whether the suffering that occurred was necessary, asking if 'the conduct which caused the suffering was for a legitimate purpose, such the purpose of benefiting the animal'. Clearly veterinary diagnosis and treatment provisionally fall into this category, provided they are done in the best interests of the patient; this ethical imperative is additionally caveated by the legal requirements that the suffering necessarily caused 'was proportionate to the purpose of the conduct concerned', and where it might occur, the 'suffering could have reasonably been avoided or reduced'.

The ethical approach outlined in the two acts mentioned is highly reminiscent of the Kantian approach in human medicine relating to patient autonomy that 'the patient is a means in themselves' not a 'means to an end'. However, humans are not 'property' in law, and this complicates the issue in relation to owners' wishes and legal rights. The late veterinary ethicist Bernard Rollin coined the phrase 'the veterinary trilemma' to discuss the ethical issues arising from ethical and legal obligations between vet, owner, and animal patient, asking whether vets should be more like car mechanics or more like paediatricians? Given the legal recognition of sentience in animals, the answer must be the latter, although exactly how this balance is achieved is not always easy. Again, the AWA 2006 provides some guidance that may be useful to the profession.

When courts consider whether suffering caused to an animal was necessary, and therefore legal, or unnecessary, and therefore illegal, the AWA 2006 suggests consideration should be given to whether 'the conduct concerned should be in all the circumstances that of a reasonably competent and humane person'. Vets are not exempt from the legal strictures of the AWA 2006 and could undergo criminal prosecution should there be doubt about their actions. Fortunately, prosecutions are extremely rare but were a general perception to arise in society that vets did not hold the prima facie principle that they should put the interests of their patient first, albeit in the light of 'all the circumstances', such as property rights, obligations to other legislative requirements, etc., the social contract between society and the profession will come under increasing strain.

The recent increase in the number of clinical ethical committees in the UK in recent years, and particularly those in teaching and referral centres where ethically contentious activities may occur because of advances in veterinary science, may go some way to reassure the public that the activity of the vets in these workplaces is indeed that of competent and humane people. Such committees can provide a more objective analysis of veterinary practice than individual vets, animal owners or business owners. Briefly outlining where controversies and ethical tensions arise in contemporary veterinary practice because of conflict with the 'best interests' principle might be useful.

3.5 POTENTIAL SOURCES OF ETHICAL CONFLICT

Detailed discussion of the sources of ethical dilemmas is the subject of much of this book, but it is worth briefly mentioning several areas where current veterinary practice, while legal, may give rise to societal concern.

Owners generally want to act in the best interests of their animal, particularly if they can afford to fund diagnostics and treatments recommended by the vet. However, unrealistic expectations of treatment options, failure to understand the aversive welfare implications of diagnostic and treatment options for the animal, and selfish attachment to the animal can lead to pressure on vets to subjugate their desire to act in what they see as the best interests of the patients. Similarly, vets have to be honest about their personal, intellectual, and technical abilities, along with their ability to access animal welfare, to prognosticate about likely outcomes for the situation an animal finds itself in, and to know when treatment is becoming futile. Doing the best for a patient requires knowing what can be done and understanding that just because something can be done does not mean it should be done, with the best interest of the patient in mind.

Vets are also not immune from selfish motives when it comes to not using the patient as a means to an end, albeit ones that may be subconscious. The desire to avoid the unpleasant sensation of failure when an animal dies in spite of their best efforts, as well as avoiding the disappointment and sadness of the owner when this happens, is understandable; however, it should be secondary to the welfare of the patient. Pressure to 'push the envelope' beyond what is objectively reasonable for a specific patient may also cause the vet to overlook a rational approach to the patient's best interests, either through the best of motives, although occasionally through vainglory, or drivers such as the need to produce publications for career advancement.

The veterinary industry is also a private industry, needing to earn an income from its activities to pay its staff and fund the equipment and premises from which it operates. However, unlike many private industries and businesses, veterinary surgeons have a monopoly on provision of veterinary care. The VSA regulates the activities of veterinary surgeons, but not of veterinary businesses, and increasingly veterinary businesses are owned by corporate bodies (ironically, also legal persons) with a fiduciary duty to their shareholders and only indirectly to their human clients and their animals. This places the employees of such businesses in an ethical dilemma, as they have duties to their employer which may conflict with their duty to look after the best welfare interests of their patient and financial interests of the owner. More diagnostic and therapeutic interventions on a patient may be in the best financial interests of the vet's employer but may not be in the best interests of the animal's welfare or the client's finances.

3.6 SUMMARY

The social contract implicit in the VSA 1966 between the profession and society and for which the profession holds its monopoly on veterinary treatment of animals is predicated on the assumption that the profession will behave ethically in upholding the 'best interests' of their patients as a prima facie principle (albeit within the confines of other legal requirements).

The VSA 1966 says virtually nothing about what the profession's governing body might construe as unethical behaviour, beyond 'disgraceful conduct in any professional respect' and 'conviction of a criminal offence which, in the opinion of the disciplinary committee, renders them unfit to practise veterinary surgery'.

If disgraceful conduct is considered as a synonym for unethical behaviour, animal welfare protection legislation other than the VSA 1966 indicates what society might expect from the profession when approaching some of the contemporary controversies and ethical dilemmas facing the profession. Failure to abide by the legal and ethical imperatives in the AWA 2006 and A(SP)A 1986 relating to the concept of unnecessary suffering will do nothing but harm the profession by undermining the legislative social contract it has with wider society, if the profession is not considered to be acting in a way society considers to be 'in all the circumstances that of reasonably competent and humane persons'.

4 Sentient Beings
Our Duty of Care: Who Are our Patients?

John Webster

'To be, and to remain enthusiastic, it is best to draw the silk curtains of facetiousness and so conserve your enthusiasm'. I confess that I have forgotten the origin of this quotation. However, throughout a long life enthusiastically devoted to animals and animal welfare, I have felt the need for a certain cheerful cynicism, if only to keep my feet on the ground. Two such thoughts have stayed with me since my student days.

'The prime function of the veterinary surgeon is to wrest the sickle from the angel of death and thrust it into the butcher's bloody fist'.

'Our students are being taught better and ever more expensive ways to prolong the suffering of geriatric pets'.

It is not easy to be a good vet. The ethics of human medicine are relatively straightforward. Medical doctors are responsible to their patients (of one species) *'not to kill but neither strive officiously to keep alive'*. Our responsibility is not just to the animals but, directly or indirectly, to One Health and One Welfare – everything and everybody involved with animals: plentiful supply of safe, wholesome food, concern for the welfare of domesticated animals and their owners, and concern for the quality and sustainability of the living environment. We acknowledge that we have a duty of care, but how can we achieve justice when we have so many conflicting demands? There are no simple answers. However, I believe that it is possible to establish a set of first principles and rules of engagement.

4.1 RIGHTS AND RESPONSIBILITIES: MORAL AGENTS AND MORAL PATIENTS

The Treaty of Amsterdam (1997) states *'since animals are sentient beings, members shall provide full regard to their welfare requirements'*. This is a worthy sentiment but of little practical help in formulating rules of engagement. Clearly, all animals are sentient, but some are more sentient than others. In my latest book in the UFAW Animal Welfare series (Webster 2022) I adopted the scientifically elegant template, the Five Skandhas of Sentience, described by the Buddha in the 6th century BC to explore the nature of sentience in different species and their implications for our moral responsibility to exercise a duty of care. The five skandhas are *matter, sensation, perception, mental formulation,* and *consciousness*. According to the Buddha, all living things, plant and animal, are sentient. Plants respond to environmental stimuli (e.g. light, temperature), but they lie in the outer circle because their response is not triggered by *sensations* such as pain, heat, etc. We recognise in law that all vertebrate species and some invertebrates (e.g. cephalopods like the octopus) have nervous systems sensitive to pain and other sensations, so they should receive protection from procedures likely to cause 'pain, suffering, disease, or lasting harm'. This list is likely to grow in the light of new knowledge.

Most of the animals with which we vets are likely to come into contact display greater depths of sentience than primitive sensations arising from stimuli, such as fear, pain, hunger, and thirst. Species that demonstrate the more profound properties of perception, mental formulation, and consciousness have *sentient minds*. Some of the emotional and cognitive expressions of sentient minds are outlined in Table 4.1. Animals with sentient minds do not just live in the present. For animals with the power of perception, fear, for example, is more than a sensation; it is a learning experience. If they learn from experience how to deal with the threat, or if they discover that their alarm is unfounded, then their fear will diminish. They learn to cope. This applies to all stresses and is the normal process of adaptation to the environment. If they discover that they cannot cope, either because the stresses are too severe, too complex, or too prolonged or because we so restrict their environment such that they are unable to perform coping behaviour, then they will suffer.

Species with the powers of mental formulation and consciousness[1] can do more than learn from experience; they can understand the principles of cause and effect. This understanding creates possibilities for education and culture. We can see this in a wide range of species throughout the animal kingdom. In my *Sentient Minds* book (Webster 2022) and on my website (www.webster.welfare.com), I give

TABLE 4.1
Emotional and Cognitive Expressions of Sentient Minds

	Emotion	Cognition
Perception	Pain and fear	Avoidance
	Hunger and thirst	Food selection
	Comfort	Nest building
	Curiosity and security	Interpret simple social signals
Mental formulation	Anxiety and depression	Understand social signals
	Pleasure, joy, hope, grief	Education and culture
Consciousness	Affiliative behaviour	Aware of self and non-self
	Empathy and compassion	Deceit

evidence for these elements of deeper sentience in a wide range of species: archerfish, bats, beavers, chickens, crows, dolphins, elephants, herons, sheep, and squid, to name but a few. These properties of deep sentience increase their capacity to make strategic decisions that increase their capacity to cope with physical and emotional challenges. However, they also increase the potential for suffering if they fail. One of the main themes that runs through my book is that evolution should not be viewed as an ascent in sentience and cognitive skills through the animal kingdom to so-called 'higher mammals', such as primates, with humans at the peak of the pyramid. Successful sentient species develop the skills that matter and neglect others. Corvid birds, for example, are better toolmakers than chimpanzees. Dogs may understand no more (human) words than a three-year-old child, but their capacity to recognise *and interpret* smells is beyond our imagination. Leon Meggison elegantly summarised the essence of Darwinism. *'It is not the most intellectual of species that survives; it is not the strongest that survives. The species that survives is the one that is able best to adapt and adjust to the changing environment in which it finds itself'*. Currently, the human species does not rate highly by these criteria.

The deeper skandha of sentience are widespread within the animal kingdom and are likely to apply to nearly all the species with which we are likely to come into direct contact. This carries the message that our responsibility extends beyond the obligation to avoid suffering by doing or failing to perform any act. Our duty is to promote their quality of life. For the vast majority of species that have escaped domestication, the message must be to leave them well and leave them alone. This is easier said than done because it implies that we should strive, so far as is possible, to preserve their natural habitat. In order to provide for quality of life in domestic animals directly under our care, we must first try to understand them.

Farm animals may, on the whole, have a harder life than pets but, at least, they live among others of their kind who share a mutual understanding. It should come as no surprise to read that most reports of behavioural disturbances in animals relate to pets, especially dogs and horses, for whom many of our actions and demands are physically inappropriate or emotionally incomprehensible.

Much has been said and written about animal rights, as set within the context of human rights. This is inevitably a biased exercise since the animals cannot contribute to the discussion. Nevertheless, I believe it is possible to approach animal rights within the context of Albert Schweitzer's immortal definition of morality: *'The great fault of all ethics hitherto has been that they believed themselves to have to deal only with the relations of man to man. In reality, the question is what is his attitude to the world and all that comes within his reach'*. Ethics is nothing other than reverence for life.

4.2 JUSTICE: THE ETHICAL MATRIX

As I have written many times, caring *about* animals, may be highly moral (and easy) but caring *for* them not only requires a great deal of understanding. It also has to be accommodated within a host of other commitments that recognise the rights and responsibilities of all parties. Inevitably, there will be conflicts between these commitments that call for compromise. The aim of practical morality in a complex world must be the pursuit of justice. Beauchamp and Childress (1994) proposed an elegantly simple approach to practical ethics in medicine, the *ethical matrix,* and Mepham (1996) adapted this to food production from animals. Two key principles of ethics are *beneficence* and *deontology.* Beneficence means to promote wellbeing. In the case of farmed animals, this equates to *utilitarianism,* or promoting the greatest good for the greatest number. However, this paternalistic (or autocratic) approach can never be enough. We must also respect the principle of deontology, which describes our duty to respect the rights of other individuals to experience the sense of wellbeing that we would expect for ourselves *(do as you would be done by).* The most obvious expression of deontology is the duty to recognise the principle of *autonomy,* freedom of choice.

Table 4.2 illustrates the application of the ethical matrix to the production of food and the practice of farming within the context of respect for all life. The principles of beneficence and autonomy are input measures and the outcome measure is justice. When applying the ethical matrix to any issue that extends beyond human relationships, we humans are moral agents with rights and responsibilities. Sentient animals, and indeed, the entire living environment are moral patients. We have responsibilities to them, but they have no responsibilities to us. Farmers and landowners are responsible for the welfare of their animals and the land. In return, they have the right to expect reasonable financial reward and pride in their work with animals and their commitment to conserve the quality of their environment. Consumers (society at large) have the right to wholesome, affordable, attractive

TABLE 4.2
Food, Farming, and the Living Environment: An Ethical Matrix

	Wellbeing	Autonomy	Justice
Moral agents			
Producers and landowners	Financial reward Pride in work	Free competition	Fair trade Good husbandry Support for sustainability
Society at large	Wholesome, affordable food	Freedom of choice	Pay more for good husbandry
Moral patients			
Farmed animals	Good husbandry	Environmental enrichment Freedom of choice	'A life worth living'
The living environment	Conservation Sustainability	Biodiversity 'Live and let live'	Respect for environment and stewards

food but the responsibility to pay more for husbandry systems that give proper respect to the living environment. Farm animals have the general right to physical and mental wellbeing and the individual right to express themselves, primarily through freedom of choice. Finally, we all share the responsibility to conserve and, where possible, to enrich the living environment.

The husbandry and welfare of farm animals is too big a subject to get into here. However, after many years, I still believe that the essence may be encapsulated within the Five Freedoms:

- Freedom from hunger and thirst
- Freedom from physical and thermal discomfort
- Freedom from pain, injury, and disease
- Freedom from fear and stress
- Freedom of choice

These present a utilitarian framework for dealing with animals *en masse*, e.g. on farms and in scientific establishments. The fifth freedom was originally written as 'Freedom to exhibit natural behaviour'. As originally defined, they may be criticised for giving insufficient attention to the need to recognise quality of life. Redefining the fifth freedom as 'Freedom of choice' gives greater respect to the principle of autonomy. In practice, it recognises our responsibility to ensure that animals are kept in a sufficiently enriched environment to ensure that they can, through their own actions, make a positive contribution to their own quality of life.

4.3 JUSTICE FOR PETS

Caring for pets nearly always means seeking to promote the quality of life for individuals, so the principle of utilitarianism does not apply. David Mellor's model of the Five Domains (Mellor et al. 2020) that recognises quality of life (the fifth domain), as the outcome of all incoming physical and emotional signals, may be a more helpful approach to structuring the understanding of our interactions with individual animals for whom we have a duty of care.

However, maintaining quality of life is not synonymous with maintaining life itself. Death is the end of life. It is also the end of suffering. Thus, being dead is not a welfare problem. Dying, especially when prolonged, is a welfare problem for the individual. Death is only a welfare problem for the living. In the wild, this usually equates to dependent members of the family (caring parents and dependent offspring), although there is good evidence that species such as elephants (and donkeys) show lasting distress at the loss of a comrade. In modern human society, pets are often regarded as members of the family. Those who suffer after the death of an old pet dog are those who cared for it and were, very often, emotionally dependent on it.

Vets can (and should) make the moral case that our primary responsibility is to the animals. However, day-to-day in practice you are faced by the need to seek just decisions based on compromise between the needs of the animal, their owner, and, of course, your own need to earn a living. I prefaced this article with the sardonic comment (not mine) that vet students are being taught better and ever more expensive ways to prolong the suffering of geriatric pets. While this is, of course, an outrageous remark, said for effect, it does serve as a cautionary tale. Euthanasia for an old, incontinent dog suffering from chronic orthopaedic pain has to be the right decision in almost all circumstances. However, there can be exceptions. When the smelly old incontinent dog is the only true companion of a smelly old incontinent man, then I believe the honourable decision would be to let them struggle on together a little longer.

I think most veterinary advice as to euthanasia can be given on the basis of what we believe is best for animal and owner in a way that is honourably free of self-interest. I am less sanguine, however, about the use of high-tech, high-cost, and possibly highly invasive treatments designed to improve health, improve appearance, restore fitness, or prolong life. We cannot escape the facts that high-tech diagnostic tools and elaborate surgical techniques are intellectually challenging, exciting, and highly profitable. Moreover, more and more owners, paying high insurance premiums, are eager to do anything for their beloved pets. When owners and vets are on the same side the balance can be heavily loaded against the welfare of the pet. Nevertheless, I repeat my central (and hardly original) message. However, the dice may be loaded, the welfare of the animal should be paramount.

This is a firm principle, but it can generate different actions in different circumstances. For example, radical surgery that leads to some post-operative distress but carries the probability of a return to full fitness and a high quality of life is likely to be a good thing, if the cost does not cripple the owner. If this is a problem, then the alternative euthanasia may appear heartless, but it will not incur suffering (to the dog). Much can depend on the general emotional state of the animal. My daughter (another Professor Webster) has an 11-year-old small Havanese dog that was born with an abnormal elbow joint on his left forelimb, has undergone several operations, and is now running around on three legs. He is and always has been incorrigibly cheerful and has never, I believe, been aware that he has a problem. In his case, I cannot conclude other than that his treatment has been a good thing, albeit horribly expensive.

The use of expensive and potentially distressing forms of heroic therapy to prolong life is hard to justify when it is carried out merely to delay the distress of loving owners. Towards the end of life, there can be little justification for any treatment that goes beyond palliative care. I would not wish for more for any of my pet animals or indeed for myself.

4.4 CODA

I repeat my opening words. It is not easy to be a good vet, especially in pet practice, where ethical decisions are inevitably linked to personal income. I should introduce a personal note at this stage. When I first entered vet school, my aim was to be a cow vet, which I then assumed would equate to farm animal practice. As it happened, my career took off in an entirely different direction. While at university, I caught the academic bug, and my subsequent career has been largely devoted to teaching and research. However, I still consider myself a cow vet who worked in a university rather than a university professor who happened to train as a vet. I have enormously enjoyed almost every day of my career and one reason for this has been that my salary has had no influence on my freedom of choice. I am therefore in no position to preach. However, the principles of beneficence and autonomy stand fast. The right to freedom of choice should be sacrosanct, but this carries the responsibility to do the right thing.

NOTE

1 In the Buddhist skandha, consciousness equates to the human facility for awareness of self and non-self.

REFERENCES

Beauchamp TL, Childress JF. *Principles of biomedical ethics*. 4th ed. Oxford: Oxford University Press; 1994.

Mellor DJ, Beausoleil NJ, Littlewood KE, et al. The 2020 five domains model: including human-animal interactions in assessments of animal welfare. *Animals (Basel)*. 2020;10(10):1870.

Mepham B. Ethical analysis of food biotechnologies: an evaluative framework. In: Mepham B, editor. *Food ethics*. 1st ed. London: Routledge; 1996. p. 101–119.

Webster J. *Animal welfare: understanding sentient minds and why it matters*. 1st ed. Oxford: Wiley Blackwell; 2022.

5 Let's all March for (Veterinary) Science

Veterinary Science in a Post-Truth Society

Tanya Stephens

The postmodern mindset which denies objective truth has had serious implications for the standing of science and veterinary science has not been immune. In a post-truth world, alternative facts replace actual facts and feelings are more important than evidence. In 2020 the World Health Organisation declared the spread of vaccine misinformation one of the top threats to human health.

Veterinarians are obligated by various codes and professional ethics to use best evidence when making clinical decisions. However, 'best evidence' may be illusionary because of concerns over the quality of some published research, an unprecedented level of retraction of published papers, and the emergence of predatory journals and 'paper mills' that sell bogus work to scientists.

Veterinary professional ethics demands that veterinarians practise 'what should be' and all veterinary procedures should be based on best evidence, be justifiable and undertaken in the best interests of animals and their owners. Veterinarians should stridently correct misinformation. In this post-truth world of fake news and the like, where science has been downgraded to mere opinion and scientists' voices are ignored, if we replace evidence-based medicine with opinion-based medicine, veterinarians lose credibility as veterinary scientists and risk losing their position as the primary source of expertise and information on animal health and welfare.

5.1 MARCHING FOR SCIENCE

'On Saturday 22nd April 2017 thousands of people rallied across Australia as part of a global movement calling on political leaders to focus more on science, to recognise the significance of science and to use scientific evidence as the basis of good public policy' (Stephens 2017).

As Professor Emma Johnston wrote in the *Sydney Morning Herald* on 14 February 2017 ('The antidote to rising populism is being grown in labs'): 'the rise of a wider "post truth" political culture means that scientists increasingly need to "pick up the baton of public intellectualism" and to counter fake news'. As we are all too aware 'anyone can speak, write, tweet and post' and that 'opinion and ideology are overriding facts'. Professor Johnston asks, 'can we counter fake news by promoting science and as scientists be the ambassadors of brand "knowledge" and brand "truth"?' Further, 'As public intellectuals our scientific qualifications and practices could, and should, be shorthand for reliability and credibility'.

The postmodern mindset, which denies objective truth, has had serious implications for the standing of science in general and veterinary science has not been immune. At its extreme, postmodernism views science as simply one among a variety of subjective explanations for the way we perceive the physical world. Science is downgraded to mere opinion, and scientists' professional voices are diminished.

According to the Oxford Dictionaries, 'post-truth' is defined as 'relating to and denoting circumstances in which objective facts are less influential in shaping public opinion than appeals to emotion and personal belief'. Postmodernist tendencies have been exploited in this post-truth world, making people more receptive of their predisposed beliefs and ideologies, producing information ghettos where these views are further polarised, a phenomenon which is actually contrary to postmodern ideals. And where we now have unprecedented access to information, post-truth has led to an age of misinformation.

It is likely that cognitive biases help explain the post-truth era where 'alternative facts' replace actual facts and feelings are more important than evidence. Human beings are not as rational as we might like to think they are, and veterinarians, who, one assumes, are well trained in the sciences but who nevertheless believe in implausible 'therapies', such as homeopathy, are an excellent example of this.

The 2010s are said to be the decade of 'bunk' and called the post-truth decade (Caulfield 2020) with social media pushing all kinds of nonsense from anti-vaccine myths, conspiracy theories, celebrity health brands, and unproven and implausible 'therapies'. The 2020s are an opportunity to counteract this threat to human and animal health and the environment and we need to do this as in 2020 the World Health Organization declared the spread of vaccine misinformation to be one of the top threats to public health.

5.2 EVIDENCE-BASED VETERINARY MEDICINE (EBVM)

The emergence of EBVM is a welcome development for practitioners, such as myself looking to use the best evidence on animals in our care. Indeed, this development has been enthusiastically adopted and led by practitioners rather than academics and supported by the Evidence-Based Veterinary Medicine Association in the USA, RCVS Knowledge, and Nottingham Veterinary School in the UK. Pre-COVID-19 there were two well attended EBVM Conferences in the UK.

Access to the best available information for veterinarians when making a clinical decision is a critical part of EBVM, which has at its heart confidence in the scientific methodology that has developed over centuries to enable us to distinguish between what is likely to be true from what is likely to be false (or unproven).

The Evidence-Based Veterinary Medicine Association defines EBVM thus:

'Evidence based veterinary medicine is the formal strategy to integrate the best research evidence available combined with clinical expertise as well as the unique needs or wishes of each client in clinical practice'.

Much of this is based on results from research studies that have been critically designed and statistically evaluated. According to RCVS Knowledge, the case for EBVM is therefore one for improving the success rates of clinical decisions, saving lives and providing better standards of care.

The use of EBVM is being driven by general practitioners such as myself, not simply because the law and codes of conduct tell us to do so but because of a genuine need to provide the best care we can. This not only leads to better health and welfare for the animals in our care but improves the wellbeing of the veterinarian who will be assured that they have made the 'best' clinical decision as the use of EBVM takes much of the guesswork out of practice.

In the '70s and '80s veterinary medicine was most definitely practised using 'opinion-based medicine' as the norm. Since then, there has been a veritable explosion of information. In 2010 alone, around 18,000 veterinary papers were published across many different scientific journals. Traditionally veterinarians have relied on personal experience and often formal scientific research, but use of this resource has been inconsistent and indirect, filtered through the opinion of experts interpreting the scientific literature. This is opinion-based medicine and often emanates from university and specialist centres and not the general practitioner.

We are very fortunate indeed that with the massive increase in scientific literature, the emergence of EBVM resources such as systematic reviews and meta-analyses has given us data to become better educated veterinarians. Additionally, practitioners can make a difference by providing data, undertaking research in practice and generally engaging in EBVM (Dean 2020). The use of EBVM has the potential to make practice even more rewarding and there are likely to be a range of non-clinical benefits, such as collegiality and interesting, relevant, and satisfying engagement in practice.

As well as supporting the production of high-quality research, EBVM promotes the dissemination of such research in a form which is practical and useful to clinicians.

Importantly, we need to be alert to human behaviour as it is said that most mistakes made by clinicians do not arise from a lack of knowledge but from cognitive biases inherent in our decision-making. Cognitive biases are more likely to create error when decision-making is automatic, as is likely in a clinical setting, and the use of EBVM aims to overcome these biases.

5.3 CAN WE TRUST THE EVIDENCE?

The use of best evidence in practice depends on good research, and good research depends on research integrity and good ethics. With vast quantities of research papers, we depend on researchers, peer reviewers, and publishers to provide us with information which is beyond reproach and in which we can trust.

In 2022 more than 2.8 million new scientific papers were published, almost 900,000 more than in 2016. With such quantity, is this at the expense of quality? Science has turned into a business, says Liam Mannix (2024), with evidence that science is delivering less actual innovation than previously. As Mannix points out, scientists want to publish more to advance their careers and gain funding, publishers want to publish more to make money, whilst governments and universities want to fund more 'quality' science. However, how 'quality' is measured has come down to the number of times a journal's studies are cited, i.e. the impact factor.

Mannix goes on to note that the average impact factor almost doubled between 1997 and 2016, and when, in 1975, the top scoring journal had an impact factor of 11.87, now it is 187.04. He asks, had science's impact really increased that much? According to Park et al. (2023), the level of true innovation in scientific papers fell by more than 90% from 1945 to 2010, and all fields of science are becoming less innovative. Quantity has overtaken quality or impact and where once one paper would do, there are three and reviews of reviews and special editions. Mannix suggests that the use of AI may lead to a further explosion in meaningless studies.

In 2023, the Australian chief scientist Dr Cathy Foley called for an overhaul of Australia's research system which can reward quantity over quality and that the 'way individuals and institutions are measured on research success is not fit for purpose and has created perverse incentives which reinforce a "publish or perish" culture'. A report found that researchers felt pressure to focus on established areas to increase their publication count at the expense of more exploratory research.

Concerns about the quality of some research is not new; however, the emergence of predatory journals and a massive increase in publications has taken this to a new level.

Questionable or unsatisfactory research practices also contribute to irreproducibility. There is an acceptance in the scientific community that some irreproducibility will occur; however, in 2018 the scale and implications of irreproducible research in Australia was seen to be particularly concerning (Stephens 2018). In addition, it has been found that well-established researchers have a much greater success rate of obtaining funding than new, young researchers.

There is also a widespread problem of publication bias which has resulted in studies with positive findings being over-represented in the published literature. Positive studies are more likely to be published, published faster, published in higher-impact journals, and more often cited, which causes the evidence base to become skewed and could sometimes result in ineffective treatments being given to patients.

A huge increase in predatory journals hasn't helped (Tramuta-Drobnis 2023). Concerns about the rise in open-access journals with questionable publishing practices were first raised in 2008 and whilst initially developed to lower publishing costs, along came the 'pay to publish' rather than the 'pay to access' model leading to predatory publishers. These publications contain incomplete or poorly conducted research, are non-peer-reviewed, or are poorly reviewed. Systematic reviews support the view that predatory journals publish poorly designed research, less valid research and incorrect papers leading to misleading or incomplete research. We like to think that peer review will detect errors; however, peer reviewers have been found to miss most scientific errors (Godlee et al. 1998).

'Paper mills', businesses that sell bogus work and authorship to scientists, are estimated to produce hundreds of thousands of articles and four times more researchers produce more than 60 papers a year than less than a decade ago. Some researchers publish a staggering new paper every 5 days. (Van Noorden 2023).

The quality of some research is highly questionable, with a reported more than 10,000 research papers retracted in 2023, an all-time record, and the rate has more than tripled in the past 10 years, with experts saying that this is only the tip of the iceberg. Publishers struggled to clean up the vast number of sham papers and peer-reviewed fraud, with Saudi Arabia, Pakistan, Russia, and China, having the highest retraction rates over the past two decades. Whilst retracted papers were mostly sham articles, they were still collectively cited 35,000 times. Retractions are rising faster than the growth of scientific papers, with total retractions passing 50,000, mostly due to scientific misconduct (Nature News 2023). The reason for the massive number is sleuthing by volunteers combing academic literature and major publishers' belated recognition that what they have been doing has made them susceptible to paper mills.

Poor research and sham publications are not harmless and falsified results can lead to incorrect treatments, sometimes with fatal consequences. Veterinary science is certainly not immune, and we should be grateful to organisations such as Retraction Watch for bringing this to our attention. We should all be wary of research findings that look too good to be true, especially those published in predatory journals.

5.4   CAREGIVER PLACEBO EFFECTS

A significant source of error in animal studies of medical therapies is the caregiver placebo effect. Using inconsistent subjective measures of response to a therapy instead of objective measures can lead to ineffective therapies appearing to be effective (Conzemius & Evans 2012). This effect explains why ineffective and implausible therapies seem to 'work' and why this is an ethical and animal welfare concern. A perceived positive effect of ineffective and implausible 'therapies' may be because the owner of the animal; undergoing acupuncture, for example, may in fact be treating the animal differently, and the animal picks up on the cues. In addition, the owner may be reluctant to tell the 'therapist' that the animal is no better after having paid for this treatment.

5.5   LIVING LONGER AND BETTER LIVES

It is said that advances in veterinary medicine have led to animals living longer and healthier lives; however, this may be primarily down to better preventative healthcare, vaccines, worming and avoidance of fast-moving cars. Certainly, in the human field, healthcare services are just one of a number of influences, and preventative medicine likely has a greater effect on longer, healthier lives than 'cures'.

These advances in veterinary medicine often point to veterinary practices, especially specialist practices, increasingly equipping themselves with better diagnostic tools, such as in house pathology, MRI, and CT machines (or 'toys' as they are called in some ads for new veterinarians), and are equated with better treatment options for animals and longer healthier lives. It would certainly be interesting to compare the effects of advances in preventative health against advances in diagnostics and treatments.

5.6 DOES THE PUBLIC TRUST VETERINARIANS?

According to the Animal Medicines Australia report 2022 veterinarians remain at 51% the primary source of information for pet-related issues followed by search engines at 39%. This was 45% in 2019 so maybe trust in 'Dr Google' has fallen. Family, friends, and neighbours were found to be a more useful source than animal welfare agencies, low on the list, as is social media and even lower veterinary expert blogs, so it would appear that influencers with pets aren't as important as we think they may be.

Ethical behaviour continues to be seen as important for society and according to the Governance Institute of Australia Ethics Index 2023 trust in veterinarians took a tumble and had a fall of 6 points from 2022. Whilst veterinarians are still in the top ten occupations, we rank below pharmacists, nurses, human general practitioners, and ambulance and fire services. It is some consolation to find that we are above the bottom ten of lawyers, politicians, and real estate agents.

Trust is of utmost importance for veterinarians to maintain their social standing and remain the primary source of information and advice on animal health and welfare. Surveys show that the community views transparency and accountability as the most important attributes, along with a commitment to animal welfare, clinical problem-solving ability, not being seen to be motivated by money, and being compassionate, open, and honest.

It would be interesting to know why trust in veterinarians has fallen although concerns about costs, lack of transparency, increasing corporatisation and a move to a business agenda are no doubt contributing factors.

5.7 SCIENCE, ETHICS, AND CLINICAL DECISION-MAKING

It is not just about knowledge and science. Veterinarians have always needed to consider ethics as well as science in making decisions about animal welfare, and it is widely accepted that scientific assessments of animal welfare involve a number of considerations that are ethical in nature.

Ethical decision-making for veterinarians does not simply involve animal ethics, which is related to concerns about animal use. Although veterinarians may need to consider the ethics of animal use, veterinary ethics are concerned with how veterinarians make decisions and act as professionals for the provision of veterinary care. The law and codes of conduct relating to veterinarians provide an ethical framework to ensure that veterinarians work in an ethical environment.

Veterinarians need to discard the perception that moral or ethical reasoning, philosophically grounded, is distant from everyday practice. In fact, daily encounters with ethical 'dilemmas' or 'challenges' or even 'choices' (which are better words as 'dilemma' suggests choosing between two issues) – be they end-of-life decision-making, pain relief for husbandry procedures, or requests to euthanise healthy animals – can serve to make the life of a practitioner more interesting and rewarding.

At the BVA Congress in London in November 2016, Franck Meijboom, associate professor at the Faculty of Veterinary Medicine and Ethics at Utrecht University, spoke about 'incorporating ethics into everyday practice'. Professor Meijboom posed a number of questions including whether vets should ignore the interests of an animal when the interests of its owner conflicted with animal welfare and instead aim for a good vet-client relationship. A majority of the audience, quite rightly disagreed, with one member of the audience commenting that pandering to a client's wishes was not a good relationship.

Regardless of whether practitioners have time to sit down and 'navel gaze', clinical decision-making is one aspect of practice that demands reflection. Have I made the right decision? Is this decision using the best evidence? Is this decision in line with codes of conduct and the law? Have I ensured that the animal is my first priority? Have I followed up to check if the animal responded to my treatment? It's clear that ethically, veterinarians need to make clinical decisions using best evidence for the best health and welfare outcomes for the animal, the owner, and the veterinarian.

5.8 VETERINARY SCIENCE IN A POST-TRUTH ERA

The post-truth era has thrown up many challenges for those of us working in veterinary practice. In a time of pseudoscience and rubbish ideas and clients who consult 'Dr Google' first, life in practice can be challenging. This is especially so if we don't have all the answers, as sometimes happens, the body of scientific research in veterinary medicine being small compared to human medicine.

Veterinary expertise is more than medical knowledge and technical competence. It is also the courage and confidence to acknowledge the limitations of knowledge and competency, which serve as a spur to increase know-how rather than as an impediment. Awareness of limitations to knowledge is an integral aspect of what it means to be a veterinary practitioner and an essential first step in the use of EBVM. As the RCVS Position Paper on EBVM states, 'in order to be considered fit-to-practice, veterinary practitioners hold the responsibility to ground their decisions on sound objective and up-to-date evidence, when available'.

Veterinary professional ethics demands that we practise what should be, not what is demanded, and all veterinary procedures should be based on best evidence, be justifiable, and be undertaken in the best interests of animals and their owners. Professionals have a special duty of care to those they serve, and they have special duties to other professionals and most importantly responsibility to society in general (Stephens 2012).

We are well aware that correcting misinformation is terribly difficult. Humans are much more complex than the average dog and prone to confirmation bias, i.e. a tendency to consume information that confirms a belief and have a need to agree with like-minded people. However, the facts can still make a difference (Caulfield 2020), silence is not the answer and has the worst effect, and a fact-filled rebuttal that corrects inaccuracies can make a difference. As Caulfield states, 'science needs to be inserted into the broader conversation in a way that will allow it to compete with the narrative-filled misinformation circulating in popular culture'.

The other avenue is to encourage critical thinking and scepticism, fact checking, and accuracy. This should start amongst veterinary students who should be able to critically assess the latest new drug or surgical procedure. They should be taught how to read a scientific paper and not be let loose into practice believing everything they read in a glossy magazine. As has been found by White et al. (2024), a minority (16%) of advertisements for veterinary therapies in veterinary magazines were accompanied by references to peer-reviewed literature. Student-directed learning instead of directed teaching may perhaps be contributing to students and new graduates cherry-picking information.

In this post-truth world of fake news and the like, where science has been downgraded to mere opinion and scientists' voices are ignored, if we replace evidence-based medicine with opinion-based medicine, we lose both credibility as veterinary scientists and risk losing our position as the primary source of expertise and information on animal health and welfare. The veterinary profession needs good scientific evidence to counteract misinformation, rubbish ideas and pseudoscience if it wants to provide best care and we should all be supporting the use of EBVM whilst at the same time being alert to the ever-increasing problem of fake research and sham science.

Let's all march for veterinary science.

REFERENCES

Caulfield T. To win the fight against health and wellness bunk, we must leave the post-truth era in the past. *The Globe and Mail* [Internet]. 2020 Jan 6. Available from: https://www.ualberta.ca/en/folio/2020/01/commentary-to-win-the-fight-against-health-and-wellness-bunk-we-must-leave-the-post-truth-era-in-the-past.html.

Conzemius MG, Evans RB. Caregiver placebo effect for dogs with lameness from osteoarthritis. *J Am Vet Med Assoc*. 2012;241(10):1314–1319.

Dean R. Launching an evidence-based veterinary medicine manifesto to drive better practice. *Vet Rec*. 2020;187(5):174–177.

Godlee F, Gale CR, Martin CN. Effect on the quality of peer review of blinding reviewers and asking them to sign their reports: a randomized controlled trial. *JAMA*. 1998;280(3):237–240.

Governance Institute of Australia. Ethics index 2023. *Governance Institute Uploads* [Internet]. 2023 Nov. Available from: https://governanceinstitute.com.au/app/uploads/2023/11/2023-ethics-index-report.pdf.

Mannix L. We've hit peak science and that's not necessarily a good thing. *The Sydney Morning Herald* [Internet]. 2024 Jan 16. Available from: https://www.smh.com.au/national/we-ve-hit-peak-science-and-that-s-not-good-20240116-p5exkb.html.

Nature News. How big is science's fake-paper problem? *Nature News* 2023 Nov 6. 623: 466–467.

Park M, Leahey E, Funk RJ. Papers and patents are becoming less disruptive over time. *Nature*. 2023;613:138–144.

Stephens T. Veterinary ethics. In: Bowden P, editor. *Applied ethics: strengthening ethical practices*. 1st ed. Melbourne: Tilde University Press; 2012.

Stephens T. Let's all march for (veterinary) science. *Aust Vet J*. 2017;95(11):23.

Stephens T. Best practice for animal use for scientific purposes. *Aust Vet J*. 2018;96(4):8.

Tramuta-Drobnis E. Are you prey to predatory journals? *Veterinary Practice News* [Internet]. 2023 Nov 20. Available from: https://www.veterinarypracticenews.com/predatory-journals/.

Van Noorden R. More than 10,000 research papers were retracted in 2023 – a new record. *Nature*. 2023;624:479–481.

White C, Basham N, Floyd S, et al. Cross sectional survey of sources of information accompanying veterinary product advertisements in two professional print publications. *Vet Rec*. 2024;194(8):e3902.

Part II

Some Ethical Challenges Facing the Veterinary Profession
Too Much Veterinary Medicine

6 Just Because We Can Doesn't Mean We Should

Polly Taylor

Technological developments have escalated beyond all recognition in the last few decades, and in both human and veterinary fields, diagnostic, surgical and medical procedures have become highly sophisticated. Such developments have undoubtedly benefited both people and animals, but they have also led to hitherto unforeseen problems that benefit neither man nor beast.

Groundbreaking, purportedly life-saving veterinary treatments are sensationalised globally and receive considerable accolade. The stray dog Monika (later rechristened Momo) lost all four limb extremities and had them replaced with endoprostheses. She was displayed on stage as a huge success story, whilst looking remarkably uncomfortable, at a Technology-Entertainment-Design, or TEDx, talk in her home country (TEDx Talks 2021). Subsequently, she was brought to Britain and ultimately euthanised as a result of prosthesis failure from infection. She was lovingly cared for in the United Kingdom (UK) but must have suffered months of pain and discomfort. Hero the Cow lost two limbs to frostbite as a calf and was given several prostheses as she grew (OnlyGood TV 2020). She was regarded as 'unusual, yes, but an opportunity' (Saul 2014) by the team working on 'the project'. An opportunity for what? Whatever the underlying reasons, publicity and accolade were part of the story.

The technological advances in materials, imaging, surgical technique and anaesthesia enabled such complex procedures to be undertaken – and regarded as successful. But what is success? The protheses worked – at least for a while – but what benefit was there to the animals concerned? Momo clearly suffered months of pain and discomfort; as for Hero, 'saving this calf may have made the rescuers feel good about themselves, but the animal's quality of life from now on will be greatly diminished' (Bussard 2014).

In the UK every veterinarian makes a declaration when becoming a member of the Royal College of Veterinary Surgeons (RCVS), which is required for them to practise legally as a veterinarian. This declaration includes the lines 'I promise and solemnly declare that . . . ABOVE ALL my constant endeavour will be to ensure the health and welfare of animals committed to my care'. Other countries have similar – although not identical – processes. Ensuring the health and welfare of animals surely means that any treatment undertaken should first of all be to their benefit – not to that of the clinician or owner.

Clever and sophisticated treatments have led to the illusion that because they are clever, modern, and groundbreaking, they must benefit the animal. This is not necessarily the case – each proposed treatment should balance up the pros and cons from the animal's point of view. Opinions will differ as to what is benefit, but we appear to have reached a point where complex and clever treatment is often not to the animal's benefit when seen from outwith the intensity and heroics of the case management.

How have we reached this sorry state – where potentially wonderful treatments are causing harm and misery? Immense advances in technology have undoubtedly contributed, making it possible to perform highly technical and complex surgical and medical treatments. However, a technically and physically successful procedure does not necessarily mean a better quality of life.

The humanisation of animals, particularly pets, has left common sense behind. Apparently, 'fur babies', not owned by but children of 'pet parents', have become surrogate people who deserve the same treatment as the rest of humankind. Failure to appreciate that a dog is a dog and a cat is a cat and neither is human leads to complete lack of understanding of the needs of each species. Even in the human world overtreatment is detrimental (Hubbeling 2022); in the animal world we are caring for creatures who cannot foresee and rationalise the future. They do not understand that the current hell of surgical suite and intensive care ward might lead to a better future.

Developments in medical and veterinary treatment options appear to have led to a widely held delusion that death can be put off for ever in modern-day medical practice; death is regarded as a treatment failure rather than a biological certainty. The inevitability of death is all the more relevant to the mistake of humanising animals. Companion animals do not live as long as people. Reality must be faced; the owner will outlive several dogs and cats in their own lifetime. To enjoy the relationship and to give pets the quality of life they deserve, they need to be accepted for who and what they are: dogs and cats who usually live for considerably less than a quarter of our own life span.

Sadly there are more reasons for clever but inappropriate treatment which does not benefit the animal. The need for original case material for postgraduate qualification or for publication supports the use of unusual treatments. The accolade for being 'the first' (Westgate 2021) or uniquely cutting-edge care (Channel 4 2024) encourages interventions for interventions' sake, with some disregard to whether the patient will actually benefit. The growth in social media has undoubtedly fuelled the reporting of clever cases for an increasing number of 'likes'. Fashion and oft-cited owner pressure to carry out an inappropriate or unnecessary procedure may account for some overtreatment. The financial reward from complex treatments is probably the elephant in the room that few will admit has any bearing on the treatment undertaken. The advent of corporate veterinary groups, aiming principally to make money for their shareholders rather than simply to mend animals, is surely evidence of this. Use of novel equipment simply to make a profit is, like it or not, a tactic not unknown within the veterinary world. For instance, laser equipment with little evidence of efficacy has been marketed with the advertising feature:

Generate Additional Income For Your Practice

Use our ROI Calculator below to find out how much additional revenue your practice can make by offering laser therapy to your clients. Start offering laser therapy in your practice and make your money back within months! Pay off the initial investment and generate profit from thereon.

(Pioneer+ Veterinary Products 2024)

The potentially high cost, in all senses of the word, underlines the question of ethics: the procedure can be done – but is it the right thing to do? For the individual case, the veterinary ethics tool (Grimm et al. 2018) offers a means of working out the best strategy for the patient where the best course of action is not obvious and runs the risk of overtreatment. A small panel represents all the stakeholders – the animal, the owner, and the clinician – and balances their points of view.

However, the overarching problem is that the veterinary profession seems to be getting carried away on a tide of apparent skill, clever treatment and even gimmicks that do not benefit our patients. It is essential that the welfare of each animal should be at the top of the list of considerations for its treatment, not how cool and innovative it may be. Better treatments for many diseases and injuries are clearly desirable and their development should be encouraged – but not at the animal's expense.

REFERENCES

Bussard J. Prosthetic legs for frostbitten calf may not be so humane. *Farm Progress* [Internet]. 2014 Feb 1. Available from: https://www.farmprogress.com/commentary/prosthetic-legs-for-frostbitten-calf-may-not-be-so-humane.

Channel 4. The supervet: Noel Fitzpatrick. *Channel Programmes* [Internet]. Undated [cited 2024 Aug 22]. Available from: https://www.channel4.com/programmes/the-supervet-noel-fitzpatrick.

Grimm H, Bergadano A, Musk GC, et al. Drawing the line in clinical treatment of companion animals: recommendations from an ethics working party. *Vet Rec*. 2018;182(23):664.

Hubbeling D. Overtreatment: is a solution possible? *J Eval Clin Pract*. 2022;28:821–827.

OnlyGood TV. Amputee cow named Hero inspires in moo ways than one. *YouTube* [Internet]. 2020 Jul 14. Available from: https://www.youtube.com/watch?v=3OTPea0WLog.

Pioneer+ Veterinary Products. Laser therapy the continuum of care. *Pioneer+ Veterinary Products Laser Therapy* [Internet]. Undated [cited 2024 Aug 22]. Available from: https://pioneervet.co.uk/laser-therapy#ihysrr.

Saul H. Rescued calf is fitted with £24,000 prosthetic legs after suffering frost bite. *Independent* [Internet]. 2014 May 23. Available from: https://www.independent.co.uk/news/weird-news/rescued-calf-hero-is-fitted-with-ps24-000-prosthetic-legs-after-suffering-frost-bite-9423146.html.

TEDx Talks. Спасти жизнь домашнему питомцу. Миссия выполнима. | Сергей Горшков | TEDxNovosibirsk. *YouTube* [Internet]. 2021 Dec 20. Available from: https://www.youtube.com/watch?v=oXU9Ogu9Lls.

Westgate J. 'World first' as UK vet treats urinary tract duplication. *Vet Times* [Internet]. 2021 Jan 21. Available from: https://www.vettimes.co.uk/news/world-first-as-uk-vet-treats-urinary-tract-duplication/.

7 Overdiagnosis

Brennen McKenzie

In human medicine, awareness of the dangers of overdiagnosis has led to widespread reductions in screening, testing of asymptomatic individuals for occult disease. Screening for even common conditions, such as prostate cancer and mammary cancer, has been curtailed, and pre-operative blood testing is not recommended for healthy people undergoing elective procedures.

Increased awareness of overdiagnosis among veterinarians would improve patient care by reducing the risks of tests and treatment that do not benefit our patients, and more judicious use of diagnostic testing would improve the usefulness of results and make veterinary care more affordable.

> Cured yesterday of my disease, I died last night of my physician.
>
> – Matthew Prior, 1714

7.1 WHAT IS OVERDIAGNOSIS?

Jake was a 5-year-old Labrador retriever who was brought to his regular veterinarian for acute-onset lameness in his right hind limb. Apart from this complaint, he was healthy in every way, with no other clinical symptoms. A routine workup diagnosed the problem as a complete rupture of Jake's right cranial cruciate ligament. The recommended therapy was a tibial plateau levelling osteotomy, and the owner agreed to proceed with this treatment.

The surgeon ordered a complete blood count and clinical chemistry, as she did routinely for all surgical patients. Jake's results were mostly normal, but his chemistry panel did show a moderate elevation in his alanine aminotransferase and a mild increase in his alkaline phosphatase levels.

Out of an abundance of caution, Jake was referred for an abdominal ultrasound, which showed a few indistinct, mildly hypoechoic nodular lesions in the liver. In order to be certain these were not evidence of neoplasia, an ultrasound-guided needle biopsy was performed. The histopathology ultimately confirmed benign nodular hyperplasia.

While this should have been good news, unfortunately, Jake died the day after the biopsy procedure. While the official cause of death was haemorrhage from the biopsy site, the real cause was overdiagnosis.

The concept of overdiagnosis is quite simple: it is the correct diagnosis of a medical condition that is truly present in a patient but that will never cause significant clinical symptoms or death. This is different from several more widely known, and feared, diagnostic errors. Misdiagnosis, for example, is incorrectly diagnosing health problems a patient does not actually have. False positive test results are often an element of misdiagnosis, though of course single lab test results in isolation should not be the only foundation for a clinical diagnosis.

Missed diagnosis is probably the most feared error; the failure to identify a condition that is present. The cardinal sin vets dread committing is not identifying a medical condition that is causing clinical symptoms or that will do so eventually.

Despite the inevitability of both misdiagnosis and missed diagnosis, so long as our scientific knowledge remains incomplete and humans remain imperfect, both of these errors are wrongly associated with incompetence in the minds of both clients and vets. This stigma, ironically, increases the chances of overdiagnosis by encouraging testing that may be overly aggressive or clearly inappropriate. We fear missed or incorrect diagnoses, but we are often blissfully unaware of the potential harm to our patients of overdiagnosis.

In human medicine, overdiagnosis has long been recognised as a common and serious problem. In 2012, a consortium of human medical specialty organisations created Choosing Wisely to help physicians and patients make better decisions and reduce overdiagnosis and treatment. Major medical journals have ongoing features devoted to overdiagnosis, such as the *Journal of the American Medical Association*'s 'Less is More' feature and the *British Medical Journal*'s 'Too Much Medicine'. Changes in clinical practice guidelines for many conditions, including highly publicised changes in practices such as screening for breast cancer and prostate cancer, have resulted from the recognition that overdiagnosis harms patients. Yet the issue of overdiagnosis remains largely unknown in veterinary medicine (McKenzie 2016).

7.2 HOW DO WE KNOW OVERDIAGNOSIS EXISTS?

A challenge in understanding and reducing overdiagnosis is that there is no perfect way to know in advance if a condition diagnosed in a particular patient is going to prove clinically important or not. This can only be known after sufficient time has passed to evaluate whether or not the condition has resulted in disease or death in the absence of treatment. And because many abnormal findings do lead to illness or even death, it is often more appropriate to treat them as if they will than to withhold further testing or treatment.

Due to economic constraints, vets may often be forced to adopt a 'wait and see' approach, and this sometimes generates evidence of overdiagnosis. For example, cases of multifocal peripheral lymphadenopathy in golden retrievers will often turn out to be clinically important diffuse B-cell lymphoma. In most cases, treatment is clearly justified as it extends health and life expectancy significantly.

However, indolent lymphomas are surprisingly common, and many of these will never cause clinical illness (Flood-Knapik et al. 2013). I have seen several patients in my career with clinical presentations typical of lymphoma, confirmed on cytology, whose owners elected no treatment, and these dogs have gone on to lives utterly unaffected by this condition. Treating such cases with chemotherapy would unquestionably have done more harm than good. Even diagnosing them at all can cause harm, especially if owners who are unable to pursue treatment elect to euthanise their pets with 'aggressive cancer' rather than waiting for them to get sick.

The challenge of identifying overdiagnosis in individual patients is a serious problem for clinicians. Fortunately, it is possible to evaluate the frequency of overdiagnosis in a population. This is how we know the problem exists, and such population data can at least give us a rough sense of the probability of overdiagnosis for specific diagnoses and patient populations. While imperfect, this information has been useful at reducing overdiagnosis in human medicine, leading to less harm to patients and less waste of resources spent diagnosing and treating clinically irrelevant conditions.

One common way of identifying overdiagnosis is by evaluating the incidence and mortality data for specific conditions and populations. For example, if the incidence of a particular fatal cancer increases, we would also expect to see an increase in the number of deaths from that cancer, assuming no new treatments are introduced right as the number of cases increases. However, if the number of cases is going up but the number of deaths is steady or decreasing, this sometimes means that we are diagnosing more non-progressive, indolent cases rather than those cases, which would actually prove fatal. In other words, we are seeing overdiagnosis.

The classic examples of this in human medicine involve screening efforts for detecting early prostate cancer or breast cancer. Screening means the testing of asymptomatic individuals, attempting to find a disease before it causes clinical symptoms. The idea is that earlier detection will lead to more effective treatment and better outcomes. However, this is not always true. More aggressive testing can also lead to detection of indolent disease that would never have become symptomatic.

Figure 7.1 shows the increase in new diagnoses for both prostate cancer and breast cancer in the 1980s. Prostate cancer diagnoses increased largely because of the introduction of a new screening test, which measured a blood-borne biomarker called prostate-specific antigen (PSA). This led to identification of many more cases that were previously found by physical examination or due to patient-reported symptoms. Breast cancer diagnoses increased around the same time due to the success of programs to increase awareness and screening.

The fact that the increase in diagnoses of these cancers was not accompanied by an increase in mortality, despite no dramatic new therapies being introduced at this time, indicates that many of the newly diagnosed cases were likely never going to progress to disseminated, fatal disease. It has since been learned that many prostate cancers are indolent and will never cause symptoms, and these would simply never have been diagnosed prior to the advent of PSA testing. Because treatment does not benefit these patients, and the diagnosis itself can cause significant harm (as discussed in the following section regarding the harm of overdiagnosis), these are perfect examples of overdiagnosis.

Screening is a particularly effective way of generating overdiagnosis. Veterinarians, like physicians, are eager to identify disease as early as possible

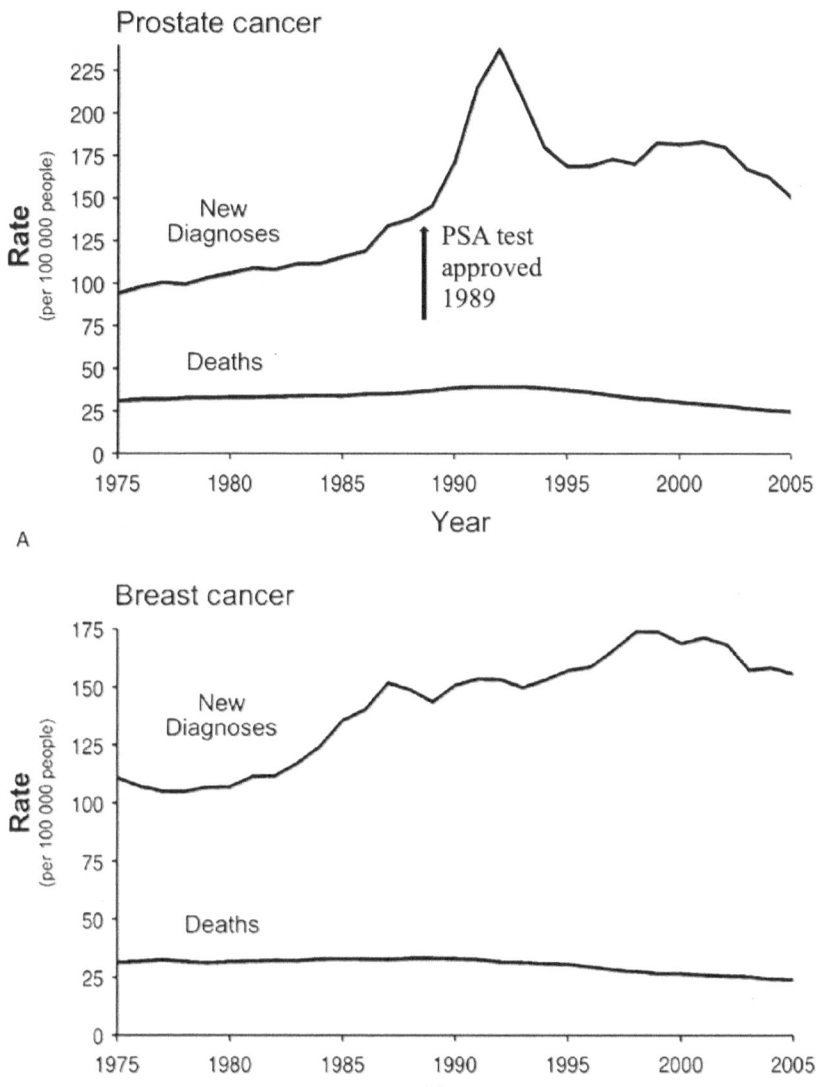

FIGURE 7.1 Incidence and mortality for prostate cancer (A) and breast cancer (B) illustrating overdiagnosis (adapted with permission from Welch HG, Schwartz LM, Woloshin S, *Overdiagnosed: making people sick in pursuit of health*, 1st ed., Boston: Beacon Press; 2011).

because we believe this will allow us to more effectively treat our patients. However, not all early diagnosis is beneficial. Being diagnosed early with a disease for which there is no effective treatment, for example, simply gives the patient more time to live with the diseases, and with any harmful effects of subsequent testing and treatment.

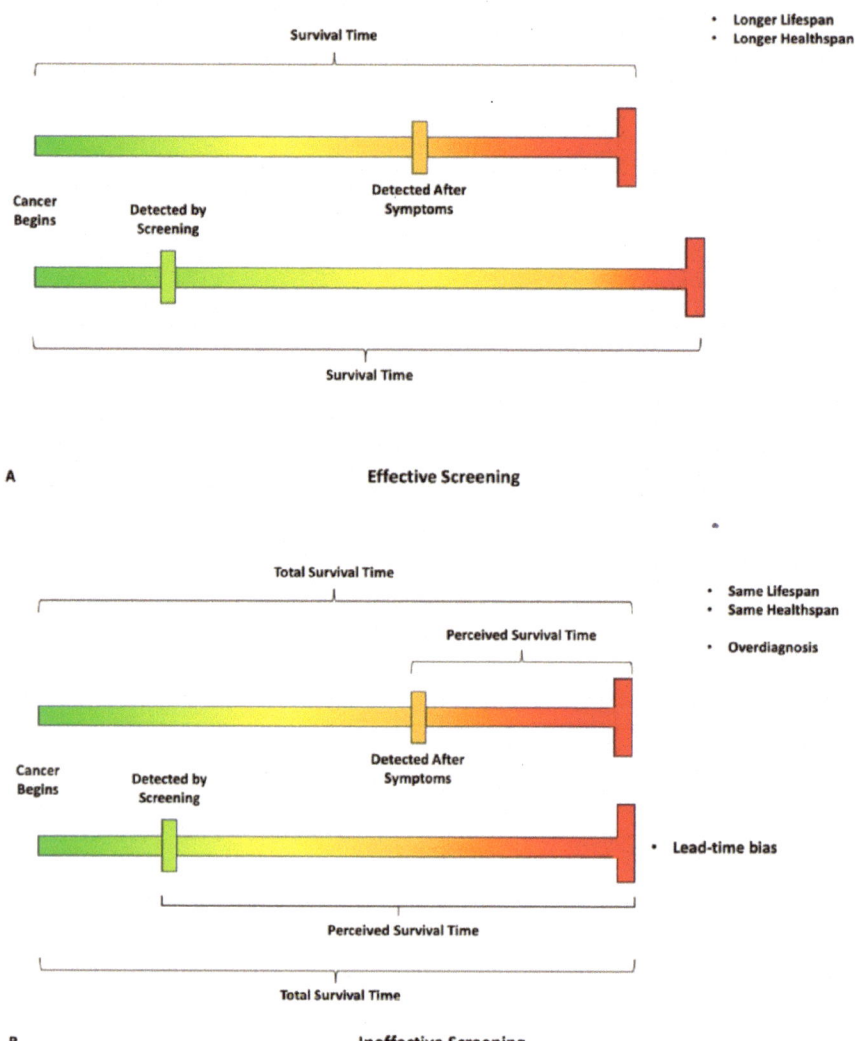

FIGURE 7.2 Illustrations of the potential outcomes of screening asymptomatic individuals for potentially fatal disease, including effective screening (A), ineffective screening with lead-time bias (B), ineffective screening with diminished healthspan (C), and harmful screening with diminished lifespan and healthspan (D).

Figure 7.2 illustrates several possible outcomes for screening of asymptomatic patients, again with cancer as the example. In the best case, screening does give an opportunity for more effective treatment and better outcomes. However, screening can also be ineffective, leading to no real change in healthspan or lifespan but a perception of better survival due to lead-time bias. Even more disturbing is the possibility that screening can lead to worse clinical outcomes.

Overdiagnosis

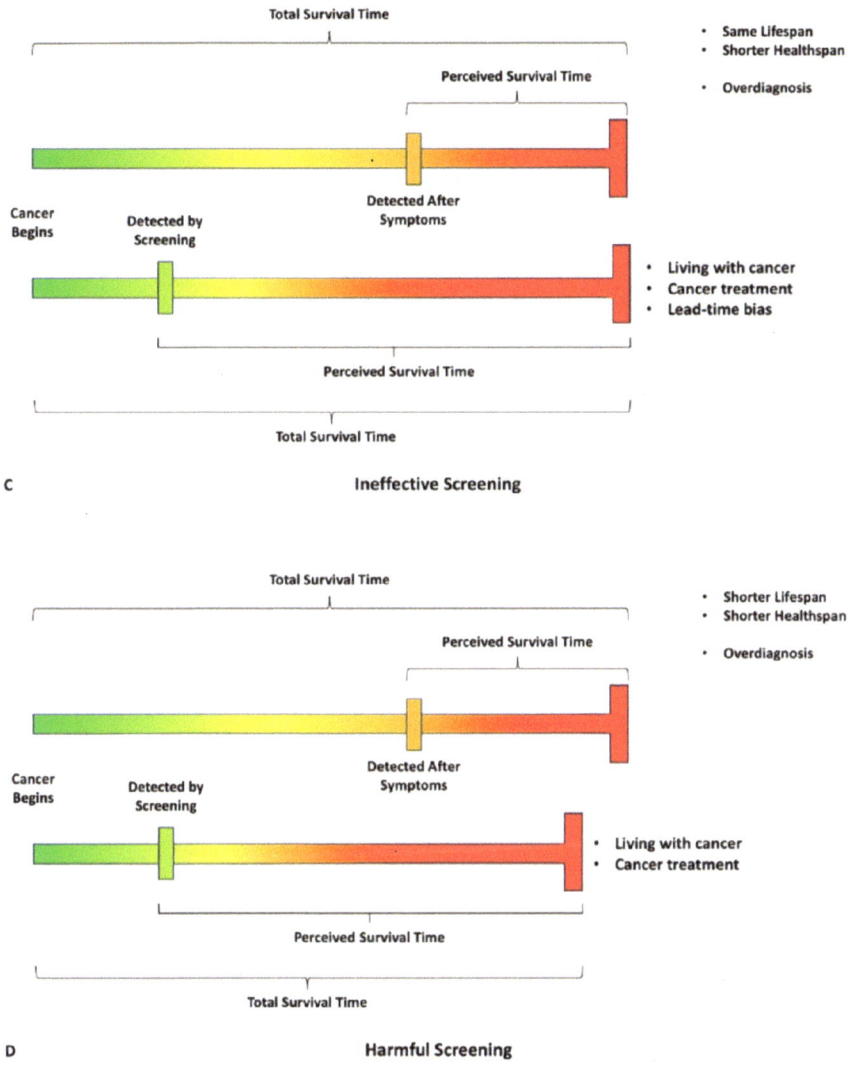

FIGURE 7.2 (Continued)

7.3 WHAT IS THE HARM OF OVERDIAGNOSIS?

The diagnosis of diseases that are unlikely to ever cause significant illness or mortality causes harm in several ways. Of course, the initial testing and any follow-up tests or treatments have financial costs. It is estimated, for example, that overdiagnosis and overtreatment of clinically irrelevant lesions detected through mammography costs $4 billion annually in the United States alone (Ong & Mandl 2015). Another study suggests that unnecessary treatment of people with mild hypertension in the US, with no benefit in terms of reducing symptoms or early mortality, may cost $32 billion annually (Martin et al. 2014).

These are only estimates for the costs of overdiagnosis for two diseases in one country, so the global financial cost is undoubtedly much greater. And despite the impulse to feel that no price should be put on efforts to improve health and treat disease, it is undeniable that such waste raises the overall costs of healthcare and reduces access for some people, all without any benefit to patients.

There are no estimates of the costs of overdiagnosis in veterinary medicine. The economic model of the veterinary profession is quite different from human medicine, and the financial costs of overdiagnosis may not impact the overall cost of veterinary care or the availability of care as dramatically. However, these costs are still a waste of client resources, and they can reduce the ability of some clients to pay for subsequent care that may be necessary or beneficial for their animals.

The financial costs of overdiagnosis, however, have not been the major driver of change in clinical practice in human medicine. This has been the physical and emotional harm to patients. Diagnostic testing and treatment of clinically benign disease can itself cause both physical injury and psychological distress.

It has been estimated that, for example, that for every death prevented by prostate-specific antigen (PSA) screening, 30 to 100 patients will be given a cancer diagnosis who would never have been clinically affected or known they had the disease. And for the majority of these men who go on to have biopsies or cancer treatment, up to 50% will experience sexual dysfunction, 30% will have urination difficulties, and one to two per thousand screened will die as a result of unnecessary treatment. Research has also shown that quality of life diminishes after a diagnosis of prostate cancer and that the risk of suicide and cardiovascular death increases immediately following such a diagnosis (Heijnsdijk et al. 2012; Fang et al. 2010). Similar evidence of physical and psychological harm from overdiagnosis is available for many other conditions in human medicine.

There has been no published research on the risks of overdiagnosis in the veterinary field. However, it is clear that such risks exist, for owners as well as patients. Owners experience significant psychological distress when caring for pets with chronic disease, and overdiagnosis may contribute to this caregiver burden. Any vet who has had to deliver a diagnosis of cancer or another potentially fatal disease knows how devastating this can be emotionally for owners.

Such diagnoses also change an owner's perspective on their pets' health and healthcare. A diagnosis of cancer, chronic kidney disease, or another serious condition may well discourage an owner from pursuing needed care even if that condition is not symptomatic and may never progress. Owners routinely use such diagnoses as a justification for eschewing other testing, dental care, pain medication for orthopaedic disease, and many other interventions that might truly benefit their pets.

Of course, just as in humans, overdiagnosis can lead to direct patient harm. Tests and treatments all have potential risks, and when the disease being identified and treated is not clinically relevant, these risks are not balanced by any benefit.

Jake died from complications caused by a test that identified an unimportant condition. Dogs and cats with indolent cancers or other non-progressive disease will suffer only the adverse effects of our treatments and gain no benefit in length or quality of life. In the worst case, owners may choose euthanasia over expensive treatment or out of a desire to avoid putting their pet through a feared decline in health and quality of life that might never actually come.

7.4 WHAT CAUSES OVERDIAGNOSIS?

Overdiagnosis is driven by numerous factors. Screening tests, imaging, and other diagnostics employed without specific clinical justification frequently lead to the detection of abnormalities. Such abnormalities are far less likely to be clinically important than those which cause symptoms, and they often represent overdiagnosis. However, once an abnormality is detected, some of the psychological harm to patients or caregivers has already occurred. And because of the anxiety induced by the finding and the desire of both clients and doctors to take some action, even when it is unclear this will benefit the patient, further testing and therapy often follow an initial overdiagnosis.

Overdiagnosis also stems from human psychology and cognitive bias (McKenzie 2014). Psychologically, doctors are prone to overdiagnosis because they are likely to be punished, in the form of blame or even litigation, for failing to diagnose a medical condition if it does eventually lead to symptoms or death. There are no sanctions, however, for unnecessarily diagnosing and treating conditions which would never have caused any harm if undiagnosed, and such an outcome is rarely even detected.

The inappropriate reliance on anecdotal evidence and clinical experience to guide diagnostic practices also contributes to overdiagnosis. Even in the face of strong evidence, for example, that mammography of women under 50 years of age leads to significantly more harm from overdiagnosis than benefit from earlier diagnosis and treatment, there has been significant resistance to the change in screening guidelines implemented to reduce this harm. Much of that resistance is justified with the use of anecdotes of women who had been diagnosed and treated for breast cancer because they and their doctors believed, rightly or wrongly, that this intervention had saved their lives.

Any doctor who believes their use of screening or other diagnostic interventions in asymptomatic patients has saved someone's life will be very reluctant to stop using those interventions regardless of the evidence that they do more harm than good. Individual stories are always more psychologically compelling than statistical data. But acting on our emotional response to such stories and ignoring the evidence regarding overdiagnosis ultimately causes more unnecessary suffering for real patients.

Patients are similarly inclined to seek diagnosis and take action on it even if the statistical evidence suggests it is in their best interests not to. Doing so gives people a sense of control over their fate or that of their animals. Even if this sense of control is an illusion, it tends to outweigh rational considerations. One survey found that 98% of people mistakenly diagnosed with cancer through screening were still glad they had had the test once the follow-up evaluation showed they actually did not have cancer (Schwartz et al. 2004). Like doctors, patients are inclined to take action rather than choosing inaction, even when inaction is demonstrably the better choice.

Finally, we cannot ignore the potential influence of financial interests on overdiagnosis. Companies selling diagnostic tools and veterinarians using them receive income from the use of these tools. And the follow-up testing and treatment of diseases, even when they are overdiagnosed, also generates revenue. While doctors are unlikely to intentionally pursue unnecessary testing and treatment purely for financial gain, it would be naive to imagine such revenue has no impact on doctors' decision-making. Federal law prohibits doctors from referring patients to diagnostic facilities in which they have a financial interest because research has shown such interests increase the number of tests done and the costs to patients (Levin & Rao 2008; Gazelle et al. 2007). There is no reason to believe veterinarians to be exempt from the same potential for financial self-interest to influence clinical decisions.

7.5 HOW DO WE REDUCE OVERDIAGNOSIS AND OVERTREATMENT?

The first step in reducing the harms from overdiagnosis is to understand the phenomenon and its causes. This includes developing the data to identify overdiagnosis of specific conditions. Because overdiagnosis can only be identified in retrospect in individual patients, we must gather and analyse epidemiologic data to recognise the level of risk for overdiagnosis of particular diseases using specific tests. We cannot safely rely on anecdotes and uncontrolled clinical experience alone to drive our diagnostic and therapeutic practices. We need data!

In the meantime, in the absence of such data, the best strategy is to understand the limitations of our diagnostic tests, including important measures such as their positive and negative predictive value, which help us to appreciate the likely significance and reliability of test results in particular patient populations. We should also ensure that we have an appropriate clinical index of suspicion for any condition before we begin testing for it. 'Fishing expeditions', 'shotgun diagnostics', indiscriminate imaging, and other such irrational diagnostic practices raise the risk of overdiagnosis (McKenzie 2021).

We must also learn to accept the inevitable uncertainty in medicine and be honest with clients about our ability to predict and control all patient outcomes. We need to recognise and disclose that testing and treatment have costs and risks as well as benefits, especially in patients without significant clinical symptoms associated with the disorders we are trying to diagnose and treat. Though it is psychologically more difficult for us, it is often wiser to avoid action when there is not good evidence to show that our actions will truly benefit our patients. Sometimes the best advice is 'Don't just do something, stand there!'

REFERENCES

Fang F, Keating NL, Mucci LA, et al. Immediate risk of suicide and cardiovascular death after a prostate cancer diagnosis: cohort study in the United States. *J Natl Cancer Inst.* 2010;102(5):307.

Flood-Knapik KE, Durham AC, Gregor TP, et al. Clinical, histopathological and immunohistochemical characterization of canine indolent lymphoma. *Vet Comp Oncol.* 2013;11:272–286.

Gazelle GS, Halpern EF, Ryan HS, et al. Utilization of diagnostic medical imaging: comparison of radiologist referral versus same-specialty referral. *Radiology.* 2007;245(2):517–522.

Heijnsdijk EA, Wever EM, Auvinen A, et al. Quality-of-life effects of prostate-specific antigen screening. *N Eng J Med.* 2012;367(7):595–605.

Levin DC, Rao VM. Turf wars in radiology: updated evidence on the relationship between self-referral and the overutilization of imaging. *J Am Coll Radiol.* 2008;5(7):806–810.

Martin SA, Boucher M, Wright JM, et al. Mild hypertension in people at low risk. *Br Med J.* 2014;349:g5432.

McKenzie BA. Veterinary clinical decision-making; cognitive biases, external constraints, and strategies for improvement. *J Amer Vet Med Assoc.* 2014;244(3):271–276.

McKenzie BA. Overdiagnosis. *J Amer Vet Med Assoc.* 2016;249(8):884–889.

McKenzie BA. Rational use of diagnostic and screening tests. *J Sm Anim Pract.* 2021;62(1):1016–1021.

Ong M, Mandl KD. National expenditure for false-positive mammograms and breast cancer overdiagnosis estimated at $4 billion a year. *Health Aff.* 2015;34(4):576–583.

Schwartz LM, Woloshin S, Fowler FJ, et al. Enthusiasm for cancer screening in the United States. *J Am Med Assoc.* 2004;291(1):71–78.

Welch HG, Schwartz LM, Woloshin S. *Overdiagnosed: making people sick in the pursuit of health.* 1st ed. Boston: Beacon Press; 2011.

8 Do You Want Bloods with That?

Tanya Stephens

Despite the fact that routine blood tests for asymptomatic human patients have been found to have no proven value and indeed occasionally found to be harmful (Shaked et al. 2019), the idea that asymptomatic, even young healthy animals, require a regular blood test, especially a pre-anaesthetic blood test, appears to taken hold in the veterinary world in Australia.

Whilst over marketing of screening tests is rife, the various promotions don't warn pet owners that this testing is of dubious value and may lead to more testing, overdiagnosis, and unnecessary and possible harmful interventions.

As well as being of dubious value and poor ethics, unnecessary testing adds to the costs of veterinary services which can act as a barrier to accessing veterinary care. From an ethical and cost perspective viewpoint it is essential to reduce the resources spent on unnecessary or ineffective tests and treatments, to use evidence-based medicine, and to adopt the strategies and tools of the human Choosing Wisely initiative in veterinary practice.

8.1 BACKGROUND

Looking online, I found that some veterinary practices in Sydney advertise the need not just for pre-anaesthetic testing but yearly wellness testing and a few even suggest 6-monthly as well with the idea that this will establish a 'baseline' value for any further testing and tell you if your pet is 'unwell'. What 'baseline' means is anyone's guess as it is never described.

These veterinary practices advertise that pre-anaesthetic testing is essential with comments such as 'some illnesses and diseases have no symptoms at all and these can be the most dangerous', which is why 'blood tests are so important', and a comment about how a blood test now will help if, a few months down the track and the pet is unwell, there is something to compare it with. One large corporate practice states that this testing is a 'normal procedure in veterinary practice'.

A pathology company website states that there are four reasons to test your pet before anaesthesia.

1. Enjoy peace of mind. Testing can significantly reduce medical risk.
2. Detect hidden illnesses. Healthy-looking pets may be hiding symptoms of a disease or ailment. Testing helps detect this kind of illness so we can avoid problems with anaesthesia.
3. Reduce risks and consequences. If the pre-anaesthetic testing results are normal, we can proceed with confidence. If not, we can alter the anaesthetic procedure or take other precautions to safeguard your pet's health.
4. Protect your pet's future health. These tests become part of your pet's medical record, providing a baseline for future reference.

Furthermore, the website states 'same day, real time blood work results decrease the risk of serious complications during induction, anaesthesia and recovery' and 'blood cell counts can change in hours or even minutes'. There are also some handy hints on how to 'get clients to say "yes" to pre-anaesthetic testing'. There are no references to support these statements.

It is easy to see why there is a veterinary 'obsession' with 'bloods' with veterinary practices, pathology companies and the purveyors of in house pathology testing machines advertising this as a 'normal' procedure, needed for best outcomes and 'peace of mind' for the pet owner as well as the veterinarian.

Whilst over marketing of screening tests is rife, the various promotions don't warn owners that this testing is of dubious value and may lead to more testing, potential overdiagnosis and unnecessary and possible harmful interventions (McKenzie 2016). In humans a Cochrane Collaboration meta-study found that routine annual health checks did not measurably reduce the risks of illness or death and conversely could lead to overdiagnosis and overtreatment.

8.2 IF ALL ELSE FAILS, LOOK AT THE ANIMAL

Apart from healthy animals, as veterinary practitioners we have all been there when considering blood tests. Vaguely unwell pet, anxious owner, waiting room full of barking dogs, noisy clients, and a flyblown rabbit. We would like to say that sometimes animals get better on their own and let's do some watchful waiting and recheck tomorrow. Owner, who is an expert user of 'Dr Google' (of course they are), says 'What about some bloods as well as some antibiotics?' (of course they do).

Maybe commission bias comes into this as well with a need to do something. Or ambiguity bias and not knowing what is wrong. Occasionally, pet owners demand blood tests for their animals to make sure they are 'healthy', and it can be difficult to dissuade them given the widespread use of blood tests in the veterinary world. This certainly happens in the human world where a patient may visit their GP demanding bloods when in fact all they really want is a chat.

However, this pre-anaesthetic testing and wellness testing is aimed at the clinically healthy animal and is a classic example of defensive medicine where testing is carried out to relieve anxieties and a concern over being reported to a veterinary board or being sued if things go wrong. Defensive medicine is poor medicine and as far as being sued is concerned, veterinarians in Australia can be assured that companion animals are objects of private property rights and only worth the cost of purchase. There is no provision for non-economic damages, such as emotional damage, and the pet owner may decide that the legal costs involved in suing to be prohibitive especially if the pet was a gift from a friend or a rescue animal.

That doesn't mean veterinarians should be careless, of course, but defensive medicine is poor medicine and particularly poor ethics. It's not just about poor medicine either as we need to take into account proper use of the client's money. Most importantly veterinarians need to avoid abrogating their professional responsibility onto the owner at the expense of the animal's welfare and the animal not the owner should always be the first priority of the veterinarian.

In my experience some specialist and emergency practices undertake blood tests the moment the animal comes in the practice door and prior to a good clinical examination with the stated aim being to 'establish baseline blood values'. This vague, meaningless, and never-defined term seems to be terribly popular. I like the wise words from one of my professors when I was a student regarding unnecessary testing: 'If all else fails, look at the animal'.

Recently a client took their dysuric but otherwise healthy young female neutered cat which clearly had feline lower urinary tract disease to an emergency/specialist practice after hours. Bloods, taken before the cat had a proper clinical examination, were 'normal', of course, and the cat was fine and just needed some basic treatment and behaviour modification, such as extra kitty litter trays. Instead of that, it had an ultrasound and the bloods and sent home with recommendations to use various supplements and other 'remedies' for which there is little or no evidence. The short trip to this practice cost the owner more than the average weekly wage and even more if there was a trip to the supplement shop, which the client was smart enough to avoid.

Next time, the owner won't be taking their unwell cat anywhere after hours. We know that as costs go up, veterinary visits go down and the client is angry. It isn't just about costs. The issue is poor clinical decision-making and poor ethical behaviour in subjecting an animal to unnecessary procedures. Surveys show that pet owners want accountability and transparency from their veterinarian and want them to care about animal welfare. They certainly don't want to feel that the veterinarian has taken advantage of their attachment to a much-loved pet.

At my practice, when I am presented with an old but clinically healthy dog, with infected painful teeth, my first priority is to make the dog pain-free and comfortable as soon as possible. Rather than carrying out pre-anaesthetic bloods, which I know will not make one iota of difference to what I do, I may instead place the dog on IV fluids, whilst I undertake the dental which I believe is a much better use of the client's money and a more ethical approach.

If I undertook the bloods, what would I do? Firstly, per surveys of other veterinarians, likely nothing different, I would still have to do something about the painful teeth and possible further testing could delay acting on what is the most important issue. The anticipated costs of all the 'extras' may condemn animals to suffer needlessly because the owner is reluctant to pay for any treatment at all.

8.3 A HYPOTHETICAL SCENARIO

I have written about this issue before in an opinion piece on bloods (Stephens 2018) where I presented a hypothetical scenario around the presentation to an inner-city practice of a female Bengal kitten for final vaccinations and to discuss desexing. The picture I painted was a typical one, common at many practices.

Physical examination of the kitten showed it to be in perfect health, and as the owners did not wish to use her for breeding purposes, the veterinarian discussed booking her in sooner rather than later for desexing as intact queens are prone to come on heat at a relatively young age.

The practice has a policy of recommending pre-anaesthetic profiles before any routine surgery even if the animal appears healthy, based on an understanding that there may be an underlying disease not evident on clinical examination, and it's best to be prepared in case of anaesthetic complications or poor outcomes. Acting defensively, the practice is concerned that if they don't carry out this testing and if anything goes wrong, they might be sued or reported to a veterinary board. In any case, it seems that all the local practices offer the same service, so this testing must conform to best evidence and current knowledge. On top of that, the practice has in-house pathology testing equipment that needs to be paid for.

The practice policy is to give the owner the option of deciding whether to have the testing done. It is, of course, an extra cost.

This is not an uncommon scenario, and pre-anaesthetic and yearly 'wellness' profiles appear to be commonplace in Australian small-animal practices.

However, what's the evidence for these tests?

Well, very little as it turns out. Pre-anaesthetic profiles are considered of little value and not routinely recommended in human medicine because the evidence suggests that they do not reduce complications or mortality rates. They also raise the risk of overdiagnosis with subsequent unnecessary or even harmful interventions. The reduction in their use in human patients is good news because overdiagnosis has grown to be a major problem in human medicine with the potential to cause the collapse of the healthcare system.

However, pre-anaesthetic screening of overtly healthy cats and dogs is commonly recommended in small-animal practice and sometimes presented as a necessary part of good patient care. Although these tests may uncover abnormalities, they have usually been found not to alter the anaesthetic plan or affect the complication rate (Alef et al. 2008; Joubert 2007; Paepe et al. 2013). As with human patients, there is always the risk that detection and subsequent investigation or treatment of diseases that would never have harmed the animal will cause more harm than good; harm may also occur because beneficial surgery is postponed indefinitely (McKenzie 2014). There are few guidelines regarding pre-anaesthetic testing in the veterinary world and those that do exist are based on opinion rather than high-quality evidence.

General blood work is designed to be used in a population that's likely to be diseased. It is also variable, depends on the level of hydration and has an accuracy range of 10–15%. It is not a screening test.

There is also the question of Bayesian probability, which is the pre-test probability of a diseased state. And if the test is abnormal (as by definition a small percentage will be) would it convince you that disease is actually present? If not, then don't do the test! If your pre-test clinical suspicion is high, then you would ignore a negative test and you'd treat anyway; again, there is no need to test. In the pre-anaesthetic scenario, a healthy animal has a low chance of disease and the test will likely not convince you even if it is abnormal. Also, 1% of tests will be abnormal, not because of a disease state but simply because the test has to define its cutoff for 'abnormal' at some statistical level.

Without a clinical indication for a test, it is only worth doing if it meets the criteria for a screening test. This might be for when there is a high prevalence of a disease that could be detected before clinical signs become apparent, when early detection improves the treatment outcome, or when the cost of widespread screening is outweighed by savings in disease costs or delayed treatment costs.

Should the client be given the option to decide on testing when there is little evidence? Is it reasonable to ask the client to make a clinical decision when we are the trained professional not them? We don't want to be overly paternalistic, but we also need to avoid abrogating our professional responsibility onto the owner at the expense of the animal's welfare. I believe the public expects the veterinarian to base recommendations on best evidence for care that goes beyond the status quo and fully informed consent is essential.

Still not convinced? Are you reluctant to abandon an integral part of your practice? Well, what about undertaking a clinical audit? Look at all your results of pre-anaesthetic or wellness testing of clinically healthy animals and see if these changed your anaesthetic technique or if there was a real abnormality detected that you didn't expect. Look at what actions were taken because of the results. Was there further unnecessary testing and treatments of no benefit to the animal?

Perhaps you could share your findings with other practitioners.

The evidence for pre-anaesthetic testing of overtly healthy animals is extremely limited and more research should be undertaken before veterinarians recommend this procedure (McKenzie 2018)

The kitten should be booked in sooner rather than later for desexing before she comes on heat.

8.4 HAVE I CHANGED MY MIND?

Has there been any further research or surveys since my opinion piece of 2018 that would make me change my mind about performing 'routine' pre-anaesthetic bloods at my practice? Or so-called wellness testing. The answer is, of course, no.

At my practice, no pathology is ever undertaken without a good clinical examination and a good idea what any testing would show and most importantly if it would make any difference to what I do.

At the moment there are no peer-reviewed evidence-based guidelines for pre-anaesthetic pathology testing of animals and in any case anaesthetic decisions are generally made based on clinical findings not pathology results (Mitchell et al. 2018). A thorough physical examination and a good history are essential and several studies in humans and in veterinary medicine continue to question the need or usefulness of pre-anaesthetic pathology testing in healthy patients. Guidelines for humans centred around a review of the patient's history and clinical examination by competent personnel are deemed the most efficient and accurate way of detecting significant morbidities.

My decision to shun pre-anaesthetic or wellness testing is well supported. A survey found that 'routine non-targeted blood tests in cats and dogs older than 8 years led to few changes in the anaesthetic management and anaesthetists correctly predicted blood test results in most cases' (Diaz et al. 2021). The cost-benefit ratio of routine pre-anaesthetic blood tests in clinically healthy animals is debatable, and the American Animal Hospital Association (AAHA) and the Australian Small Animal Veterinarians (ASAV) anaesthesia guidelines recommend evaluating specific concerns and risk factors to determine the need for testing.

However, Dell'Osa and Jaensch (2016) found significant changes in the blood of 6.2% of dogs and 19.2% of cats, which were considered to be in good health based on history and physical examination, and concluded that 'biochemical and haematological testing as part of regular preventive health checks may facilitate early detection of diseases before they present clinically allowing earlier intervention and better health outcomes'. 'Significant abnormalities included anaemia, inflammation and evidence of liver, kidney and pancreatic disease'.

I have a number of concerns with this study. Firstly, of course, this is just one study which has not been peer-reviewed, and as a clinician, I can't understand why these animals were deemed to be 'healthy' on clinical examination, with anaemia, for example. The study is at odds with other studies which show that clinicians are able to accurately assess the health status of animals on clinical examination. In addition, what does 'regular preventative health checks' mean? Once a week perhaps? Certainly not specified. The statement that results will uncover diseases before they present clinically makes no sense and is not explained.

John Inns (2017) responded to this paper, pointing out there was no conflict of interest statement included in the paper despite the corresponding author giving their address as IDEXX Laboratories and asked 'if a company with a vested interest in obtaining positive results from "wellness" testing had funded the study'. In addition Inns wrote that the authors provided no evidence to the assertion that regular preventative health checks may allow better health outcomes, they didn't provide any follow-up on the subsequent health status of these tested animals and that 'in the case of liver enzyme elevation . . . the statement that further evaluation would be warranted if supporting clinical signs develop . . . suggests that there was little point in performing this test in a healthy dog'.

As Inns rightly points out, wellness testing is not a benign procedure. It can have significant health, welfare and financial costs and there is little published guidance available on the interpretation of abnormal results in a clinically normal animal. Inns asks if dogs and cats benefit from wellness testing or is it being performed to increase practice profitability or for medico legal reasons?

Warne et al. (2018), authors of 'Standards of Care anaesthesia guidelines' use this Dell'Osa and Jaensch (2016) paper to support the use of pre-anaesthetic pathology for clinically healthy animals whilst also acknowledging that their guidelines had not been peer-reviewed and that the main author Dr Warne received personal fees from the pathology company IDEXX during the conduct of the study. In addition one of the co-authors is employed by IDEXX.

These guidelines state that 'when faced with financial or technical limitations that prevent extensive pre-anaesthetic biochemical and haematological testing', as being the only impediment to testing. In this situation, the authors suggest that minimal pre-anaesthetic testing be mandatory to include packed cell volume, blood glucose, total solids, blood urine nitrogen, urine-specific gravity, and peripheral blood smear thrown in for good measure if major surgery is going to be undertaken.

8.5 GOOD GUIDELINES WOULD BE USEFUL

Apart from being of dubious value, unnecessary testing adds to the costs of veterinary services, and there is a growing and significant animal welfare issue of veterinary costs as a barrier to accessing veterinary care. It is essential to reduce the resources spent on unnecessary or ineffective tests and treatments and adopting the strategies and tools of the human Choosing Wisely initiative in veterinary practice.

There are few evidence-based guidelines in veterinary medicine, and there is an urgent need to develop clinical guidelines for veterinarians which are peer-reviewed and based on best evidence using appraisal tools as is employed in human medicine. Guidelines in human medicine have arisen from an increasing recognition that having knowledge is not enough to provide good care and that critically appraised clinical guidelines are important in changing the approach to healthcare, preventing overdiagnosis, improving outcomes and ensuring efficient use of resources.

In human medicine the overuse of tests and medicines paradoxically exists alongside evidence-based medicine driven by defensiveness among health professionals who fear being sued, gaps in knowledge, erroneous beliefs, and lack of meaningful consultations with patients. Overdiagnosis in the human health world has the potential to cause the collapse of the healthcare system where it has been found that many common tests and treatments are often unnecessary, ineffective, or worse still, harmful.

As pets have increasingly become part of the family, pet owners expect the same level of healthcare for their pets as they have, and it is easy to see why some veterinarians and pathology companies are happy to take advantage of this mindset, and in this way, veterinarians are abrogating their professional responsibility onto the owner at the expense of the animal's welfare. Testing to ease our anxieties or because of concerns about being sued is not appropriate for a professional aiming to provide best care and trying to do what is right.

To change practitioners' behaviour starts with education. A good understanding of the use of evidence-based veterinary medicine would help alongside how to read a scientific paper. Of course, a seasoned practitioner such as myself would throw in common sense, which is unfortunately not as common as we think it is, and good clinical decision-making of course.

Given the widespread promotion of pre-anaesthetic pathology testing, it can be tricky to counteract this in practice without suggesting that the practice in the next suburb which undertakes this testing is somewhat substandard or wrong. After all, collegiality and avoiding criticism of fellow practitioners is an essential aspect of professional ethics.

However, the other and more important aspect of professional ethics is to act in the animal's best interests, have the animal as the first priority, and use the best evidence and current knowledge which is part and parcel of legislation and codes of conduct pertaining to the practice of veterinary science.

Furthermore, veterinary professional ethics demands that veterinarians do what is right and not what is asked for, and ethical decision-making and ethical behaviour are essential in upholding the integrity of the profession and maintaining a social contract with the public. If trust in our profession fails and the public feel we are not doing what is right, then we may no longer be seen as the primary source of information on animal health and welfare.

REFERENCES

Alef M, von Praun F, Oechtering G. Is routine pre-anaesthetic haematological and biochemical screening justified in dogs? *Vet Anaesth Analg* 2008;35:132–140.

Dell'Osa D, Jaensch S. Prevalence of clinicopathological changes in healthy middle-aged dogs and cats presenting to veterinary practices for routine procedures. *Aust Vet J.* 2016 Sept;94(9):317–323.

Diaz MDM, Kaartinen J, Allison A. Pre-anaesthetic blood tests in cats and dogs older than 8 years: anaesthetists' prediction and per-anaesthetic changes. *Vet Anaesth Analg.* 2021 Nov;48(6):854–860.

Inns J. Letter to the editor re 'clinicopathological changes in healthy middle-aged dogs and cats presenting to veterinary practices for routine procedures'. *Aust Vet J.* 2017;95(1–2):3.

Joubert KE. Pre-anaesthetic screening of geriatric dogs. *J S Afr Vet Assoc.* 2007;78:31–35.

McKenzie BA. Veterinary clinical decision-making: cognitive biases, external constraints, and strategies for improvement. *J Am Vet Med Assoc.* 2014;244:271–276.

McKenzie BA. Overdiagnosis. *J Am Vet Med Assoc.* 2016;249:884–889.

McKenzie BA. Why do we run diagnostic tests? *Veterinary Practice News.* 2018 Feb 7.

Mitchell K, Barletta M, Quandt J, et al. Effect of routine pre-anaesthetic laboratory screening on pre-operative anaesthesia-related decision-making in healthy dogs. *Can Vet J.* 2018;59(7):773–778.

Paepe D, Verjans G, Duchateau L, et al. Routine health screening: findings in apparently healthy middle-aged and old cats. *J Feline Med Surg.* 2013;15:8–19.

Shaked M, Levkovich I, Adar T, et al. Perspective of healthy asymptomatic patients requesting general blood tests from their physicians: a qualitative study. *BMC Fam Pract.* 2019;20:article number 51.

Stephens T. Do you want bloods with that. *Aust Vet J.* 2018;96:6.

Warne L, Bauquier SH, Pengelly J, et al. Standards of care anaesthesia guidelines for dogs and cats. *Aust Vet J.* 2018;96(11):413–427. Available from: https://doi.org/10.1111/avj.12762.

9 Oncology and Ethics

Tanya Stephens

Thanks to better nutrition, preventative health care and doting owners, companion animals are living longer. This means they are increasingly subject to the ravages of old age and this includes diseases such as cancer which is a leading cause of death in dogs. In addition, with the emergence of the 'fur baby' and greater economic value, pet owners are prepared to spend more on their pets.

It is not surprising that oncology has become a specialty in veterinary medicine in high- and middle-income countries, with a multitude of treatment options from surgery to chemotherapy to radiation therapy, plus other add-ons, such as special nutrition, palliative and hospice care, and rehabilitation.

Despite the emergence of oncology as a specialty, there has been little in the way of an ethical debate on oncology and animals. This particularly applies to chemotherapy as, unlike other treatments, chemotherapeutic agents are carcinogenic, mutagenic, or teratogenic, require special handling, and may involve multiple procedures.

As oncology continues to grow as a specialty, it is imperative that veterinarians consider the ethics of therapies for cancer and whether these are always in the best interests of the animal and their owners.

9.1 BACKGROUND

This chapter is based on a published paper, 'The Use of Chemotherapy to Prolong the Life of Dogs: The Ethical Dilemma' (Stephens 2019) and further references can be found on that paper.

Thanks to better nutrition, vaccination, disease control, confinement, avoidance of fast cars, a comfy bed and doting owners, companion animals are living longer. This means they are increasingly subject to the ravages of old age, and this includes diseases such as cancer.

Many years ago, at my small-animal practice, I used chemotherapy to treat a number of dogs with lymphoma, one of the more common types of cancer in dogs. I would do regular blood smears on the spot, for example, and the drugs could be ordered in small amounts.

Sadly, whilst all the dogs survived for up to a year, they all relapsed, and the owners questioned why they had bothered as did I as well. In addition, my staff felt uncomfortable being around chemotherapeutic agents and were not prepared to use them. This meant that if I was treating a dog, I couldn't have a break away from work. On top of that the company that supplied the drugs stopped supplying them in small amounts and I would need to buy in bulk.

I decided at that time to stand back and assess what I had been doing. It became clear to me that there was an ethical issue with using chemotherapy on animals if all I was doing was extending their lives for the sake of the owners and my own professional satisfaction – especially if that longer grip on life involved multiple trips to the practice and the side effects of chemotherapeutic agents, exclusion from the family at times and the risks the drugs posed to the owners and my staff.

Now, when I see an animal at my practice with a cancer that may be amenable to chemotherapy and the owner is very keen on specialist care, I refer them to an oncologist. There are plenty to choose from. In Australia, as in other middle-to-high-income countries, veterinary oncology as a specialty is now well established.

A good friend, a paediatric oncologist, had a number of dogs with lymphoma that were treated, and she pondered on the fact that she had good 'cure' rates in children with cancer, yet treatments for lymphoma using chemotherapy in dogs hadn't progressed. Sadly, the good friend died of leukaemia, and I often wonder if a lifetime of exposure to chemotherapeutic agents contributed to her demise.

It is not surprising that oncology has become a specialty in veterinary medicine with a multitude of treatment options from surgery to chemotherapy to radiation therapy, plus other add-ons, such as special nutrition, palliative and hospice care, and rehabilitation.

In addition, as companion animal ownership has increased in economic value and owners are prepared to spend more on their pets, and as companion animals are increasingly seen as members of the family, there may be an expectation by owners that their pets are entitled to the same level of healthcare as human members of the family, including treatment for cancer.

9.2 PROGNOSIS

There have certainly been some amazing advances in treating the human animal with cancer; however, the success rate in animals is variable and I wonder how 'success' is really measured in animals. After all, animals, unlike humans, can't give consent and can't visualise a cancer free future or want to live another week to see a long lost relative before they die.

Cancer represents one of the major causes of death in dogs. It accounts for approximately half of the deaths in dogs over the age of ten, and approximately one in four dogs will develop cancer during their life. In the USA cancer is said to be the leading cause of death in dogs more than two years of age.

Cancer in companion animals may be amenable to a range of treatment options from surgery to radiotherapy and chemotherapy, depending on the type of cancer with variable outcomes. Lymphoma, a common cancer in dogs accounting for 8% of cancers, is particularly susceptible to chemotherapy. The dog will not be cured by chemotherapy but may have its life prolonged from 2–24 months. The dog may feel better still suffering from the cancer or it may suffer from the side effects of the treatment. Untreated dogs have an average survival time of 4–6 weeks. Although up to 90% of dogs will go into remission, remission is not a cure (defined as elimination of the disease entirely), so in effect chemotherapy is a form of palliative care and palliation rather than a cure is a major goal of chemotherapy in veterinary oncology.

Best et al. (2023) looked at long term remission and survival in dogs with high grade B cell lymphoma treated with chemotherapy with or without sequential body irradiation. They found that whilst the remission rate with chemotherapy is 80–90% for 9–10 months, the remission rate for greater than 2 years is just 5–10%, and long-term remissions are infrequent. This hasn't changed in dogs over a great many years despite significant improvements in long term remission rates in humans. Irradiation may increase survival time in dogs; however, more research is needed to support this.

9.3 ONCOLOGY, CHEMOTHERAPY, AND ETHICS

Despite the emergence some years ago of oncology as a veterinary specialty, there has been very little in the way of an ethical debate on oncology or the use of chemotherapy in companion animals. Bley (2017) suggests that ethical decision-making in oncology be made using the four principles of biomedical ethics by Beauchamp and Childress. However, this approach, which was developed for ethical decision-making for humans, depends on using the principles of autonomy and justice, which are not applicable for animals.

In addition, there is a concern that owner autonomy may have a negative impact on animal welfare, and there may not be adequate consideration of the legal standing of animals. Whilst animals, at least in Australia, are objects of private property rights, legislation for the protection of animals recognises that animals suffer when ill-treated and therefore have intrinsic interests regardless of their property status; i.e. there is a limitation of personal property rights in order to uphold the interests of animals.

Chemotherapy raises particular ethical issues as, unlike other treatments, chemotherapeutic agents are carcinogenic, mutagenic, or teratogenic and may be irritant and require special and careful handling. In addition, chemotherapy is more likely to be labelled palliative compared to other treatments for cancer such as surgery.

Furthermore, chemotherapy may involve multiple trips to the veterinarian, multiple procedures, and periods in isolation. Cancer-associated pain has been shown to be underdiagnosed, leading to inadequate pain management and diminished quality of life. Fatigue, pain, and dyspnoea, which can be made worse by hypercalcaemia and anaemia, are commonly encountered in animals dying of cancer. An additional concern is the public health risks associated with chemotherapeutic drugs with evidence of lack of care in handling them in veterinary hospitals. And aftercare of an animal undergoing chemotherapy may place an added burden that the owner should take into consideration.

Although veterinarians, particularly veterinary oncologists, may view cancer as just another disease of animals that can be treated, animal owners, in the light of their own experiences or that of their relatives, are likely to view cancer and chemotherapy from a different perspective.

Human patients, when considering their own health, tend to overestimate intervention benefit, so it is not surprising that pet owners generally overestimate the effects of chemotherapy on treatment survival times with potential false expectations. Importantly, owners can make quality-of-life assessments on the animal undergoing chemotherapy based on their subjective observations rather than functional tasks, personality expression or changes in behaviour which aligns with what is known about the caregiver placebo effect.

The decision to use chemotherapy to extend the life of an animal involves balancing the risk of adverse events versus benefits. If animals have no concept of the future and are likely to suffer some serious adverse events with such treatments, consideration should be given as to whether it is ethical and whether it is in the animal's best interests to use chemotherapy. In balancing the interests of the owner, animal, and veterinarian, there is the added dimension that there has been limited research on treatment decision-making by owners of animals diagnosed with malignancies.

There are other significant concerns with the use of chemotherapy in companion animals. Owners of animals undergoing chemotherapy may be poorly informed, and despite the fact that chemotherapy is becoming a more common therapy, there have been no large-scale studies on the prevalence and incidence of side effects associated with this treatment.

Informed consent is essential and pet owners would benefit from a better understanding of the pros and cons of using chemotherapy before treatment is initiated and may not truly understand all the implications of various treatment options. As well, we know from studies, human nature being what it is, veterinarians want to give good news, and the pet owner naturally wants to hear good news which can adversely affect appropriate decision-making.

Consideration should be given as to whether it is ethical and appropriate to use chemotherapy to prolong the life of a companion animal when they have no concept of the future and may suffer adverse effects with such treatment and whether it is in the best interests of the animal. As chemotherapy is not generally considered curative, it is in effect palliative care.

9.4   IS PALLIATIVE CARE IN THE BEST INTERESTS OF AN ANIMAL?

The emergence of veterinary hospice and palliative care as distinct areas of veterinary practice has brought a new dimension to end-of-life decision-making. Whilst it has been argued that hospice care is 'not giving up too soon', it can also be argued that the establishment of veterinary hospices panders to 'misguided' anthropomorphism'. And who benefits most – the owner, the animal, or the veterinarian?

Palliative and hospice care have emerged in veterinary practice alongside longer living pets and the 'humanisation' of pets, which are increasingly referred to as 'fur babies' of pet 'parents'. Dogs have evolved from wolves to sleeping in backyard kennels to an animal that sleeps indoors on the owner's bed. Although to be fair, there is plenty of historical evidence that some dogs have always enjoyed that privilege. Archaeological evidence suggests that little dogs, which served no useful purpose as working dogs, were traded across the Mediterranean over 2000 years ago.

In humans, hospice care is defined as going to a hospice and takes over from palliative care when nothing more can be done. Hospice care is, however, poorly defined in veterinary medicine as animals are unlikely to be hospitalised to spend their last days in a hospital cage and die peacefully. Palliative care is defined as treatment that relieves the symptoms of a disease or condition without dealing with the underlying cause and can be understood to give owners time to come to terms with losing a pet.

If we look at theories underpinning the assessment of animal welfare, the hedonism, preference, and perfectionism theories, we can argue that to have a good life an animal should have a life with more pleasure than pain, where positive experiences outnumber negative experiences, where the animal's preferences are satisfied, and the animal is able to realise significant species-specific potential.

This may not be possible if the animal is likely to be confined and unable to engage with the family because of human health risks with chemotherapy. In addition, there is no consensus on the most appropriate way to measure quality of life with ageing which is important given that many cancers occur in older pets.

In the decision-making process, veterinarians need to be aware that their own moral views may differ from those of their clients, and to avoid overruling these views, it is important in any discussion leading to a decision regarding the euthanasia of an animal, to be conscious of and take account of alternative ethical considerations about the value of an animal's life. The owner may have a religious viewpoint that is against euthanasia and pet owners can reach radically different conclusions when judging an animal's quality of life. Clients may have false expectations, can be over optimistic about the benefits of treatment, want good news, and have been found to be largely disempowered by consent forms.

If we consider that animals live from instant to instant and have no self-awareness, then it is unlikely they would choose to suffer if they could not imagine a future without suffering. It has been argued that death is not a welfare issue, and if an animal has no concept of death and no explicit desire to stay alive, then the quality of life is more important than the quantity of life. This perspective is supported by animal welfare legislation, which protects the welfare of animals.

There is no evidence that an animal can perceive future benefits against current suffering, and they cannot understand that withstanding current painful interventions will lead to a pain-free future.

The moral views of pet owners, veterinarians, and others have an impact on how palliative care and euthanasia is viewed. Those with an animal rights viewpoint would claim that the animal has the right to any available treatment regardless of the emotional and financial burden on the owner and the animal's welfare. This view is of course unrealistic and can lead to poor animal welfare. A utilitarian view would be a cost-benefit analysis taking into account the animal's welfare, the owner's quality of life, and the welfare of other affected parties. This is of course what mostly happens. Then there is the relational view with a belief that the relationship between the owner and the animal is unique and the human-animal bond must be maintained. This bond can be affected by the loss of emotional attachment because of suffering, and so it can be easier for the veterinarian to suggest euthanasia, unless of course the owner views caring for the terminally ill animal as emotionally rewarding.

9.5 SHOULD WE BE EUTHANISING CANCER PATIENTS?

This is the question posed by Ware et al. (2019) in response to an article by Elliott and Alderson (2019) on managing cancer pain in cats and dogs. They commented that euthanasia is briefly mentioned at the end of the article and seems to be suggested only after exhaustion of other measures despite the article making it clear that cancer-associated pain is a 'real dilemma'. Ware et al. comment that 'going to extremes with non-curative interventions in terminal patients may prolong quantity of life while sacrificing quality' and the patient's best interests should be put first.

In a similar vein to Elliott and Alderson, Repetti et al. (2023) discuss palliative care for cancer patients and note that animals may suffer from systemic spread of the tumour and paraneoplastic syndromes, which result in pain and suffering, which may not be easily treated. They state, 'When palliative care is performed, the option of euthanasia is not completely ruled out, but is not the only alternative in cases of a terminal diagnosis'.

Euthanasia is one of the most frequently mentioned challenging situations in small-animal practice although I personally see it as a privilege to be able to euthanise a suffering animal. I find it interesting that the expressions of gratitude by my clients are few and far between for saving an animal's life but are quite abundant for kindly ending it.

To assist in euthanasia decisions, an ethical matrix could be used such as that suggested by Bley (2017) or based on quality-of-life assessment tools. These are useful but still require the veterinarian to make individual judgements as a one-size-fits-all solution to euthanasia would risk oversimplifying a highly complex case. Additionally, as welfare assessment is subjective, the idea of a perfect quality-of-life measure is unrealistic, especially in older animals, although a checklist to guide decisions is useful for both the veterinarian and the owner. In practice I tend to ask pet owners if their pet can still run around and smell the roses and to make a list of everything the animal used to enjoy and is no longer able to do.

There is no shortage of research on the stresses and strains of euthanasia decision-making affecting pet owners and veterinarians. For veterinarians, there is the moral stress described by philosopher Bernie Rollin regarding the tension between the aim of veterinarians to protect and sustain the life of an animal and the reality of the practice of euthanasia.

This stress contributes to the 'burnout' syndrome and can be associated with leaving the decision to euthanise too long rather than euthanising too soon. Pet owners wishing to continue treatment despite poor animal outcomes were rated the most stressful for veterinarians, and veterinarians have been found to be more stressed thinking about euthanasia than actually doing it. To add to the problem, there is burden transfer with the clear link between client distress and stress and burnout in veterinarians and empathetic distress where veterinarians share the negative experiences of others.

A survey in Australia (Nestadt 2022) found that a refusal to euthanise was infrequent, that less than 20% of veterinarians use quality-of-life assessment tools, and one-third of pet owners said they left the decision too late. The main reason for euthanasia decisions was found to be pet illness and poor locomotion, followed by cost, with owner income a factor in euthanasia decisions. For the pet owner, there is anticipatory grief and caregiver burden. Caregiver burden is the biggest predictor of euthanasia after an animal's quality of life, with age-related decline having an impact on human caregivers and caring for a pet with a chronic or terminal illness associated with higher levels of stress, anxiety, and depression compared to having a healthy pet. There is some evidence that owners who have decided to have their pets euthanised experience less grief than owners whose pets die naturally.

The concept of 'shared care' is mentioned in euthanasia decision-making. Whilst balancing the interests of all parties is essential and veterinarians have sensibly shifted from a paternalistic approach, a move to owner autonomy can detract from the veterinarian's ability to exercise their professional autonomy over decisions using a patient centred approach. Heistand (2022) discusses how 'owner autonomy' has negative consequences on animal welfare and a strong patient advocate concept recognises that veterinarians are obligated to their patients and this aligns with veterinary codes of professional conduct.

On a positive note, Matte et al. (2019) found that when 'veterinary professionals successfully navigate euthanasia decisions and help shepherd pets through a good death, their sense of wellbeing and that of their clients' improves'.

Legally and ethically the primary responsibility of the veterinarian is to the animal and not the owner, and promoting healthy decision-making around euthanasia is important for the veterinarian's wellbeing, humane outcomes for animals, maintaining the human-animal bond, and maintaining the reputation of the profession.

9.6 SUMMARY

Cancer is a common disease in dogs and cats, and the decision to treat raises ethical issues for the owner, society, and veterinarians. There is a need to balance the welfare of the animal, the owner's interests, the role of the veterinarian, and societal expectations.

Despite the emergence of oncology as a specialty, there is a lack of sufficient discussion around the ethics of cancer treatments, especially chemotherapy, and whether they are always in the best interests of the animal. Even in humans, there is a growing concern around 'burdensome care' in terminally ill patients where actions are undertaken that result in little or no benefit and use up precious time and opportunities at the end of life.

That there is even a place for oncology in veterinary medicine has been questioned; as the philosopher Bernie Rollin points out, 'an animal cannot weigh the benefits of being treated for cancer against any suffering it may entail and cannot affirm a desire to endure current suffering for the sake of future life'.

Unfortunately, some pet owners attach themselves to an unrealistic view of medicine as a panacea for all ills and can place impossible demands on the veterinarian. This is supported in some cases by the media with depictions of heroic treatments. Veterinarians need to be assertive for the best interests of the animal and avoid abrogating their professional responsibility onto the owner at the expense of the animal's welfare, and they must not see euthanasia as a bad welfare outcome or a failure on their part; as Grimm et al. (2018) state, 'although moral stress is likely, we argue that facing this moral stress is inherent to the professional's responsibility'.

As the specialty of veterinary oncology continues to grow and as the use of chemotherapy becomes more commonplace in the treatment of animals with cancer, it is imperative that there be an ongoing ethical debate on oncology, particularly on the use of chemotherapy in animals.

REFERENCES

Best MP, Straw RC, Gumpel E, et al. Long term remission and survival in dogs with high grade B cell lymphoma treated with chemotherapy with or without sequential low-dose rate half-body radiation. *J Vet Intern Med.* 2023 Sept 12;37.

Bley CR. Principles for ethical treatment decision-making in veterinary oncology. *Vet Comp Oncol.* 2017 Aug;16.

Elliott J, Alderson B. Managing cancer pain in dogs and cats. *In Pract.* 2019 Oct;41:361–367.

Grimm H, Bergadano A, Musk GC, et al. Drawing the line in clinical treatment of companion animals: recommendations from an ethics working party. *Vet Rec.* 2018 Jun 9;182(23):664.

Heistand K. The autonomy principle in companion veterinary medicine: a critique. *Front Vet Sci.* 2022;9.

Nestadt C. *Experiences of euthanasia in veterinary clinics in Australia.* Proceedings of the Australian Veterinary Association Conference, Gold Coast; 2022.

Repetti CSF, Rueda JR, Porto CD, et al. Palliative care for cancer patients in veterinary medicine. *Vet Med Czech.* 2023;68(1):2–10.

Stephens T. The use of chemotherapy to prolong the life of dogs suffering from cancer: the ethical dilemma. *Animals.* 2019;9(7):441.

Ware J, Clutton E, Murphy K, et al. Should we be euthanising cancer patients? *Vet Rec.* 2019;185(18):574.

10 Small-Animal Overtreatment
Intensive Care

Peter Fordyce

In recent years, spectacular technical advances in veterinary medicine, coupled with owners' expectations and ability of finance such treatment, have made the veterinary intensive care unit 'VICU' a place of great hope, but also a place of potential great suffering. Avoiding unnecessary suffering is a moral, professional, and legal imperative for those involved in intensive care. It often involves complex decisions about whether the degree of suffering an animal is enduring is proportionate to the reasonably predicted likelihood of the patient leaving to have a life worth living. This involves recognising when treatment is becoming 'futile', and ending the patient's life at that point, so 'unnecessary suffering' is avoided. Difficulties associated with defining and quantifying animal suffering have not kept pace with advances in medical technologies that keep animals alive, and this has complicated rational decision-making about when 'enough is enough' for the patient. Failure to recognise human interests that are antithetical to the patient's best interests can further complicate such decisions.

10.1 INTENSIVE CARE

Recent advances in veterinary medicine have, in many ways, been breathtaking. while not quite paralleling those in human medicine, it is now possible to do things for (and to) animals as part of veterinary treatment that would have been difficult, if not impossible at the turn of the millennium. Consequently, many animals have lived longer lives, and with a better quality of those lives, in the face of disease processes which would have either ended their lives earlier, or degraded the pleasures that they enjoyed from being alive. Such improvements in the quality of the lives of animals in recent years have come from advances in understanding the pathology that causes disease processes, along with advances in pharmacology, diagnostic methodologies, and new and improved surgical techniques and materials – both from within veterinary medicine and imported from the human field. Dissemination of this new knowledge has been assisted by improvements in communication, such as the Internet, making information much more readily available to vets (as well as affordably cheaper), along with increasing professional requirements for continuing professional development by professional bodies such as the Royal College of Veterinary Surgeons (RCVS) and the European Board of Veterinary Specialisation. The latter also require the publication of peer-reviewed scientific veterinary medical research as a condition of college entry and continuing membership, leading to an increasing body of 'evidence-based medicine' supporting clinical reasoning, and hence helping achieve the best health outcome for patients. Increasing levels of knowledge and skill within the profession, has permeated all areas of veterinary practice, including the veterinary intensive care unit (VICU). Here, an animal's life may hang in the balance because of pathological changes and states that compromise its physiology to the point that, without intensive veterinary intervention, it would die.

While great advances in technology and skills have enabled animals in the VICU to survive when they would not have done so 20 to 30 years ago, VICUs are also places where there is the potential for great suffering to occur. While mitigation of patient suffering is a key role of the veterinary team supporting a patient through the VICU, (be that suffering resulting from a disease process such as infections or trauma, or supporting the post operative period following surgery) suffering will occur, and this needs to be balanced against the likelihood of the patient surviving to go on and have a good life in the future. However, with the increased availability of VICU medicine comes the possibility for larger numbers of animals to be exposed to the risk of inappropriate suffering, if the degree of suffering the animal must endure is not appropriately balanced against the prognosis for that patient.

While the availability of new technical information discussed above has been an important driver in the development of VICU medicine in recent years, it is not the only factor that driven such advancement; the ability and willingness to fund such treatment has also played an important role. A brief comparison between 'production animal' medicine, and 'companion animal' medicine may be enlightening in helping explain potential causes for some of the ethical dilemmas that occur in the small animal VICU.

Developments in 'production animal' intensive care have not parallel those in companion animal intensive care. Given that the relationship between a production animal and its owner is predominantly predicated on the instrumental value of the animal in terms of the profit the owner can make for it, if the cost of treatment in the VICU is likely to exceed the market value of the animal, euthanasia will be the rational outcome. VICU treatments are expensive, and market value of production animals limits options for treatments.

The situation regarding companion animals is often different as the relationship is not primarily predicated on the animal's financial/market value, but on the pleasure the owner gets from the companionship from their animal(s). Such pleasure incurs a sense of duty towards that animal's sense of wellbeing, with many companion animals being regarded as surrogate family members. The' relational value' that a companion animal owner places on their animal is often much greater than the animal's 'objective' market value, and is therefore much harder to quantify. Given the funds to pay for care in a VICU, owners of companion animals will pay for treatments if they are available, even if the cost exceeds the market value of the animal. Hence, while a farmer might reasonably complain if they were not informed that euthanasia might be the best way to cut their losses regarding a patient, suggesting to a pet owner that it would be 'cheaper to kill their pet and buy another one' would almost certainly result in a breakdown in the relationship with the veterinary surgeon. In short, desire to act in what the owner considers to be in the 'best interests' of a companion animal in the VICU drives treatment that would be limited by the animal's objective market value if it was a 'production animal'.

Companion animal owner motivation, coupled with increasing technical veterinary abilities in intensive care medicine have pushed advancement of intensive care treatment options forwards. The advent of veterinary insurance has also been a significant enabler in facilitating owner's wishes to 'do the best' for their animal, given the high costs involved in running a VICU.

The desire of owners to 'do the best' for their animals, coupled with the ability to pay for the advanced techniques now available, has coincided with a wider knowledge in the pet-owning population of what it might be possible to do for their animals. The television and social media are full of stories about the amazing success that can be wrought by modern medicine, and understandably, if it can be paid for, owners would want that for their animals. Not surprisingly, given the ethical imperative that vets swear on admission to the RCVS that their 'constant endeavour will be to ensure the health and welfare of animals committed to my care', vets will strive to facilitate this.

Where then might 'ethical dilemmas' arise in this new era of technically advanced and affordable high impact intensive care medicine? The answer lies in part in dissecting out the patient's best interests from the potential motivations of those involved in the decision-making processes, problems associated with objective scientific analysis of how much an animal is suffering, and is likely to suffer, and a realistic assessment of prognosis.

Defining what 'the best interests' of the patient are will vary with individual cases, but broadly might be considered as allowing the animal to leave the VICU and go on and have a reasonable length of 'life worth living', having endured a level of suffering that was proportionate to that aim, and minimised as far as possible in terms of severity and duration. Such an interpretation would co-inside with the societal ethic underpinning Section 4 on the Animal Welfare Act 2006 (as devolved) on the legal imperative of not causing 'un-necessary suffering' to animals. The problem comes with practical interpretation of the above definition of 'best interests'.

While there are valid measures for assessing some forms of animal suffering, recognition and quantification of suffering in human intensive care medicine and 'end of life care' is far more advanced than in veterinary care. Similarly, given the intrinsic problems associated with prognosis in medicine, attempting to balance degree of suffering with potential prognostic outcomes in terms of deciding what are proportionate actions becomes very complex. Recognising this complexity in discussions about what might be the best way forward when acting in the best interests of the patient is important in avoiding un-necessary suffering for a patient, particularly when euthanasia may be a valid option. Avoiding 'futile treatment' is therefore an important ethical imperative in the VICU (Futile treatment being defined as 'a medical treatment whose success is possible, but reason and experience suggest that it is highly improbable).

Just because treatment options are available, and can be afforded, this does not mean continuing treatment is necessarily in the best interests of the patient. For example, if the animal has a 95% chance of survival while enduring a short period of minimal distress, treatment should obviously continue as the harm-benefit ratio is clearly in favour of continued treatment. The situation is clearly reversed if the animal has a 5% chance of survival while enduring extreme distress. Attempting to decide what would be the actions of a 'reasonably competent and humane person' for cases that lie between the above two situations can often lead to ethical dilemmas and moral distress within the VICU care team as failure to reach a rational decision that is based on scientifically validated clinical and welfare parameters about what the best interests of the patient are, can lead to inappropriate euthanasia or, because it is futile, overtreatment.

While failures to recognise the difficulties of patient welfare assessment and clinical prognosis can contribute to ethical dilemmas in the VICU because of differing perceptions of what is a proportionate way forward in the patient's best interests, an acceptable ethical outcome is also dependent on those involved respecting the Kantian principle that the patient should be an end in themselves, and not a means to an end. This means decision-makers should not (consciously or unconsciously) put their own self-interest above those of the patient's welfare, and which may result in ether futile treatment, or over-treatment of the patient. (Over-treatment be defined as 'inappropriate medical interventions that are not in the best interest of patient').

While the desire to 'do more' for the patient is clearly virtuous and understandable, and particularly where the funds are available to do so, it is also important to recognise that in some circumstances the motivations for decision makers to act in certain ways might be contrary to the best interests of the patient.

The subject of analysis of suffering in animals, and the recognition of possible motivations for actions that result in futile treatment and overtreatment and now discussed in more detail.

10.2 THE PROBLEM OF RECOGNISING WHAT SUFFERING IS IN ANIMALS, AND QUANTIFYING IT

Recognition of what constitutes suffering in animals is philosophically difficult, as they are not able to verbalise their emotions in the way that humans can; therefore, it must be inferred through behavioural, physiological, and pathological changes measured in them. While this is not dissimilar to the way the human medical profession approach the issue of suffering in non-verbal humans (such as infants

Small-Animal Overtreatment

and mentally incapacitated adults), the situation with animals has the additional complexity of interpreting the mentioned criteria in a species that is different from us, and with different evolutionary needs and evolutionary driven responses. Much has been accomplished in the field of animal welfare science in recent years to provide defendable validated methodologies to rationally approach the issue of some forms of suffering in animal, but much still remains unknown in comparison with the situation for humans in intensive care situations.

The AWA 2006 does not provide a definitive statement of what animal suffering is, defining it broadly as "physical or mental suffering and related expressions shall be construed accordingly". This allows courts to make their own decision as to whether an animal has suffered, (and if it has, whether that suffering was un-necessary, or not). However this is not particularly helpful for an animal in the VICU as it provides no practical guidelines at to what forms of suffering the patient may be enduring, or their degree, and hence whether the suffering is proportionate to the aim allowing the animal to survive their stay in the VICU, and have a life worth living after it.

Unlike the AWA 2006, the Animals (Scientific Procedures) Act 1986 (A(SP)A 1986) provides much more detailed advice on what constitutes animal suffering, and the egregiousness of that suffering, to the government agency that regulates the use of animals for biomedical research. The Act regulates what can and can't be done to animals in relation to harms caused to them which are of no benefit to them. Within this act, the government agency (Home Office) is required to make a 'harm- benefit analysis' to determine whether the harms caused to the animals can be ethically justified by the benefits sought by causing those harms. To do this, types and degrees of harms must be quantified, so a rational decision can be made about whether 'the end justifies the means': guidance notes are provided in regulations, with specific examples of harms, and the degree of severity of those harms.

Acts of veterinary surgery, including diagnostics and treatments conducted in the VICU, are exempted from A(SP)A 1986 as they are for the benefit of the individual patient. While many clinicians working in and with VICUs will have had excellent training in pain recognition and management, they may have had limited training in the methodology of assessing the degree other forms of suffering exemplified in A(SP)A 1986, potentially undermining assessment of the proportionality of medical interventions and the suffering they cause the patient in relation to a reasonable clinical assessment of prognostic outlook. Such a failure may result in futile or over-treatment occurring, particularly where euthanasia or the patient may have been a more ethical outcome.

While information and methodology embedded in the legislation associated with A(SP)A 1986 may be a useful way for clinicians in the VICU to approach assessment of suffering in their patients, there is also the 'Donald Rumsfeld Problem' in relation to how animals might suffer (i.e. there are things we know we know, and things we know we don't know, but also things we don't know we don't know'). In the context of suffering in the VICU, there is much we don't know, and much we don't know we don't know about the experiences of the animals we treat.

Looking at the human experience of surviving time in intensive care may help indicate areas that need further consideration when conducting a harm-to-benefit ratio calculation for veterinary patients in the VICU.

Analysis of statements from people who have survived time in human ICUs suggest that there are causes of suffering and distress which are rarely (if ever) considered in the VICU. Space precludes detailed discussion, but unpleasant sensations such as thirst and a dry mouth, hunger, nausea, abdominal bloating and/or constipation, urinary discomfort, muscle cramps spasms and stiffness, thermal distress (burning up/shivering), photophobia, noise hypersensitivity and aversion, fear, anxiety, tiredness and exhaustion, dysphoria, along with deeply unpleasant sensations such as choking and 'air hunger' associated with airway compromise or other causes of respiratory distress are all reported.

Such experiences are thought to contribute to 'post-traumatic stress disorder' seen in some human ICU patients, but the extent to which these are recognised, quantified, and factored into considerations about what an animal might reasonably be expected to endure in the light of a given prognosis in the VICU is probably minimal, and if so, will contribute to the risk of futile or overtreatment, when euthanasia might be in the best interests of the patient.

To summarise, the potential lack of scientific knowledge about how, and how much animals may be suffering in the VICU has not kept pace with the ability to keep animals alive in the VICU, making an assessment over whether the suffering they endure is proportionate to the aim of them returning home to live a reasonable life difficult. Further research in this field is needed to enable clinicians to be able to defend the ethical acceptability of their actions in relation to the proportionality of their actions, whether the debate about this comes from within, or from outside of the VICU team.

10.3 CONFOUNDING HUMAN FACTORS POTENTIALLY OBSCURING THE PATIENT'S BEST INTERESTS

As discussed above, prognostication and assessment of suffering is intrinsically difficult, but hopefully future publication of information in these areas will help clinicians come to more evidence-based appropriate decisions about the point at which treatment is becoming futile (or at least unreasonable), and where further treatment would be seen as overtreatment. However, avoiding overtreatment also involves an understanding of human motivations that might drive overtreatment, and recognising them when they occur. Three examples might include avarice, the curse of 'gold standard treatment', and pathological altruism.

Avarice is defined as an extremely strong desire to acquire money or possessions. As previously mentioned, veterinary services in the UK are predominantly provided by private businesses, and increasingly corporate ones with fiduciary duties to their owners. While no sane person would argue that a sound or ethical business policy for a veterinary business would be to 'screw every last penny out of an animal in the VICU before it either dies, or the insurance money runs out', changes within the way veterinary services are supplied to the public in recent years have brought about a more financially driven approach to veterinary medicine.

Clearly, businesses need to remunerate their staff properly, and investors obtain a return on their investment, but when a monopoly is involved (as created over veterinary treatment by the Veterinary Surgeon's Act 1966), the ethical issue becomes one of what is a reasonable approach to financial return, and where are its boundaries.

Financially driven targets with financial bonuses for employees achieving them are part of the corporate world and are already infiltrating the veterinary profession. The duty of a veterinary employee to maximise the profit for the shareholder may therefore be at variance with their duty to the client and welfare of the animal in their care. Put simplistically, should vets view the client holding the animal in front of them as (a) a person asking them to do the best for their animal or (b) a marketing opportunity? So long as veterinary surgeons remember their primary obligation to act in the best interest of their patients, and can navigate and withstand the competing financial pressures from employers, the veterinary patient will not suffer unnecessarily.

Understanding this is especially important in the context of the VICU, where much profit can be made from an insured animal but where failure to recognise the risks of harms to the patient from any financially driven overtreatment can be egregious for the patient's welfare. Fortunately, there is no evidence to suggest greed is a significant factor in overtreatment in the VICU, but awareness of the potential pressure to cause it is important if the public is to maintain its trust in the profession.

A second, and perhaps a more insidious potential cause for overtreatment in the VICU is the problem of the concept of 'gold standard care'. 'Gold standard' is a term originating from the finance industry, and now adopted by the human medical profession to define an idealised perfect option for treatment; increasingly, it is used in veterinary medicine to imply that this is, by default, 'the optimal and preferred option for veterinary case management'. Taken at face value, why would clients not want gold standard care for their animals, and veterinary surgeons not want to provide it? Why should the concept be a problem? Two potential reasons exist.

The first is the use of the term as a justification to increase profits for the organisation by carrying out procedures on the animal that are of equivocal benefit for the patient's welfare, on the basis that to do so is the 'gold standard' treatment, i.e. 'we provide the best possible care for your animal based on scientific evidence'. However, 'the 'best possible care' is/should usually be nuanced and contextualised to the individual patient's clinical situation, along with their wider social situation; it is not the unthinking application of diagnostic and treatment algorithms gleaned from textbooks.

The second driver for applying 'gold standard care' relates to the potential for litigation from clients, should VICU treatment fail to provide the outcome the client desired; there being an understandable perception that not following 'gold standard' might make the VICU team more vulnerable to professional and legal criticism. Following 'gold standard' might provide a defence in the event of complaint, and might be in the best interests of the patient in some circumstances, but in other circumstances this might not be so.

The term and approach inferred by 'gold standard care' has increasingly come under criticism from members of the veterinary community concerned with animal welfare, particularly those concerned with the ethics of high-impact invasive medicine, such as that in the VICU. While it would be unfair to suggest that those who advocate for this approach have been educated beyond their intelligence, opting for a rigid approach to management of a case by following 'gold standard care' protocols, rather than actively considering the most appropriate management options based on the individual circumstances of the animal (including clinical, welfare and social contexts), is difficult to defend ethically. If 'gold standard treatment protocols' are applied inappropriately in an individual patient's circumstances they will risk a patient's welfare because of over-treatment. Additionally, they may undermine the relationship between the profession and the client if the latter perceives their use to be a way to generate profit at the cost of their animal's welfare.

In addition to failing to recognise the pressures arising from financial drivers and an uneducated approach to the application of 'gold standard' techniques, other human frailties may result in harms to patients from over-treatment if not honestly recognised and addressed. There are of course many, but the concept of 'pathological altruism' bears discussion here.

Pathological altruism can be interpreted in varying ways but can be used to describe behaviour where the superficial and overtly professed intent of the action of a person is altruistic, but their actions result in harm either to the altruist, or more commonly to the supposed beneficiary of the altruist. (The situation of people suffering from the psychological illness of 'cat hording' would be a good example from the area of wider animal welfare concerns). In the context of the VICU, problems of pathological altruism can occur in dealings with the owner of the patient, as well as within the VICU team.

Owners understandably want their animals to survive the time in the VICU, allowing the patient to return home and enjoy the relationship they had before the animal needed veterinary help. Such a desire is often strengthened by the emotional and financial sacrifice they have made to get them to that point. However, most owners also do not want their animals to suffer unavoidably, and will want to avoid overtreatment if it causes further suffering because such treatment has become futile.

Unfortunately, some owners will wish to persist with treatment that is becoming futile, rather than face having to decide to end the life of their animal. While the desire to help an animal live a long life is clearly altruistic, when treatment is extended in the face of an extremely guarded prognosis, and such overtreatment is clearly futile, then the altruism becomes pathological if it causes the animal to suffer longer than necessary.

In this situation, clear ethical and clinical reasoning processes need to be communicated to the client, and a scientifically based assessment of the nature and degree of suffering that the animal is enduring, coupled with evidence-based prognostication, can help. Resisting the psychological (and potentially legal) pressure from owners can be difficult for clinicians in this situation. Placating the client by continuing treatment beyond what the VICU team consider to be in the best interests of the patient may be a temptation, as it is the easiest way out for the humans involved; however, the resulting over-treatment would clearly not be in the best interests of the patient.

Recognising that trying to avoid the distress caused to clients by providing bad news about the prognosis for a patient, and the degree of suffering an animal is enduring, can also be important driver for pathological altruistic behaviour. Informing owners that treatment is failing, further treatment would be futile, and euthanasia would be the kindest option for the patient is not a pleasant experience. Owners will be upset, and both owners and the VICU team may suffer unpleasant emotional states associated with loss of the patient, and sensations of guilt about the failure to achieve the desired outcome. This can be particularly true when clients and clinicians have been heavily invested in the success of the outcome of a case, and the animal has endured much suffering to reach this point.

Continuing to persevere with treatment beyond the point at which it is proportionate because of a pathologically altruistic desire not to upset the feelings of the humans involved in the decision-making process will clearly result in overtreatment. The concept of a 'sunk cost fallacy' (putting good money after bad in an attempt to recover the loss) is a recognised pitfall in the science of economics. In the case of the VICU, it is the patient that will suffer the cost to it's welfare because of over-treatment if owners and clinicians fail to recognise when treatment is becoming futile, despite the financial and emotional investment that has been invested in the patient's care to bring the patient to this point.

10.4 WHAT MIGHT BE DONE TO HELP AVOID OVERTREATMENT IN THE VICU?

Veterinary professionals, owners, (and if they had a voice- veterinary patients) would all want to avoid overtreatment in the VICU because of the adverse impact on the welfare of the animal involved, and the un-necessary suffering that it engenders. Further research into the nature and degree of different types of suffering that animals might be experiencing in the VICU, along with training in recognition and mitigation of these aversive mental states will undoubtably assist accessing the proportionality of any suffering the patient experiences when weighed against the likely success of the patient going on to have a good life with their owner. Similarly recognising that there are factors un-related to the clinical situation that the patient is in is important in avoiding overtreatment, as, once recognised, they can be addressed.

In the last few years, the potential adverse effects on animal welfare that inappropriately applied cutting-edge technology and/or intensive interventions used in veterinary medicine, and particularly the VICU, have been increasingly recognised. As a result many larger veterinary centres are now setting up clinical ethics committees to provide support and advice to members of the VICU teams where a concern is raised concerning the morality of the animal's treatment plan, and particularly the problem of over-treatment. Along with improved understanding of the issue of recognising how animals may be suffering when in the VICU, and improved knowledge of clinical prognostic indicators, by learning from experience, these committees can provide a forum for objective analysis of what to consider when asking the question 'what is in a patient's best interests?'. Identifying reasons why overtreatment may be occurring, should be part of their remit, as is perhaps more importantly, asking the question from section 4(3)(e) of the AWA 2006, i.e. "whether the conduct concerned was in all the circumstances that of a reasonably competent and humane person".

Part IIB Research on Companion Animals

11 Innovation versus Experimentation
Experiments on Pets?

Polly Taylor

11.1 FIDO

In 2013, Fido, a young adult, 25 kg labrador sustained a ruptured cruciate ligament (CLR) and was treated with a new type of cruciate surgery: CORA-based levelling osteotomy (CBLO). This surgery attempts to improve upon the better-known tibial plateau levelling osteotomy (TPLO). Both procedures involve cutting the tibia, rotating it to alter the architecture of the joint and placing implants to put it back together. Fido's surgery was not successful, and he was euthanised due to intractable pain some months later but not before a number of further surgical interventions were made to try to rescue the joint.

In 2013 the CBLO was innovative, not proven as a viable treatment for cruciate ligament repair; nor is it now. However, Fido was subjected to this surgery with the owner understanding that this was a 'minimally invasive arthroscopic cruciate repair' considered the best current type of surgery for the condition. There was no indication that this surgery was a novel technique and that Fido's surgery was effectively an experiment to see whether CBLO was in fact an improvement on the TPLO.

11.2 INNOVATION VERSUS EXPERIMENT

Innovation is defined as 'a new idea or method' while experiment is defined as 'a test done in order to learn something or to discover if something works or is true' (Cambridge Dictionary 2023). Experimentation is a necessary step of innovation.

There is no doubt of the benefits to society from innovation, for instance, say the wheel, the telephone and the computer; in most fields, innovation is usually hailed as beneficial progress. However, innovation does not always equate with benefit; experiment is required to discover whether the innovation really is beneficial. Innovation that transfers to clinical treatment requires research and validation before it can be regarded as effective and recognised as an acceptable treatment for the condition for which it was developed. Innovative veterinary diagnostics and interventions should be tested in regulated clinical trials before they are carried out in routine clinical practice. That way, harms and benefits can be identified before putting patients at large at risk. As Theranos whistleblower Tyler Shultz said in an interview, the 'move fast break things kind of model just does not work in healthcare' where patients' lives are at stake (CNBC Television 2022). This must also apply to veterinary healthcare, where patients are particularly vulnerable and the potential for adverse consequences is high. Animals can't speak to report problems, caregiver placebo effect and enthusiasm may come into play, and protection is often non-existent (Taylor & Meyer 2023).

11.3 EXPERIMENTS ON PETS

Clinical trials are experiments on real patients to evaluate a new treatment for a naturally occurring disease or injury. The outcome of the treatment is expected to be of benefit but, as the subject of the investigation, is unknown. This dilemma is the very reason an independent ethical review body is required to authorise any such clinical trial.

Evaluation of treatments for naturally occurring disease is surely best carried out on patients suffering naturally from that disease. Causing a disease in an otherwise healthy animal in a laboratory when the natural disease exists in the real world is morally questionable. The response to treatment of that natural disease in its normal environment is also more likely to be truly representative of the real world than in the laboratory. This has led to the suggestion that pets, particularly dogs as they live in similar environments to their human owners, should be exploited more widely in medical research (Anonymous 2016). Whilst the benefits are apparently considerable (Lascelles et al. 2022), the vulnerability of the subjects themselves, not to mention their caregivers, necessitate stringent regulation to ensure these animals are not harmed.

Experiments to evaluate innovative procedures in pet animals may be conducted in two entirely distinct circumstances – first, as for Fido described earlier, for a condition occurring in the species concerned and, second, for use of the pet as a model for a similar condition in the human species. Both require regulation to safeguard the welfare of the animal concerned.

In the first circumstance, experiments evaluating treatment of a condition occurring in the pet species itself, innovative veterinary procedures are often accoladed as heroic, life-saving, 'a first', and so forth (Fearon 2010). However, they may be unsuccessful, cause harm and lead to Fido's scenario. Further mischief stems from inadequate owner consent that is not 'informed' as the unknown outcome and potential for harm may be glossed over. This is not to say that innovation should not happen, but that the proposed procedures need to be evaluated under regulations that protect the animal and its owner from harm.

Regarding the second circumstance, pets as models for human disease, the lack of translation of basic research in laboratory animals into therapeutics for treatment of a variety of conditions in humans is well recognised. Pets, particularly dogs, are often advocated as a better model. Lascelles et al. (2018, 2022) reviewed translational research in companion animals for pain therapy. They outline the benefits of better reflection of the complex genetic, environmental, temporal and physiological influences present in humans. However, whilst in most countries research on laboratory animals is governed under strict regulation safeguarding the animals' welfare, no such regulation exists for pet animals where the treatment under investigation is disguised as clinical benefit. Lascelles et al. (2018, 2022) do point out that the animals cannot provide consent themselves and advocate that each study should be reviewed by an ethics committee and that informed, signed owner consent should be obtained after full review of the risks and benefits. However, an editorial in *Nature* (Anonymous 2016) advocated that the rules for pet trials should be loosened to reduce the very restrictions that safeguard the animals concerned. No mention is made of the fact that whilst the new treatment for, for example, cancer may be of benefit, it may itself cause serious harm. Indeed, the laboratory animal used for pure scientific research has better protection than the pet undergoing, for instance, a newly devised surgical procedure.

Client-owned companion animals are being used to generate foundational data for a number of diagnostic and interventional procedures with the aim of translation to the human market. Pet owners often appear to be unaware of this, may be unduly influenced by hype, and allow their pets to be subjected to what is in effect research for the human species. This leads to the ridiculous inconsistency of a negative reaction to laboratory animals being used for regulated research but not to companion animals being used for unregulated research (or no research but straight clinical practice) under the guise of 'innovation'.

Prevalent practices and entrenched convictions, legal and regulatory loopholes that can be exploited, and an apparent reluctance to have difficult conversations challenging the *status quo* may perpetuate the notion that it is acceptable to experiment on client-owned animals without the safeguards of controlled, clinical trial research (e.g. ethical review, informed consent, specific enrolment criteria, early stopping rules). Implantation of an intraosseous transcutaneous amputation prosthesis (ITAP) (Fitzpatrick et al. 2011) provides one such example of experimental surgery disguised as clinical treatment. An ITAP was fitted in four dogs whose distal limb neoplasia was treated by amputation. No external ethical review was reported and, although it might be argued that this treatment was to the benefit of the individuals concerned, it was clearly to inform the potential for developing this technique for limb salvage *per se*. The facts that metastasis had probably already occurred and life expectancy was relatively short adds weight to the need for external review of the planned procedure. Surgery of this calibre is not trivial, and for an animal that cannot foresee that this might be of benefit, the whole process is devastating. However good the pain relief, it is difficult to see the numerous substantial interventions and periods of hospitalisation interspersed throughout the remaining limited life span as benefiting the dog. Hiestand (2022) reminds us that 'therapeutic interventions are rarely, if ever, pleasant for animals, with even seemingly benign treatments requiring transportation, handling, confinement, discomfort, and fear, all of which present welfare compromise to patients who cannot understand the purpose of their experience'.

Experimental surgery is intended to lead to a procedure becoming established as an appropriate treatment for the condition. However, such experimentation also has the potential for harm. The TPLO was developed in this way (Slocum & Devine 1984; Slocum & Slocum 1993) and this procedure now has a good track record as appropriate treatment for cranial cruciate ligament rupture (Pegram et al. 2024). Slocum took an unconventional approach (Ness 2002) and got lucky; this is no justification for the process to be repeated 30 or more years later. Degeling (2010) observed that 'the history of veterinary responses to canine cruciate injuries indicates that as idealisation replaces analogical reasoning in the design of interventions, the performance of the biotechnological ideal – rather than the pathophysiology of the average patients' injury – increasingly becomes the basis for innovation . . .'. We must ensure that what seems a brilliant idea to the innovator is still subject to proper scrutiny of scientific method and ethical justification; the potential for harm as well as good must be acknowledged before the experiment begins.

11.4 CLINICAL VETERINARY RESEARCH

Clearly there is a need to resolve the balance between progress and stifling the development of new clinical treatments. The contrast between pure experimental research and clinical treatment must be acknowledged. Scientific experimental animal research (EAR) has no benefit to the test subjects themselves, e.g. rodent models of conditions in humans. Clinical treatment should benefit the individual animal concerned and stems from evidence that the therapy works. In the United Kingdom (UK), the distinction between EAR and clinical treatment is clear: scientific experiment is carried out under the Animals (Scientific Procedures) Act (ASPA) 1986 and clinical treatment under the Veterinary Surgeons Act (VSA) 1966. Clinical treatment is deemed Routine Veterinary Practice (RVP) by the governing body of practising veterinary surgeons, the Royal College of Veterinary Surgeons (RCVS). Equivalent guidance from authorities in other countries exists, although the approach is not identical. What is consistent, however, is that EAR is generally well regulated and laboratory animals are well protected, whereas research on pet animals disguised as clinical treatment has no such control and the potential for harm is significant.

Clinical veterinary research (CVR) falls in the void between routine clinical treatment and EAR. Medical clinical research involving human subjects is guided internationally by the Declaration of Helsinki (DOH), a framework of ethical principles developed to protect human clinical research subjects. No such guidelines exist for CVR in animals whether they be companion animals, farm animals or exotics.

The authorities which govern veterinary professionals require them to uphold minimum standards of care; veterinary diagnostic and interventional procedures require evidence to support their use as routine veterinary practice. In the United States and elsewhere, the regulatory pathway to new drug or device approval for humans is much more difficult and expensive than for animals. Somebody has to pay the price for innovation. In regulated clinical trials, the sponsor of the new procedure typically funds experiments and may offer incentives to participants. Outside the auspices of regulated clinical trials, the animal patient and the owner usually bear the burden, potentially without lawful research protection. This includes not only the costs for the unsubstantiated procedure but also any complications endured and treatment thereof. Moreover, the ultimate outcome of yet-to-be-proven 'innovative' procedures could be worse than with accepted standards of care; this further underlines the need for regulated clinical research in animals.

The line distinguishing RVP and CVR is hazy. In both cases, patients undergo veterinary treatment for their disease condition. Procedures undertaken as RVP have evidence and experience of sufficient safety and efficacy for successful outcome. For CVR, the treatment intervention itself is under investigation. The incentive to conduct CVR is likely to have arisen from observations made during everyday clinical practice or the wish to improve a current method or device. Hence, CVR is likely to develop from progression of a simple minor adjustment in a routine procedure performed for the benefit of the individual patient. A pilot or proof of concept study may come next, ultimately leading to a full investigation of the impact of the intervention itself. At this point it is clearly true CVR, particularly if randomisation is required. Informed owner consent and independent review of both the ethics and the science are now essential, particularly if there is potential for significant harm to the patient.

Clinical trials evaluating new drugs are also CVR. Veterinary clinical drug trials are usually an exception as new drugs are generally much better regulated than clinical evaluation of, for instance, a new surgical procedure involving orthopaedic implants. In the UK, for example, new drugs are evaluated under an Animal Test Certificate (ATC) issued by the Veterinary Medicines Directorate (VMD 2022). The ATC is issued on the basis of evidence of likely safety and efficacy as well as approval by an ethics committee.

Regulation of CVR is not consistent internationally. In the UK, CVR falls under the VSA and is governed by the RCVS. This results in confusion as the RCVS Guide to Professional Conduct contains mutually incompatible guidance (RCVS 2022):

> Clinical Veterinary Research (CVR) is when *routine procedures* are undertaken for the benefit of the animal/s, with the concurrent intention to generate new knowledge that benefits animals, such as *developing new procedures,* improving a diagnosis, changing a routine procedure, or comparing existing procedures.

'Routine procedures' and *'developing new procedures'* are mutually exclusive. In the US, federal agencies such as the Food and Drug Administration (FDA), Environmental Protection Agency (EPA) and Department of Agriculture (USDA) regulate new veterinary drugs, parasiticides and biologics, respectively, but not necessarily new veterinary devices and certainly not new veterinary procedures. Regulation of standards of care (i.e. RVP) generally falls to state veterinary boards, none of which appear to have statutes or rules governing CVR.

11.5 INDEPENDENT ETHICAL REVIEW

It is clear that CVR is neither EAR nor RVP. Although there should be some evidence for the procedure's likely safety and efficacy for a clinical trial to be undertaken, the outcome is still unknown and indeed may cause harm. Independent ethical review is essential to assess the harm:benefit ratio of each individual trial and decide whether the balance is sufficiently on the side of safety of the test subjects. The makeup of the ethical review committee is vital. As well as having appropriate expertise to evaluate the proposed study protocol, it must be independent and not be biased by the aspirations of the originator of the investigation. Colleagues and especially employees of the originator cannot be regarded as independent. The clinician originating a clinical investigation must believe the treatment works and may be over optimistic as to its likely success. Independent review is essential to highlight potential problems and to apply restrictions, such as formal evaluation at an early stage, before any harm or potential for harm is beyond a previously identified acceptable point. The more invasive the treatment, the more important is specified early review of the process.

11.6 INFORMED OWNER CONSENT

The owner or caregiver of the animal subject of the clinical trial must understand the full picture of the process, its likely outcome, the potential for harm, and the physical, emotional, and financial burden on themselves. Only if these points are emphasised with the option to withdraw freely is this consent 'informed'. Enthusiasm for the impact of an innovative procedure must not be allowed to sway the owner/caregiver into consenting to an untried procedure masquerading as a wonderful new and assured treatment.

11.7 WHERE NOW?

In this age of social media and astonishing developments in technology, it is easy for owners and clinicians alike to be blinded by apparent clinical excellence and to ignore the effects of high-tech treatment on the patient. So-called 'advanced' veterinary diagnostics, medicines, and surgical procedures may be used in clinical practice even if they have not been definitively proven to advance the field. In best-case scenarios, they may eventually be proven to benefit patients. In worst-case scenarios, they may continue to be used without question or evidence, or they may eventually be proven to harm patients – in either case medical reversal could take years to accomplish. Stem cell therapy is one such example of a novel intervention that lacks evidence from prospective, regulated studies yet has been used for years (McKenzie 2021). Although stem cells may have sound clinical rationale, this so-called innovative therapy is often carried out at considerable burden and expense to patients and clients despite the dearth of robust and reproducible data to substantiate use.

To characterise new approaches that lack evidence as innovative when they are, in fact, experimental, constitutes not only misrepresentation potentially leading to undue influence, but it raises other serious ethical concerns. Investigations disguised as clinical practice can slip through without ethical approval. The best starting point to address these issues would be to close companion animal research loopholes via enforceable legislation. This is not to say that the clinical trial should be disallowed but simply that it needs alternative regulation, forming a separate tier between EAR and normal clinical treatment.

What happens if such investigations are carried out without ethical review and informed owner consent? The most direct answer is that publication should be denied. Journals variously adhere to ethical standards and most will not publish the results of CVR without evidence of ethical review committee approval. The DOH for animals proposed by Ashall et al. (2023) would provide just such regulation if it could be adopted globally. A universal DOH for animals to which all veterinary journals subscribe would go a considerable distance to improving this situation. A DOH for animals and reliance on ethical review would go a long way to preventing the harms some pets experience in pushing forward the frontiers of science.

REFERENCES

Anonymous. Pet projects need a helping hand. *Nature.* 2016;540:169–170.

Ashall V, Morton D, Clutton E. A declaration of Helsinki for animals. *Vet Anaes Analg.* 2023;50(4):309–314.

Cambridge Dictionary. 'Innovation' and 'experiment'. In: *Cambridge dictionary definitions* [Internet]. Undated [cited 2023 Oct 31]. Available from: https://dictionary.cambridge.org/us/.

CNBC Television. Theranos whistleblower disappointed Holmes found not-guilty for defrauding patients. *YouTube* [Internet]. 2022 Jan 4. Available from: https://www.youtube.com/watch?v=WAZUMk1msVg.

Degeling C. Cutting a bone to heal a ligament: idealized animals and orthopaedics. *Med Stud.* 2010:2:101–119.

Fearon R. Does heroic treatment need tonic? *Vet Times* [Internet]. 2010 Nov 1. Available from: https://www.vettimes.co.uk/article/does-heroic-treatment-need-tonic/.

Fitzpatrick N, Smith TJ, Pendegrass CJ, et al. Intraosseous transcutaneous amputation prosthesis (ITAP) for limb salvage in 4 dogs. *Vet Surg.* 2011;40(8):909–925.

Hiestand KM. The autonomy principle in companion veterinary medicine: a critique. *Front Vet Sci.* 2022;9:953925.

Lascelles BDX, Brown DC, Conzemius MG, et al. The beneficial role of companion animals in translational pain research. *Front Pain Res (Lausanne).* 2022;3:1002204.

Lascelles BDX, Brown DC, Maixner W, et al. Spontaneous painful disease in companion animals can facilitate the development of chronic pain therapies for humans. *Osteoarthritis Cartilage.* 2018;26(2):175–183.

McKenzie B. Stem cell therapies in veterinary medicine: where are we now? *SkeptVet* [Internet]. 2021 Apr 4. Available from: https://skeptvet.com/Blog/2021/04/stem-cell-therapies-in-veterinary-medicine-where-are-we-now/.

Ness M. Taking time out of practice to pursue a unique learning experience. *In Pract.* 2002;24(5):282–284.

Pegram C, Diaz-Ordaz K, Brodbelt DC, et al. Target trial emulation: does surgical versus non-surgical management of cranial cruciate ligament rupture in dogs cause different outcomes? *Prev Vet Med*. 2024;226:106165.

Royal College of Veterinary Surgeons (RCVS). New RCVS guidance to help profession navigate clinical and ethical judgements. *RCVS News* [Internet]. 2022 Jun 24. Available from: https://www.rcvs.org.uk/news-and-views/news/new-rcvs-guidance-to-help-profession-navigate-clinical-and/.

Slocum B, Devine T. Cranial tibial wedge osteotomy: a technique for eliminating cranial tibial thrust in cranial cruciate ligament repair. *J Am Vet Med Assoc*. 1984;184(5):564–569.

Slocum B, Slocum TD. Tibial plateau leveling osteotomy for repair of cranial cruciate ligament rupture in the canine. *Vet Clin North Am Small Anim Pract*. 1993;23(4):777–795.

Taylor P, Meyer RE. Veterinary clinical research or experiments on pets. *Vet Anaes Analg*. 2023;50(5):383–385.

Veterinary Medicines Directorate (VMD). Animal test certificates. *GOV.UK* [Internet]. 2022 Aug 25. Available from: https://www.gov.uk/guidance/animal-test-certificates#types.

12 Veterinary Ethical Review – A Multitude of Questions

Stephen N. Greenhalgh

12.1 INTRODUCTION

The principle of ethical review is well-established and mandatory in many settings – human healthcare, sociological research involving human participants, and experimental animal use, for example. Ethical review in the clinical veterinary setting has largely been modelled on practices in human healthcare, particularly when considering clinical research involving animals. However, as is so often the case with ethics in general, there are many grey areas surrounding ethical review in a veterinary setting. A questioning approach may highlight some of these uncertainties and prompt a constructive debate around the role of ethical review as applied to non-experimental animals.

12.2 WHY (SHOULD ETHICAL REVIEW BE UNDERTAKEN)?

Unfortunately, many requests for ethical review may arise primarily or solely because those seeking it are obliged to – that is to say, the funder or publishing journal or institution has or will request it. It may therefore be perceived as a hurdle to overcome rather than an important nay essential element of our 'moral contract' when we, as humans, elect to interact with our non-human animal counterparts.

Assuming, or even acknowledging the possibility, that (some) animals have moral standing, also referred to as ethical status, prompts us to accept that by using animals we are exerting power over them (Mullan & Quain 2017). Ethical review helps us fulfil our obligation to consider how we use this power and whether it is right or acceptable to do so in the manner we propose.

Appropriate, independent (more on this later) ethical review should, in its broadest remit, assess what is being proposed in relation to four areas of potential ethical risk (Adami et al. 2023):

  i. the animal (or its data) and any other animals that may be affected, directly or indirectly;
  ii. the owner (in the widest sense) of, or those with responsibility for, the animal or its data;

iii. the humans involved (whose actions may inadvertently expose themselves to physical, psychological, moral or reputational injury);
iv. the institution from which those proposing the actions originate (if applicable) and wider society.

The general goal is to weigh up what is being proposed, its harm or potential for harm, against the potential benefits of the proposed actions. This is the cornerstone of the harm-benefit analysis that is undertaken when assessing experimental animal use (Laber et al. 2015; Brønstad et al. 2016; Animals In Science Committee 2020; Home Office 2015). In clinical research it is often referred to as risk-benefit analysis. The harm or risk of harm should ideally be non-existent or, at the very least, as low as reasonably possible. In a non-experimental setting, the utilitarian approach carries far less weight. If harms are envisaged to any individual involved (animal or human), the potential benefit(s) to that individual (or its immediate cohort) must outweigh these. This is tricky enough to describe in general terms; making this harm-benefit assessment in context can be extremely challenging (Eggel & Grimm 2018; Coleman 2021). However, rather than dismissing the whole endeavour as futile, this strengthens the case for a wider consideration of the proposed actions by a plurality and certainly by more than the person(s) directly involved.

12.3 WHAT (SHOULD UNDERGO ETHICAL REVIEW)?

It is widely accepted that proposals for prospective research involving animals, be they experimental or clinical, should undergo ethical review before the research begins. However, there are numerous other scenarios where humans interact with animals or use material or data derived from them. Prior ethical review is likely to be beneficial to the animals, humans, and society in most, if not all, such cases. Box 12.1 lists scenarios where ethical review could (or should) be considered.

> **BOX 12.1   WHAT SHOULD UNDERGO ETHICAL REVIEW?**
>
> Retrospective, or secondary, use of (clinical) data
> Retrospective, or secondary, use of tissue or previously collected samples (including those obtained historically)
> Observational research
> Interventional research
> Zoological or wildlife research
> Conservation or management practices
> Obtaining data about animals from humans
> Secondary use of tissue (or data) from experimental animal research
> Clinical case management
> Use of animals in teaching and education
> Use of animals for food production, clothing, sport, work, and service etc.

12.3.1 Retrospective, or Secondary, use of (Clinical) Data

Although often considered of low ethical risk, it is still important to evaluate how the data were collected and what use is proposed. Is there appropriate consent for the proposed use? Or can the use without consent be justified? Are the data appropriate for the proposed use and will they be handled appropriately after extraction? Might the user (intentionally or otherwise) be proposing to use the data for an ethically questionable purpose? For example, extracting dog breeds and owner postcodes from a clinical database to test a hypothesis that supposedly 'less intelligent' breeds are owned by people living in more socio-economically disadvantaged areas.

Furthermore, in the absence of ethical review of retrospective data use, unscrupulous individuals might consider generating and collecting the data they need prospectively (without prior ethical review) and then undertaking a retrospective evaluation (again with no ethical assessment).

12.3.2 Retrospective, or Secondary, use of Tissue or Previously Collected Samples

Justifications for ethical review of proposed secondary use of previously obtained tissues or samples include all those stated in relation to the retrospective use of data. Additionally, biological samples may be a rare or finite resource, in which case assessment should be made as to whether any 'destructive' use of the sample is justified by the potential benefit.

Proposals to use historically obtained samples, which may not have been obtained according to current standards, warrant particular consideration, especially in relation to what consent was obtained for acquisition, storage, and future use.

The use of tissue *post mortem* from animals that have been killed (or have died) for other reasons (for example, meat production, hunting for sport, or population control) also merits consideration. The defence that 'it's dead anyway' oversimplifies the potential ethical concerns with obtaining and using animal tissue from such a variety of sources. The demand for tissue may inadvertently drive supply, making the use no longer truly opportunistic. The manner by which the sample or tissue was originally obtained may be illegal in, or morally repugnant to, the society in which the secondary use will be undertaken. For example, tissue obtained from whaling or poaching. The proposed use may give cause for ethical concern. For example, harvesting of cells to undertake controversial genetic engineering techniques.

12.3.3 Observational research

Studies involving animal observation alone are not immune from ethical critique. The act of observation has potential to cause distress, disturb habitats or disrupt normal behaviours. On occasion, what is observational research in methodological terms may involve an 'intervention' to obtain the required measurements. This may be non-invasive (for example, an ultrasound scan or use of a weigh tape) or invasive (for example, taking a rectal temperature or a nasal swab).

12.3.4 Interventional Research

It is widely accepted that prospective interventional studies, such as those to assess the efficacy of a potential new therapy, require prior ethical review (Morton & Allen 2024; RCVS 2012, 2016). Independent review has been listed as one of the 'universal' requirements of ethical clinical research in humans (Emanuel et al. 2000).

12.3.5 Zoological or Wildlife Research

In addition to the considerations already introduced, it should be highlighted that, although wild animals may not have 'owners' in the usual sense, this does not negate the need for the ethical consideration of any proposed interactions with and by humans for research purposes. It is still necessary to evaluate whether consent is necessary to undertake the proposed research (for example, in the form of permits from relevant authorities). Arguably, interacting with undomesticated species has greater potential for ethical concern than research involving domesticated species.

12.3.6 Conservation or Management Practices

The potential benefits and harms of interventions such as species reintroduction or culling programmes requires pre-emptive consideration.

12.3.7 Obtaining Data about Animals from Humans

This is usually regarded as social science research and the involvement of human participants is the primary driver for ethical review. However, there may be animal or veterinary considerations that arise from the data collection that should not be ignored. For example, a questionnaire to owners of geriatric dogs asking how easily their pet can jump in and out of the car might inadvertently result in owners carrying out this 'test' and risking injury to their animal.

12.3.8 Secondary Use of Tissue (or Data) from Experimental Animal Research

In the UK, the Animals (Scientific Procedures) Act 1986 (ASPA) controls the conduct of regulated procedures on protected species (see Chapter 13 by Ngaire Dennison for further information). Any proposal to carry out procedures on experimental animals that fall under the purview of the Act undergoes an extensive ethical review. However, this review may not extend to all potential uses of the data or tissues arising from the project, particularly if it does not fit within the programme of work described in the licence permitting the experimental work under ASPA. Further, tissue or data may arise from experimental animal use that is not regulated under ASPA (or its legislative equivalent in other jurisdictions) – for example, if the animals or the procedures involved do not meet the 'threshold' for regulation. In any case, it should not be assumed that a *carte blanche* exists to do whatever one wants with these tissues or data.

12.3.9 CLINICAL CASE MANAGEMENT

While most veterinary clinical procedures can be regarded as commonplace or routine, some may be new cutting-edge techniques or involve specific patients, or there may be combinations of factors that increase both the complexity of the case itself and the ethical considerations pertaining to it (Yeates 2016). As such, the management of these cases needs more stringent ethical consideration, involving more than just the attending (or primary) clinician and the animal's owner.

12.3.10 USE OF ANIMALS IN TEACHING AND EDUCATION

The use of animals in the education and training of veterinary surgeons, physicians, allied healthcare professionals, and wider society may be considered under a single large umbrella. Some uses of little or no ethical risk will contrast with other uses that are highly contentious. Examples include zoological parks, the use of animals in displays, the dissection of cadavers, and undertaking training procedures (which may be non-invasive or highly invasive) on dead or living animals.

12.3.11 USE OF ANIMALS FOR FOOD PRODUCTION, CLOTHING, SPORT, WORK, AND SERVICE ETC.

The list of human interactions with animals that *might* benefit from ethical review is extensive. An ethical analysis of such uses is beyond the scope of this chapter and the remit of this book. The acceptability of such interactions (following varying levels of ethical review) is generally determined at a societal or governmental level, with legislation ultimately prescribing the circumstances, boundaries, and protections related to the use in question. However, this does not preclude such uses from future ethical review. Societal sensitivities will change and our understanding of the species in question will increase. In particular, new or significantly different uses of animals, for example, the intensive farming of the octopus for human consumption, should be subject to an ethical assessment.

12.3.12 SETTING THE BAR FOR ETHICAL REVIEW

The consideration as to whether ethical review is required in a particular situation is analogous to undertaking a diagnostic test. While the perfect diagnostic test has both high sensitivity (identifies true positives) and high specificity (does not produce false positives), in reality it is often necessary to prioritise one over the other. Given the potential ramifications of overlooking a scenario that is of ethical concern, it is preferable that our 'test' of whether ethical review is required has a high sensitivity, even at the expense of low specificity.

This may result in cases being identified that ultimately are of no ethical concern but still meet the threshold for ethical review. Undertaking 'unnecessary' ethical review in such cases is far preferable to the opposite scenario of not undertaking ethical review when it is warranted. In short, the number of ways in which humans interact with and use animals, and the variety of ethical considerations that might arise as a result, justifies setting a low bar when deciding which interactions merit ethical review.

A few simple questions may assist in determining the need for ethical review:

1. Am I proposing research that will involve the use of animals or their data? If yes – ethical review is required.
2. Is the veterinary or husbandry procedure I am proposing considered routine practice and uncontroversial? If no – ethical review should be undertaken.
3. Is the intention to do something with animals or their data that does *not* have a widely accepted 'societal licence' for its undertaking? If yes – ethical review is required.

12.4 WHEN (SHOULD ETHICAL REVIEW BE UNDERTAKEN)?

Having identified which animal-based interactions require ethical review, the question arises as to when this review is undertaken. The safest answer is always *before* the proposed use commences, which is to say, prospectively. Retrospective ethical review may not always be redundant: it can offer an opportunity for reflection and identify learning for future similar uses. However, beyond this, it is often plagued with difficulties that greatly limit its utility. Primarily, it precludes the opportunity to prevent unethical practices from commencing in the first place. It restricts or wholly denies the option of refining the proposed use or adding or improving ethical protections. When the proposed use has already been completed or is already underway, those acting as ethical reviewers may feel pressured into signing off on something even if they have ethical concerns about what is being or has been done. Raising these concerns, or going so far as to provide an unfavourable opinion or deny ethical approval, creates an unwelcome limbo in which the way forward is not easily navigable. The reviewers are largely disempowered because they cannot undo what has already been done. In finding themselves in a difficult situation, disappointed proposers may simply dismiss the verdict and continue regardless. Importantly, the animals involved are inescapably disenfranchised by the whole process. Finally, knowing that the option of retrospective ethical review exists may, consciously or otherwise, foster a culture of it being 'better (or more expedient) to ask for forgiveness than permission'. This may be appropriate in other situations but is unacceptable in the context of ethical use of animals.

12.5 WHO (SHOULD UNDERTAKE THE ETHICAL REVIEW)?

The question of who undertakes ethical review in a given scenario depends primarily on the scenario itself, although there are a few guiding principles. There is a reasonable body of literature on the appropriate composition of ethical review committees which considers this question in greater detail (Baneux et al. 2023; Ashall et al. 2023; Adami et al. 2023; Oates et al. 2021; WHO 2011).

Ethical review requires more than a single person because multiple viewpoints reduce the chance of oversight while providing a breadth of perspective. Decisions based on a consensus may be made and accepted with greater confidence than those made unilaterally. This is particularly important because many aspects of ethical assessment are not easily nor definitively categorised into 'right' or 'wrong', particularly when scenarios are complex. No single individual should have the power to determine whether what is proposed is ethically acceptable or not.

The ethical review body must contain members who are knowledgeable on the subject of the proposal under consideration, and they must be able to weigh up potential ethical considerations that are pertinent to the animals, any owners, the proposers (researchers, clinicians, etc.), and the institution (and wider society). This can be challenging to achieve. Beyond some expertise in ethics itself, knowledge of the species involved, current practices surrounding their management or treatment, knowledge of relevant legislation (which may be territory-specific for international projects), data laws and data ethics, study design, and so on may be required.

Those undertaking the review should ideally not have a direct or vested interest in the scenario under consideration. This sounds obvious, but it can be challenging to ensure in many circumstances. Concerns with conflicts of interest tend to focus on direct participation in the proposed activity or the potential for direct financial benefit. However, indirect conflicts of interest may exist if reviewers have their own agenda about what is permissible. Some may have professional relationships with the applicants, while others may benefit when proposal approval leads to institutional profit or kudos. It may be difficult to abolish such potential conflicts entirely. However, all potential conflicts must be declared to the group so that their potential to introduce bias into the decision-making process may be recognised.

The involvement of lay people in ethical review has been advocated (Legood 2005; Jennings & Smith 2015; WHO 2011). However, what constitutes 'lay-ness' is not always clear. For example, at what point of education, experience, or expertise does the layperson become a subject expert? Taken to extremes, when is the lay representative on a given committee relieved of their responsibilities because 'they came to know too much'? It is important to acknowledge that those offering, or willing, to act as lay representatives in ethical review may have some interest or related expertise, for example, as a 'disinterested' scientist. While this does not preclude them contributing to the ethical review process, it may undermine their credentials as the *vox populi*. (Can any single voice 'represent society'?) This is not to argue against the inclusion of laypeople: independent voices and alternative perspectives are essential to effective ethical review. However, these points are set out here to temper expectations. The designation of 'layperson' on an ethical review committee is not a panacea, nor does it instantly confer added value. Conversely, the absence of laypeople does not automatically devalue any ethical review.

Some training in ethics or animal welfare science is desirable for at least some members of the review committee and should be encouraged. Such training can help provide a framework for the review, support a process for navigating challenging situations in a dispassionate fashion, and increase the chances that all matters requiring consideration receive it. Equally, a lack of training should not preclude individuals from contributing their expertise or experience to the decision-making process nor devalue their contribution. To do so risks making the ethical review process exclusive or being perceived as such.

The number of people available for ethical review often depends on practical considerations, including the rapidity with which decisions are required. This is commonly cited as a key challenge for ethical review of proposals for the treatment of challenging clinical cases (Quain et al. 2022; Yeates et al. 2013). While consideration of such cases does not align well with an ethical review structure involving 20 individuals meeting quarterly to consider a multi-page application document, to conclude that ethical review is impossible in such scenarios is defeatist. Modern technology has facilitated rapid convening of individuals in distinct geographical locations. Consequently, even lone-working veterinarians are not excluded from contemporaneous consultation with a wider group. Several strategies for ethical review of clinical cases exist (Quain et al. 2022). What is most important in such cases is that an overt consideration of the ethics surrounding what is being proposed is undertaken, using the guiding principles previously outlined. That is to say, at the very least, more than one person, without direct involvement and with some expertise, should weigh up the ethical considerations at play and assist in reaching a consensus decision around what constitutes one or more acceptable ways to proceed. Although veterinarians should at all times put the welfare of their patients first, this does not bestow them with ethical autocracy.

Perhaps surprisingly, the Royal College of Veterinary Surgeons' (RCVS') Code of Professional Conduct for Veterinary Surgeons does not contain a single direct mention of 'ethics' or 'ethical' as it relates to clinical veterinary practice. However, the supporting guidance *does* contain text that considers ethics more directly, albeit pertaining to specific circumstances such as clinical veterinary research, experimental research involving animals, and kidney transplant in cats. One sentence is noteworthy (emphasis added):

> What is regarded as routine in relation to a specific veterinary clinician, clinical setting, patient, species or condition at one point in time, **may not be regarded as ethically acceptable**, nor constitute, routine veterinary practice if carried out by a different veterinary clinician in a different clinical setting, in relation to a different patient, species or condition, and/or at a different point in time.
>
> **Code of Professional Conduct for Veterinary Surgeons and Supporting Guidance, Royal College of Veterinary Surgeons.**

As this implies that not a single element of routine veterinary practice is ethical by default, it would seem prudent that due ethical consideration is given to all but the simplest and most straightforward of routine practices. Further, given that the 'specific veterinary clinician' is listed as one of the factors relevant in determining the ethical acceptability of the proposed practice, perhaps this same clinician should not be the sole individual determining whether their intended actions are acceptable or not.

In conclusion, while there are guiding principles and recommendations about who should form the ethical review panel, the fact that overt and intentional ethical review occurs is more important than the precise composition of the collective that undertakes it.

12.6 WHERE (SHOULD THE ETHICAL REVIEW BE CARRIED OUT)?

Whether the ethical review is undertaken in-house or by an external committee depends on several factors. Smaller organisations may not have the staffing nor caseload to support their own ethical review committee. There may also be concerns about how independent in-house review will be. Although larger institutions, particularly academic ones, usually have both numbers and expertise, neither insulates them from the accusation that they are 'marking their own homework'.

Ideally, ethical review would be undertaken by an entirely independent committee. In the UK, the RCVS has set up an Ethics Review Panel 'to provide a mechanism for practice-based researchers, who may not normally have access to such through university or industry connections, to gain ethical review for their work'. Although a welcome initiative, providing independent review for those working in practice and without access to existing ethical review committees, it currently would be unable to cater for all UK-based veterinary ethical review. Neither does it presently review all the scenarios outlined earlier for which ethical review may be indicated, particularly that of clinical cases.

There are other challenges to consider for those advocating an entirely independent system of ethical review. How does one ensure that there is appropriate local and contextual knowledge to aid the understanding and assessment of what is being proposed? And that decisions are aligned to the ethos of the host organisation? Who covers the cost of the review? If applicants pay for ethical review, a client-supplier relationship may be generated, which is likely to produce conflicts of interest. If applicants have a choice as to where they submit their proposals, then the possibility of 'ethical tourism' emerges whereby applicants shop around until a favourable opinion is obtained. Some possible solutions, or at least mitigations, to these concerns would be to promote greater alignment between the various UK-based ethical review committees. This is the primary aspiration of the recently formed Association of Veterinary Ethics Committees. Potentially, the harmonisation of current ethical review practices and guidelines could then lead on to cooperation between ethical review committees, perhaps reviewing one another's caseloads. Until such a point is reached, it is important to recognise the potential limitations of the local, semi-independent review that is the current norm. There should also be the facility to refer challenging scenarios for review elsewhere, or at least the option to seek a second opinion or expert advice.

12.7　HOW (SHOULD THE ETHICAL REVIEW BE CARRIED OUT)?

The detail and depth of the ethical review process will depend on the scenario being assessed. Proposals to use previously acquired clinical data in retrospective research will inherently be of lower ethical risk than a prospective randomised controlled trial. It is important that the review is proportional to promote buy-in from all stakeholders, including applicants and reviewers.

Applying an agreed framework can be extremely helpful in ensuring consistency and transparency of decision-making. This needs to be tailored to the scenario under consideration. Several frameworks and guidelines have been published to support ethical assessment in various clinical and research settings (Baneux et al. 2023; Quain et al. 2022; Campbell 2021; Grimm et al. 2018; Brink & Lewis 2023). The structure of the review may also be supported by committee-specific application forms, guidance (to applicants and reviewers), and review checklists.

One non-negotiable element to the ethical review process is that reviewers must be able to offer a candid opinion without fear of recrimination or retribution. A relatively straightforward way to encourage this is to maintain reviewer anonymity when feeding back a decision and comments to the applicant. However, this may not always be practical in small organisations. In such cases, additional protections are required, equivalent to those offered to whistleblowers. The culture supporting the importance of ethical review needs to be led from the senior leadership of the organisation. This is particularly important to ensure that there cannot be pressure, real or imagined, on more junior staff to arrive at certain decisions.

12.8　CONCLUSION

Ethical review must be an integral part of human-animal interactions in their broadest sense. It is required to ensure that proposed uses are ethically acceptable from the perspective of animals, their owners, those who will directly use the animals or their data, and the organisations of which they are a part (the 'why').

All potential uses of animals or their data should be considered for ethical review in some way, shape, or form (the 'what'). Such uses extend to far more than just the use of animals in clinical or experimental research.

Ethical review should always be undertaken before the proposed use commences (the 'when') and by more than a single individual. This collective should have the appropriate training and expertise to assess the pertinent ethical considerations relevant to the proposed use (the 'who'). A number of factors will determine whether the review is undertaken internally or externally (the 'where'). Irrespective of this, conditions should be in place to ensure that the review is proportionate to the ethical risk, as independent as possible, and allows reviewers to provide an honest opinion without fear of reprisal (the 'how').

There are many scenarios in which pre-emptive ethical review should be considered highly advisable, if not mandatory. Rather than denying this or explaining away its absence because the perfect conditions for ethical review cannot be met, ethical review should instead continue to be embedded across the gamut of animal use by humans. Acknowledging any imperfections or inadequacies in the review process will itself drive evolution and improvement. All will benefit.

REFERENCES

Adami C, Murrell J, Fordyce P. Ethical considerations in clinical veterinary research. *Vet J.* 2023;300–302:106026.

Animals In Science Committee. Review of harm benefit analysis in the use of animals in research: summary of recommendations for animal welfare ethical review bodies (AWERBS). *GOV.UK* [Internet]. 2020 Dec. Available from: https://assets.publishing.service.gov.uk/media/5ff459308fa8f53b7e43fc99/HBA_summary_for_AWERBs.pdf.

Ashall V, Morton D, Clutton E. A declaration of Helsinki for animals. *Vet Anaesth Analg.* 2023;50(4):309–314.

Baneux PJR, Bertout JA, Middleton JR, et al. Perspectives on implementing veterinary clinical studies committees. *J Am Vet Med Assoc.* 2023;261(9):1–6.

Brink CB, Lewis DI. The 12 Rs framework as a comprehensive, unifying construct for principles guiding animal research ethics. *Animals (Basel).* 2023;13(7):1128.

Brønstad A, Newcomer CE, Decelle T, et al. Current concepts of harm-benefit analysis of animal experiments – report from the AALAS-FELASA Working group on harm-benefit analysis – part 1. *Lab Anim.* 2016;50(1 Suppl):1–20.

Campbell MLH. An ethical framework for the use of horses in competitive sport: theory and function. *Animals (Basel).* 2021;11(6):1725.

Coleman CH. Risk-benefit analysis. In: Graeme L, Dove E, Ganguli-Mitra A, et al., editors. *The Cambridge handbook of health research regulation.* 1st ed. Cambridge: Cambridge University Press; 2021. p. 130–138.

Eggel M, Grimm H. Necessary, but not sufficient: the benefit concept in the project evaluation of animal research in the context of directive 2010/63/EU. *Animals (Basel).* 2018;8(3):34.

Emanuel EJ, Wendler D, Grady C. What makes clinical research ethical? *JAMA.* 2000;283(20):2701–2711.

Grimm H, Bergadano A, Musk GC, et al. Drawing the line in clinical treatment of companion animals: recommendations from an ethics working party. *Vet Rec.* 2018;182(23):664.

Home Office: Animals in Science Regulation Unit. The harm-benefit analysis process: new project licence applications (advice note 05/2015). *GOV.UK* [Internet]. 2015 Dec. Available from: https://assets.publishing.service.gov.uk/government/uploads/system/uploads/attachment_data/file/487914/Harm_Benefit_Analysis__2_.pdf.

Jennings M, Smith JA. *A resource book for lay members of ethical review and similar bodies worldwide.* 3rd ed. Horsham: RSPCA Research Animals Department; 2015.

Laber K, Newcomer CE, Decelle T, et al. Recommendations for addressing harm-benefit analysis and implementation in ethical evaluation – report from the AALAS-FELASA working group on harm-benefit analysis – part 2. *Lab Anim.* 2015;50(1 Suppl):21–42.

Legood G. The recruitment and role of lay members. *Res Ethics.* 2005;1(4):135–138.

Morton DB, Allen K. The importance of practice-based clinical veterinary research and its legal and ethical controls. *Equine Vet J.* 2024 Jul 26;56. Published online.

Mullan S, Quain A. *Veterinary ethics: navigating tough cases*. 1st ed. Great Easton: 5m Publishing Ltd; 2017.

Oates J, Carpenter D, Fisher M, et al. BPS code of human research ethics. *British Psychological Society* [Internet]. 2021 Apr. Available from: https://doi.org/10.53841/bpsrep.2021.inf180.

Quain A, Mullan S, Ward MP. 'There was a sense that our load had been lightened': evaluating outcomes of virtual ethics rounds for veterinary team members. *Front Vet Sci*. 2022;9:922049.

Royal College of Veterinary Surgeons (RCVS). Code of professional conduct for veterinary surgeons and supporting guidance. *RCVS Advice & Guidance* [Internet]. 2012 Apr 1. Available from: https://www.rcvs.org.uk/setting-standards/advice-and-guidance/code-of-professional-conduct-for-veterinary-surgeons/.

Royal College of Veterinary Surgeons (RCVS). Ethical review for practice-based research: a report of a joint RCVS/BVA working party 2013. *RCVS Document Library* [Internet]. 2016 Mar 16. Available from: https://www.rcvs.org.uk/document-library/rcvs-bva-ethical-review-working-party-report-2013/.

World Health Organization (WHO). *Standards and operational guidance for ethics review of health-related research with human participants*. Geneva: WHO Press; 2011.

Yeates J, Everitt S, Innes JF, et al. Ethical and evidential considerations on the use of novel therapies in veterinary practice. *J Sm Anim Prac*. 2013;54(3):119–123.

Yeates JW. Ethical principles for novel therapies in veterinary practice. *J Sm Anim Prac*. 2016;57(2):67–73.

13 Can Considering Laboratory Animal Legislation Improve Animal Welfare in Innovative Veterinary Practice?

Ngaire Dennison

13.1 BACKGROUND

Humans exploit animals for food, clothing, and companionship. In the United Kingdom (UK), livestock farming uses over a billion animals per year providing more than 4.2 million tonnes of meat in 2022 (Department for Environment, Food & Rural Affairs 2023). Around 57% of households contain a total of approximately 38 million pets (UK Pet Food 2024). The number of animals used in research is far fewer: 2.76 million scientific procedures involving living animals were carried out in Great Britain in 2022 (Home Office [Statistics] 2023a). Despite this, using animals for research has always caused controversy. Therefore, controls on such use have been in place in the UK (in the form of the Cruelty to Animals Act) since 1876. This Act made it an offence to perform experiments on a living animal that would cause pain, unless for advancing physiological knowledge, saving or prolonging life, or alleviating suffering. These controls were revised and strengthened with the introduction of the Animals (Scientific Procedures) Act (ASPA) in 1986. The ASPA was amended in 2013 to bring the UK in line with the requirement of EU Directive 2010/63.

13.2 THE LEGISLATION

In the UK, animal research is controlled by the Animals (Scientific Procedures) Act 1986, known as ASPA. The law regulates the use of 'protected animals' (all vertebrate animals other than man and cephalopods) in experiments other any other scientific procedure that may cause pain, suffering, distress, or lasting harm that is equivalent to, or more than, the discomfort caused by the insertion of a needle in line with good veterinary practice.

The ASPA provides three levels of regulation – with a requirement for licences to be in place at the level of the place (establishment licence), the project (project licence), and the person (personal licence). Licences are only granted after the Competent Authority (Regulator), the Animals in Science Regulatory Unit at the Home Office deems that appropriate housing and care will be provided, that all individuals performing experimental procedures will have the requisite training and skills, and for each project, that the likely benefits will outweigh the potential harms via a harm-benefit analysis (HBA) (Home Office 2015). No project can last more than 5 years without being updated and gaining a new authorisation.

13.3 HARM BENEFIT ANALYSIS

The estimate of benefits being realised in a scientific project considers the expertise of the applicant, the funding available (including source and whether the work has been peer-reviewed), the success of previous research (including number and quality of peer-reviewed publications), and the facilities available.

Evaluation of potential harms considers the numbers and types of animals, the sort(s) of procedures each animal will receive, what mitigations are in place to minimise the harms, and how the harms experienced by the animals may accumulate.

In addition to the overall HBA, an estimate of the worst-case scenario for the harm to any animal used in a protocol is set in advance, giving a prospective severity classification for each protocol. Limits are placed on what can happen to the animals by the setting of legally enforceable humane endpoints. Since January 2013, there has been a requirement for reporting the 'actual severity' of harm for each individual animal at the end of the animal's use. The actual severity reports the highest degree of harm experienced by the animal at any point in the study; i.e. it is not an 'average'.

13.4 ASPA; OTHER LEGAL REQUIREMENTS

There is detailed mandated training for those working under ASPA (Home Office [Guidance] 2023b) which includes experimental design and ethics for those designing studies and/or performing procedures on animals.

Each establishment that breeds, supplies, or uses animals in research must employ key *named* individuals, each of whom has specific legal responsibilities. These people include

   I. a person responsible for overseeing the welfare and care of the animals kept at the place specified in the licence (the Named Animal Care and Welfare Officer, or NACWO),

Considering Laboratory Animal Legislation

> II. a veterinary surgeon with expertise in laboratory animal medicine to provide advice on the welfare and treatment of those animals (the Named Veterinary Surgeon, or NVS),
> III. a person responsible for ensuring that the persons dealing with those animals have access to any information they need about the species concerned,
> IV. a person to be responsible for ensuring that the persons dealing with those animals are adequately educated and trained and are supervised until they have demonstrated the requisite competence, and
> V. a person to be responsible for ensuring that the conditions of the licence are in compliance.

The NACWO and NVS, whilst working collaboratively with the researcher, have primary roles as independent advocates for the animals.

13.5 THE 3Rs (Table 13.1)

The ASPA requires that the principles of the 3Rs are applied at all times. These principles, replacement, reduction, and refinement, were published in 1959 by Drs William Russell and Rex Burch in *The Principles of Humane Experimental Technique*. The 3Rs are now considered an ethical framework for improving the welfare of laboratory animals around the world.

TABLE 13.1
Definition of 3Rs

	Basic definition	Updated NC3Rs* definition
Replacement	Avoiding or replacing the use of animals in areas where they otherwise would have been used	Accelerating the development and use of predictive and robust models and tools, based on the latest science and technologies, to replace the use of animals in addressing important research questions
Reduction	Minimising the number of animals used consistent with scientific aims	Appropriately designed and analysed animal experiments that are robust and reproducible and add to the knowledge base
Refinement	Minimising the pain, suffering, distress, or lasting harm that research animals might experience	Advancing laboratory animal welfare by exploiting the latest *in vivo* technologies to minimise pain, suffering, and distress and improving understanding of the impact of welfare on scientific outcome

* The National Centre for the 3Rs (NC3Rs) is a UK body established in 2004 to accelerate advances in replacing, reducing, and refining the use of animals in research and testing.

13.6 AWERBs

Before a project can be submitted to the regulator, it must be reviewed by a local Animal Welfare and Ethical Review Body (AWERB). The tasks of this body include

I. advising the staff on the welfare of animals in relation to their acquisition, accommodation, care, and use;
II. advising the establishment licence holder whether to support project proposals;
III. advising on the application of the 3Rs, including ensuring protocols are as refined as possible by establishing humane endpoints (see the following);
IV. ensuring there are appropriate internal operational processes as regards monitoring, reporting, and follow-up in relation to the welfare of animals;
V. following the development and outcome of projects by considering the effect on the animals used and identifying and advising on what could further contribute to replacement, reduction, and refinement;
VI. providing a forum for discussion and development of ethical advice to the establishment licence holder on all matters related to animal welfare, care, and use;
VII. promoting a culture of care; and
VIII. reviewing all projects using one or more protocols that involve potentially 'severe' procedures. The researchers who hold the licence for such projects must provide a formal retrospective assessment of the work. This is reviewed by the AWERB before being submitted to the Regulator.

13.7 CALCULATING STUDY OF HARMS UNDER ASPA

In compliance with the regulation, researchers have developed detailed systems for considering all potential harms to the animals being used. Considerable emphasis has been and is placed on the total lifetime experience of the animal and how harms may accumulate (Honess & Wolfensohn 2010; NC3Rs Innovation Platform 2021; Mellor et al. 2020).

An idea of how a local AWERB might consider the harms of a study may be gained using an example of a murine arthritis model, which is being used to identify a potential treatment for similar conditions in humans (and animals). A common assessment approach by the AWERB for considering the accumulation of harms would be to consider:

I. The *acquisition* of the animal. Was it bred on site or was it transported from a breeding establishment?
II. The process of *acclimatisation/habituation*. Are there approaches that can help to mitigate against any potential pain or distress during subsequent procedures?
III. How will the animal be *housed*. Does the study require any limitations on best practice for housing? For example, does it need to be housed on its own rather than with cage-mates? And can it still have (and use) a full

Considering Laboratory Animal Legislation 113

  range of natural behaviours/interaction with the environment, or will the procedures being undertaken mean these become limited?
IV. The *creation of the model* (in this case surgery to destabilise a joint). Is analgesia being applied? How will the analgesia be applied? Can voluntary intake be used, or will animals need to be dosed (injected/gavaged) to deliver the analgesic? How effective is the peri-operative analgesic regimen, considering the type of drug(s) that can be used within any limitations imposed by the type of animal and the scientific requirements of the study, the frequency of dosing required, and any possibility of pain breakthrough? What are the post-surgical housing conditions? What level of monitoring and support are available/possible?
V. What (if any) treatment is being given to *modify* the extent of arthritis? Is there a likely difference in the possible pain for different experimental groups (for example, is there a control group that won't receive analgesia)?
VI. What is the likely *duration* of clinical signs?
VII. What is the *fate* of the animal? Is humane killing at a fixed time point irrespective of the clinical signs, or are animals killed if clinical signs progress beyond a specific level that has been agreed prospectively as the maximum ethically acceptable?

The review will involve researchers who are not involved in the study and the NVS and NACWO. The named individuals are independent of the study and their legal purpose is to protect animal welfare. The work will most often be funded by a peer-reviewed grant. There is no financial benefit to anyone serving on the AWERB as to whether the study goes ahead or not. This approach avoids conflicts of interest. The regulator will also review all these factors, applying for additional independent scrutiny.

13.8 PREDICTING STUDY SUCCESS AND SUBSEQUENT BENEFITS UNDER ASPA

The regulator must establish the likelihood of study success and whether the benefits anticipated by the licence applicants are likely to be realised. This will have been considered by the AWERB. This is assisted by answering the following questions.

  I. Has consideration been given to design of the study? What are the criteria for success/failure? If it fails, what are the next steps (modify the procedure in this animal, change procedure in another)?
 II. Has the accumulation of harm been considered and humane endpoints been agreed in advance? (That is, when will the procedure be considered to have failed/how much suffering is too much?)
III. How is the knowledge gained from the procedure going to be disseminated (are both successful and unsuccessful results to be reported)?
IV. Are the limitations of any conclusions drawn from the work clearly described? For example, will consideration be given to how applicable

the conclusions are for the general population if only a limited number of animals/a single or few breeds or ages/or only a single sex has had the procedure performed?
V. What are the benefits? Who benefits? For example, are the benefits to gain knowledge (fundamental science) or to people, the environment, or other animals (translational research). When will the benefits be realised? Are there different short-, medium-, and long-term benefits?

13.9 HARM–BENEFIT ANALYSIS UNDER ASPA

Detailed consideration of the potential harms and the likely benefits will then yield a HBA (Home Office 2015; European Commission Working Group 2013). For the HBA, the balance is deliberately 'tilted' in favour of the animal in that *possible* harms are considered against *likely* benefits. A HBA is performed by the local AWERB and the regulator. Non-technical summaries from all granted projects are available on a designated UK government's website.

13.10 HOW SIMILAR PROCEDURES ARE RESTRICTED BY THE VETERINARY SURGEONS ACT

When the surgical reconstruction of a joint is conducted by veterinary clinicians on a client-owned animal then the governing legislation is the Veterinary Surgeons Act 1966 (VSA). However, when the surgical reconstruction is untested, or innovative, i.e. borders on the experimental, then the regulatory boundaries become blurred. Given the priority must be the health and welfare of the animal, the important question then becomes 'Would using an ASPA-based approach to consideration of procedure, i.e. a formal HBA, be most likely to give the best outcome for the animal?' An equally important question is 'When does an innovative procedure become an experimental one?' because the answer will determine which regulatory conditions apply. Whether innovative procedures planned for a client's pet are regulated by the VSA or ASPA depends on whether the procedure is deemed to be 'routine' (or as was previously designated-recognised) veterinary practice (RVP) or something else?

13.11 ROUTINE VETERINARY PRACTICE

There is some concern that the Royal College of Veterinary Surgeons' (RCVS) advice on what constitutes routine veterinary practice (updated in January 2023) is open to interpretation, and that the line between what is RVP and what goes beyond this is obscure. RVP is defined as 'procedures and techniques performed on animals by veterinary surgeons (or veterinary nurses under their direction . . . which ensure the health and welfare of animals committed to their care'. 'These can be thought of as the routine, established procedures undertaken on animals every day' (see section 25.7 of the RCVS Code to Professional Conduct). However, in the associated FAQs, RVP is 'the clinical investigation and management of the health and welfare of animals is generally considered to be routine

Considering Laboratory Animal Legislation 115

veterinary practice when it involves a procedure or technique that is likely to be of direct benefit to the individual animal', which appears to offer a far broader scope.

The FAQs *do* make it clear that development of any new procedure or technique must 'reasonably be expected to result in a similar or better outcome than that following conventional treatment' and that 'it would not be acceptable for a veterinary surgeon to use an animal in the development of a new or improved veterinary procedure or treatment where it has not previously been made available to the veterinary profession and there is no background evidence to predict a clinical application in the species or other veterinary benefit (parallel evidence in humans may be acceptable)'. However, there are published cases where transfer of procedures between dissimilar species *have* been performed as RVP, and in these cases, the designation of 'routine', the predictions of success, and the identification of potential harms have been made by clinician(s) directly involved in the case. This facility to 'mark one's own homework' offers major advantages to the clinicians involved – and major disadvantages to the animal and its owner – by significantly 'tipping' the balance of power to the clinician.

If a procedure is judged to be 'routine' veterinary practice:

I. There is *no requirement* for *independent ethical consideration*. This lack of a former structure allows inconsistent decision-making.
II. There is *no legally required independent advocate* for the animal.
III. The surgery will be funded by the owner or an insurance company, where decisions on whether the treatment proceeds or not will be based on the advice of a vet who is likely to be personally involved in the surgery. Therefore, this is a considerable potential for a *conflict of interest*.
IV. There is *no formal process* for considering the 'whole animal experience', i.e. *harms*. Consider: the journey to the practice may be stressful far an animal unused to car travel. After admission, the animal may be left in an unfamiliar environment with possible adjacency to unfamiliar animals. Later, the animal will undergo surgery after which – it is hoped – it will receive post-operative analgesia. It will then be observed in a recovery ward for one or more days. After discharge, post-operative progress will be assessed by multiple trips to and from the clinic, where negative peri-operative associations may prove particularly stressful. In the event of post-operative complications, further surgery may be required, repeating and aggravating the animal's unpleasant experiences.
V. There is no formal process for assessing the *benefits* of innovative procedures. The veterinary clinician may benefit by having the satisfaction of 'curing' a patient (which may be a biased perception as the procedure may be a success but much of the 'harm' may be unobserved by the clinician). They will also gain new knowledge and, in the process, they or their practice will gain financially. The owner may benefit from more time with a beloved companion. The animal may benefit from an extended life, but part of assessing the benefits should be a consideration of quality (PDSA 2021), rather than just quantity, of life.

13.12 CONFUSION OVER CLINICAL VETERINARY RESEARCH

The RCVS definition of clinical veterinary research (CVR) is 'a routine procedure being undertaken for the benefit of the animal(s), with the concurrent intention to generate new knowledge that benefits animals, e.g. developing new procedures, improving diagnoses, changing a routine procedure, or comparing existing procedures'. To establish whether something is CVR or not examines not only the procedure itself but the 'intention' for undertaking it, as well as the overall context. The RCVS state that what is regarded as 'routine' in relation to a specific veterinary clinician, clinical setting, patient, species, or condition at one point in time may not be regarded as ethically acceptable, nor constitute, routine veterinary practice if carried out by a different veterinary clinician in a different clinical setting, in relation to a different patient, species, or condition and/or at a different point in time. This leaves the potential for major differential interpretation between clinicians. (See Chapter 12 by Stephen N. Greenhalgh.)

Veterinary schools should have an ethics committee that considers CVR (in addition to a considerable range of animal-based investigations described by Stephen N. Greenhalgh). Unfortunately, these are unavailable to veterinary practitioners. The RCVS Ethics Review Panel (ERP) is a subcommittee reporting to the RCVS Standards Committee (RCVS 2020) whose function is to provide a mechanism whereby practice-based researchers, denied straightforward access to university or industrial boards, can gain ethical review for their work. Unfortunately, the ERP only reviews proposed clinical trials – not individual cases and, importantly, its consultation is in no way mandatory. Consequently, individuals who do not believe their intended actions constitute CVR are not obliged to seek any form of approval. Furthermore, many ERPs are unable to make prompt decisions in urgent cases (although exceptions are made by the RCVS ERP) allowing untested life-or-death innovations to evade review. In contrast, establishments working under ASPA are usually able to make ethics-based decisions in urgent situations within hours.

Several papers have identified concerns relating to the ethical assessment of certain veterinary procedures or some veterinary clinical trials (e.g. Hernandez et al. 2018; Quain et al. 2021; Bertout et al. 2021), and concerns exist that there are differences between approaches within the veterinary profession (Clutton 2009). The RCVS itself says that 'even where a procedure is usually deemed to be routine veterinary practice, this does not automatically mean that it is ethically acceptable in all circumstances' (see section 25.12 of the Code for Professional Conduct). Similar concerns have been raised elsewhere, e.g. in at least three of the British Veterinary Association's Animal Welfare Foundation discussion forums (Taylor 2019). At one, the question whether clinical innovation raised welfare concerns was answered with 95% of the audience agreeing at the debate's end that it did.

13.13 CAN ASPA ASSIST IN CLINICAL DECISION-MAKING?

In response to these concerns, the European Society for the Laboratory Animal Veterinarians (ESLAV), the Laboratory Animal Veterinary Association (LAVA), and the University Federation for Animal Welfare (UFAW) jointly held a series of three online meetings in January, March, and April 2021 to investigate how laboratory and clinical vets might support each other in decision-making, with attendees from across laboratory and clinical veterinary sectors. The major concerns raised by attendees at the ESLAV/LAVA/UFAW meetings were as follows.

13.14 LACK OF TRANSPARENCY IN ETHICAL DECISION-MAKING IN VETERINARY PRACTICE

Many attendees felt that a more transparent approach within practice could be achieved by adopting similar review structures as those undertaken by AWERBs under ASPA (and similar European legislation). Such systems would (i) require that consideration be given to the whole life experience of the animal, (ii) mean an estimation of the severity of harms that procedures will cause (both in advance of a procedure going ahead and a review of the actual post-procedural harm), (iii) require an assessment of the estimated benefits the procedure will deliver, and (iv) ask whether any steps can be taken to make future procedures less harmful.

Before novel procedures are considered in client-owned animals, additional questions to be answered include (i) what the likelihood of success of the novel procedure is and (ii) whether the age, concurrent disease status, and the individual animal's ability to cope, e.g. with separation from owner, kennelling, transport, etc., been considered.

13.15 LACK OF INDEPENDENT OVERSIGHT OF DECISIONS

The limited or absent independent ethical oversight of decision-making in veterinary practice concerning novel procedures contrasts starkly with procedures involving laboratory animals or human patients facing uncertain hospital treatments. Ethics committees meeting similar requirements for independence are tasked with similar responsibilities in veterinary schools (although the independence of some has been questioned). Although ethical panels may exist in other clinical practice situations, identifying where these exist and in what circumstances they are used is not easy.

Ensuring the ethical treatment of laboratory animals is a legal requirement of the AWERB and involves a range of people with varying perspectives. AWERB members must include independent researchers with animal experience, a NACWO and an NVS. The regulator also expects all AWERBs to include a lay person and most AWERBs will additionally incorporate (or co-opt) statisticians (or other experimental design experts), scientists with no animal experience, and personnel external to the home establishment. There are no specific requirements for ethics panels for clinical research stipulated by the RCVS.

All concerns raised by AWERB members will be considered and, when disagreement exists, the chair, who will be independent of the research being undertaken, will have the final say. Review within a practice situation should consider the concerns of the whole team and thought given to a system whereby an independent expert has the final say as to whether a proposed treatment goes ahead or not. When applied in veterinary practice, an ethical appraisal requires that the overall experience of the animal be considered, and this is best done by an independent evaluator whose primary responsibility is to evaluate the procedure *only* in respect of its potential to benefit the animal. In many situations, both the owner and the surgeon/surgical team have potential 'vested interests': the owner has emotional attachment and may feel pressure to accept an 'advanced' treatment while the veterinary team may be focused on trying a new/modified procedure.

13.16 LACK OF A ROBUST SYSTEM EVALUATING THE ANIMAL'S OVERALL EXPERIENCE

The severity classification used under ASPA provides a way to understand an animal's likely experience. The system requires that potential harms are classified as 'mild', 'moderate', or 'severe' (See Table 13.2).

Factors considered in assigning severity in individual cases include the type of manipulations involved; handling methods; the nature of pain, suffering, distress, or lasting harm caused by (all elements of) the procedure; the intensity of pain; its duration and frequency; the multiplicity of techniques employed; the cumulative suffering within a procedure; and the extent to which natural behaviours are curtailed, including restrictions on housing, husbandry, and care standards. The experience of the animal due to individual factors (age, sex, personality) will also be considered where these could change the level of suffering for that animal.

In clinical practice, the ultimate goal/eventual outcome can usefully become the basis for discussion and future improvement. Under ASPA, a more formal severity classification must be undertaken. This will be based on the animal's greatest level of suffering at any time during the study, rather than the end result – which is the case in clinical practice. This is an important distinction because clients often only see the positive end-result of veterinary treatment, rather than the unpleasantries their animal experiences during hospitalisation. While the final prospective severity classification is set by the regulator, the researcher must initially propose one that satisfies the AWERB. This means that the NACWOs and NVSs will be involved, both of whom will have ethical training or at least experience in ethical decision-making. The requirement for assigning an actual severity allows better review of whether the estimated harms were accurate and is used by researchers, named people, and the AWERB to inform approaches to future studies.

Many of the complex clinical innovations that have been described in the literature (or featured on TV) would be classified as 'severe' under the ASPA because animals can take a considerable time for pre-interventional physiological and behavioural indices to be restored. Many are likely to experience significant and prolonged discomfort (or pain) and may require lengthy or frequent hospital stays. Under ASPA, such procedures would demand a very high benefit in order to achieve ethical acceptance and, for some species, i.e. primates, dogs, cats, and horses, an additional level of review will be imposed by an independent national committee (Animals in Science Committee 2024).

TABLE 13.2
Severity Classification Used under ASPA

Severity classification	Description (Home Office 2014)	Examples
Mild	Procedures where any pain or suffering experienced by an animal is, at worst, only slight or transitory and minor so that the animal returns to its normal state within a short period of time.	Subcutaneous, intravenous, or intramuscular injection of substances (assuming the competence of those performing the procedure and adherence to best practice guidelines for volume, needle size, etc.). More than one injection may remain 'mild' if there are no cumulative effects.
Moderate	Procedures which cause a significant and easily detectable disturbance of an animal's normal state (assuming appropriate monitoring is conducted by trained and competent staff). The disturbance is enough for an animal to show discomfort, abnormal behaviours, significant weight loss or other indicators of poor welfare, but does not prevent normal feeding and drinking or other normal activities other than for short periods or to a limited extent for longer periods.	Pain of any significant intensity, if no longer than a few hours duration and not considered to be severe, as judged by species-specific criteria. Example 1: an animal receives a known irritant and shows overt signs of pain for a prolonged period without improvement (by persistently licking the affected part for more than three hours) justifies a severe, rather than a moderate, classification. Example 2: a situation in which a rodent show signs of obvious illness, e.g. piloerection, huddled posture, reluctance to move, and isolation from the group, which are *promptly* detected and lead to the animal being killed immediately, could be classed as moderate. If animals remain in this condition for more than 24 hours, this classification would be inappropriate.
Severe	Procedures causing a major departure from the animal's usual state of health and wellbeing, e.g. long-term diseases where assistance with normal activities, such as feeding and drinking, are required or where significant deficits in behaviours/activities persist. This would include any state that a person would find difficult to tolerate, or a disease where clinical signs are such that they threaten life.	Surgical and other interventions under general anaesthesia which are expected to result in severe or persistent moderate post-operative pain, suffering or distress, or severe and persistent impairment of the general condition of the animals.

13.17 ANIMAL ADVOCACY

An important difference between laboratory animal and companion animal practice is that in the former, the NVSs and NACWOs are required to act as animal advocates. In the latter, owners may not be appropriate advocates for numerous reasons: they may be emotionally overwhelmed, they may not fully understand the treatment proposed (nor the potential consequences), and they may have conflicting concerns around financial costs and providing 'the best care' for their pet. Some owners may feel under pressure to accept any treatment, however expensive or unlikely to succeed, until they have tried every possible option to save their pet. The definition of 'best care' frequently seems to focus on the method of 'cure' rather than the animal's experience during treatment.

Another fundamental difference between animals used for research and pets is that any 'severe' event a pet animal endures should be for its long-term benefit. In the research setting, any harms are not (usually) for the good of the individual but are permitted in order to secure a scientific benefit. However, the legal structure of ASPA means that the degree of suffering any animal can endure must be set in advance, via the establishment of pre-emptive humane endpoints (HEPs) and the requirement to avoid unnecessary pain, suffering, distress, or lasting harm. Whether such endpoints are used in general practice is unknown. If they are, to be effective, they must be agreed upon before treatment begins and exist within the confines consented to by the owner/carer. Consent must be based on the owner having received a full explanation of all possible complications arising from treatment. There seldom seems to be an agreed formal 'humane endpoint' established before innovative clinical procedures are begun. One reason for this is that veterinary innovators eager to promote novel treatment may be reluctant to discuss with clients the possibility that complications or treatment failure might cause their animal to suffer and necessitate repeated treatments or euthanasia.

Setting HEPs for animals protected under ASPA means that all parties have agreed to the conditions when an established action will be taken. This expedites decision-making and minimises the duration of a laboratory animal's potential suffering. In clinical cases, HEPs may not be established because the vet and the owner may believe different endpoints are justified, in which case there is a high risk of disagreements prolonging an animal's suffering until a course of action is decided.

13.18 MIXED MESSAGES: THE PROFESSION AND THE PUBLIC

There appear to be many misconceptions concerning treatments that have been promulgated on social media and more standard media forums. These encourage a focus on the technique(s) and (sometimes) the practitioner performing it and not the experience of the animal and the ultimate (rather than the immediate) outcomes. There is an increasing number of cases of crowdfunding of extreme procedures. There needs to be a more balanced dialogue within the profession, and between it and the public, and specifically better communication around the subject of euthanasia, which should be considered as a potentially positive outcome for an animal, to end suffering, rather than a 'failure'.

Considering Laboratory Animal Legislation 121

13.19 INADEQUACY OF CURRENT SYSTEMS

Many delegates felt that the current control of veterinarians conducting questionable innovations were inadequate, being too slow, too limited in scope, and lacking in clarity as to where some types of studies sat within the legislation. Even where a study can be seen clearly to be CVA, delays in ERP review can impact on being able to perform the study, which can ultimately delay approval of new treatments. It was felt that the grey areas between the VSA 1966 and ASPA were too expansive.

13.20 LACK OF CLARITY IN CRITICAL TERMINOLOGY

It was felt that confusion over meanings facilitated the growth of grey areas and created additional loopholes for innovators to exploit. Amongst numerous examples, the term 'RVP' attracted the greatest concern. (This term has since been updated by the RCVS but appears to have done little to limit the grey areas or collapse the loopholes).

13.21 WHAT CAN BE LEARNED FROM LABORATORY ANIMAL PRACTICE?

The ESLAV/LAVA/UFAW meetings concluded that numerous principles used routinely in laboratory practice to protect animals could help veterinary clinicians and their clients, especially in the area of innovative treatment. Consequently, several general recommendations were proposed.

I. There should be **more guidance/training on ethical assessment to support better decision-making in clinical veterinary practice**, especially where novel techniques are being considered.
II. **At least one independent person should be involved in ethical assessment**. The need for independence is an ASPA requirement and a fundamental pillar of human medical ethics. The EU Ethics Review for Human Research mandates that the principal medical investigator must not be responsible for a patient's treatment and care. Independent oversight of clinical trials, which is recommended by the Medical Research Council (MRC) Guidelines for Good Clinical Practice, is typically provided by an independent advisory Data Monitoring Committee (DMC) and an independent executive committee.
III. **A framework for assessing suffering should be developed** using the expertise of those who have developed such frameworks, along with ethicists and animal welfare scientists. The framework should include objective severity guidelines/quality-of-life (QoL) assessments and should be developed for each discipline. They should facilitate the estimation of total (accumulated) suffering and so consider duration and psychological (as well as physical) suffering. For example, suffering arising from exposure to strange environments with unknown carers and behavioural

restriction should be incorporated. The framework should address how HEPs can be determined, discussed, and agreed with owners. Additionally, **an explanation of the effects of treatment(s) and how these and other adverse effects accumulate must be made clear**. Assessment of likely long-term outcomes should be mandatory under this framework. QoL assessment tools are currently being developed to support clinicians (Malkani et al. 2022), although additional tools may be required. The language of ASPA (for example, talking about mild, moderate, and severe suffering) may help with owners' ability to improve advocacy.

IV. There should be a **robust assessment of the design of clinical veterinary research studies**. Experimental design is not taught in detail, if at all, in veterinary courses, so training should be provided for veterinarians undertaking clinical trials and/or wishing to perform procedures falling under CVR. This training should include experimental design and analysis techniques.

V. **Humane endpoints should be discussed in advance with animal owners** to help consider when 'enough is enough' and when euthanasia rather than further treatment would represent the animal's best option.

VI. **A more formal and transparent system of harm-benefit analysis should be developed** for application in the clinical environment.

VII. **Ethical decision-making needs to be agile**; the current ERP system is alleged to be too slow.

VIII. **A retrospective review of all novel procedures should be required** in order to provide reflection and/or audit of case outcome. There should be a method for **publishing negative results/adverse events**, particularly when new surgical methods and/or novel devices are involved.

IX. The **RCVS ERP should make their opinions known publicly** in a non-technical way. Such transparency would usefully inform the public while assisting future decision-making amongst veterinary clinicians.

13.22 SUMMARY

Lifetime experience is a critical concept in the evaluation of the overall harms experienced by any animal. Whilst ASPA is not faultless, the structures it embodies allow for independent scrutiny and consider the likely harms for the animals against the potential short-, medium-, and long-term benefits of the research. Most importantly, ASPA protects animals who cannot consent to or readily evade what they experience as laboratory animals.

A system that would allow similar protections for companion animals would be desirable. Independent ethical consideration and/or independent 'animal advocacy' would be beneficial in helping owners consider the potential harms their animal may experience against the likely benefits of the proposed procedures. This would then allow more informed decision-making when alternative approaches – including euthanasia – are to be considered. Such considerations are particularly important when novel techniques and treatments are being proposed.

REFERENCES

Animals in Science Committee. Appointments and reappointments to the animals in science committee. *GOV.UK* [Internet]. 2024 Mar 12. Available from: https://www.gov.uk/government/news/appointments-and-reappointments-to-the-animals-in-science-committee.

Bertout JA, Baneux PJR, Robertson-Plouch CK. Recommendations for ethical review of veterinary clinical trials. *Front Vet Sci*. 2021;8:715926.

Clutton RE. Clinical studies, pain and ethics. *J Small Anim Pract*. 2009;50(2):59–60.

Department for Environment, Food & Rural Affairs. Agriculture in the United Kingdom 2022. *GOV.UK* [Internet]. 2023 Jul 13. Available from: https://www.gov.uk/government/statistics/agriculture-in-the-united-kingdom-2022.

European Commission Expert Working Group. Working document on project evaluation and retrospective assessment. *Publications of the European Union* [Internet]. 2013 Sept 18–19. Available from: https://op.europa.eu/en/publication-detail/-/publication/7a2f43a1-2550-11e9-8d04-01aa75ed71a1/language-en.

Hernandez E, Fawcett A, Brouwer E, et al. Speaking up: veterinary ethical responsibilities and animal welfare issues in everyday practice. *Animals (Basel)*. 2018;8(1):15.

Home Office. Advisory notes on recording and reporting the actual severity of regulated procedures. *GOV.UK* [Internet]. 2014 Jan 1. Available from: https://www.gov.uk/guidance/animal-research-technical-advice#recording-and-reporting-the-actual-severity-of-regulated-procedures.

Home Office. The harm-benefit analysis process: new project licence applications. *GOV.UK* [Internet]. 2015 Dec. Available from: https://assets.publishing.service.gov.uk/media/5a759e39e5274a545822ce88/Harm_Benefit_Analysis__2_.pdf.

Home Office. Statistics of scientific procedures on living animals, Great Britain: 2022. *GOV.UK* [Internet]. 2023a Nov 9. Available from: https://www.gov.uk/government/statistics/statistics-of-scientific-procedures-on-living-animals-great-britain-2022/statistics-of-scientific-procedures-on-living-animals-great-britain-2022.

Home Office. Guidance for training and continuous professional development under the animals (scientific procedures) act 1986. *GOV.UK* [Internet]. 2023b Dec. Available from: https://assets.publishing.service.gov.uk/media/6581c8b4fc07f300128d44ed/Guidance_for_training_and_CPD_under_ASPA_FINAL1912.pdf.

Honess P, Wolfensohn S. The extended welfare assessment grid: a matrix for the assessment of welfare and cumulative suffering in experimental animals. *Altern Lab Anim*. 2010;38(3):205–212.

Malkani R, Paramasivam S, Wolfensohn S. Preliminary validation of a novel tool to assess dog welfare: the animal welfare assessment grid. *Front Vet Sci*. 2022;9:940017.

Mellor DJ, Beausoleil NJ, Littlewood KE, et al. The 2020 five domains model: including human-animal interactions in assessments of animal welfare. *Animals (Basel)*. 2020;10:1870.

NC3Rs Innovation Platform. Animal welfare assessment grid (AWAG). *NC3Rs* [Internet]. 2021 [cited 2024 Sept 14]. Available from: https://nc3rs.org.uk/crackit/animal-welfare-assessment-grid-awag.

People's Dispensary for Sick Animals (PDSA). How can I tell if my pet still has good quality of life? *PDSA Pet Help and Advice* [Internet]. 2021 [cited 2024 Sept 14]. Available from: https://www.pdsa.org.uk/pet-help-and-advice/looking-after-your-pet/all-pets/how-can-i-tell-if-my-pet-still-has-a-good-quality-of-life.

Quain A, Ward MP, Mullan S. Ethical challenges posed by advanced veterinary care in companion animal veterinary practice. *Animals (Basel)*. 2021;11(11):3010.

Royal College of Veterinary Surgeons (RCVS). *Ethics review panel: role of the panel.* RCVS [Internet]. 2020 [cited 2024 Sept 14]. Available from: https://www.rcvs.org.uk/who-we-are/committees/standards-committee/ethics-review-panel/.

Royal College of Veterinary Surgeons (RCVS). Code of professional conduct for veterinary surgeons 25: routine veterinary practice and clinical veterinary research. *RCVS Advice & Guidance* [Internet]. 2023 Jan 11. Available from: https://www.rcvs.org.uk/setting-standards/advice-and-guidance/code-of-professional-conduct-for-veterinary-surgeons/supporting-guidance/routine-veterinary-practice/.

Taylor P. The Animal Welfare Foundation 2019 discussion forum: clinical excellence – or overtreatment? *AWF YouTube Channel* [Internet]. 2019 Mar 28. Available from: https://www.youtube.com/watch?v=YAYi-ZdgrCc&list=PLZEA50ttXGWIteM0ILcK4dpMYX5k96qup&index=7.

UK Pet Food. *UK pet population: UK pet industry statistics* [Internet]. 2024 Mar. Available from: https://www.ukpetfood.org/information-centre/statistics/uk-pet-population.html.

Part IIC Evidence-Free Veterinary Medicine

14 Why Believe in Magic? *The use of Ineffective Therapies has Welfare and Ethical Implications*

Tanya Stephens

Whilst quackery and pseudoscience have been around for a long time, it is concerning that any veterinarian, trained in the sciences, engages in Complementary and Alternative Veterinary Medicine (CAVM) given the lack of evidence and the health, welfare, and ethical concerns of using implausible and ineffective 'therapies' on animals. Of additional concern is the association of CAVM with anti-vaccination sentiments.

Veterinary regulators should initiate and enforce restrictive codes and veterinary professional associations should not only disassociate themselves from pseudoscience and CAVM but actively condemn it to maintain professionalism and a social contract with the public.

14.1 INTRODUCTION

When I was a veterinary student those who dabbled in so-called alternative/complementary/holistic/integrative (take your pick) 'therapies' were dubbed 'snake oil salesmen'. We were aware of a general thirst for knowledge in the profession and the great need for scientific evidence to guide veterinarians towards best treatment options, especially in companion animal medicine. How gratifying it has been to see such amazing advances over the last 20–30 years in veterinary medicine as a result of this and the welcome emergence of evidence-based medicine. How depressing to find that some veterinarians would discount this by choosing to use 'treatments', not because they are supported by scientific evidence but because they are supposedly 3000 years old and for that reason are thought to be effective.

My interest in this topic was ignited some years ago when a complementary and alternative veterinary medicine (CAVM) practice opened up which offered acupuncture and homeopathy and various herbal therapies. They also offered free initial consultations. One day, an old client called into my practice with her very old dog which was lame and in pain. There was a palpable painful swelling over the femur and an x-ray confirmed osteosarcoma. As costs were an issue, the client had decided to try out the new practice and take advantage of the free consultation for her lame dog.

At the 'alternative' practice the dog was diagnosed with 'arthritis' and the client was offered acupuncture, at a cost, which she agreed to and of course it didn't do anything for the dog. I contacted the practice to obtain a history and was curious as to how the diagnosis of arthritis was made and why they carried out acupuncture on a dog which clearly had something seriously wrong with it.

The practice informed me that they didn't undertake 'traditional' Western medicine, only alternative Eastern medicine, and didn't x-ray the dog. My first thoughts were, what a waste of a veterinary degree and how awful to leave an animal in pain because of an ideology. I had already euthanised the dog of course.

Up until this point I had been fairly ignorant of the use of CAVM by veterinarians and wanted to see if there was anything I could do about it. I was disturbed by the animal health and welfare impacts and the ethics of using ineffective and implausible 'treatments'. After all, whilst some pet owners and a few veterinarians may believe in CAVM, I was pretty sure that 'Fluffy' wouldn't and would 'choose' a treatment that worked, especially for pain relief, rather than be subject to needless needling. (Stephens 2018)

Serendipitously the Australian Veterinary Association was holding its annual conference in Hobart, Tasmania, the next year (2007) and one of the guest speakers was veterinarian David Ramey. David had already co-authored a book with the philosopher Bernie Rollin on CAVM. I had to go, and I was inspired by David to jump on the anti-CAVM bandwagon.

There is plenty of CAVM to choose from – homeopathy, Bach flower remedies, acupuncture, herbal medicine, reiki, crystal healing, spiritual healing, chiropractic, animal reflexology, the list goes on. Each has its own jargon, but many have in common a belief in 'vitalism'. This is the qi of the acupuncturist, vital force of the homeopath, and the innate intelligence of the chiropractor. Oddly, practitioners of one aspect of CAVM will often embrace other aspects of CAVM even though they appear contradictory. Homeopathy seems to be on the list of modalities of a surprising number of CAVM practices in Australia. It seems to me that you really have to believe in magic to think that homeopathy is a valid 'therapy'.

There are a number of excellent books and resources to educate veterinarians on CAVM, such as David W. Ramey and Bernard E. Rollin's *Complementary and Alternative Veterinary Medicine Considered*, Niall Taylor and Alex Gough's *No Way to Treat a Friend*, Brennen McKenzie's *Placebos for Pets*, the SkeptVet, and a journal article by Manuel Magalhaes Sant'Ana 2019.

14.2 COMPLEMENTARY AND ALTERNATIVE VETERINARY MEDICINE (CAVM): WHERE IS THE EVIDENCE FOR INCREASING DEMAND?

Practitioners of complementary and alternative veterinary medicine (CAVM) state that there is an increasing demand for their services and there is certainly a growing band of CAVM practitioners here in Australia, but I wonder if it's true about increasing demand. I'm rarely asked by my clientele about CAVM and requests for histories to be sent to CAVM practitioners are non-existent, which is interesting as my practice is in an inner-city area with a human alternative/wellness/naturopath/chiropractor/acupuncturist on virtually every corner.

An analysis of the bibliometric outputs of non-conventional therapies (NCT)/CAVM revealed an increase in NCT terms over the last 20 years. A substantial increase in studies refers mainly to plant extracts, medicinal plants, and essential oils with references to Traditional Chinese Medicine and herbal medicine also increasing but at low numbers. References to acupuncture decreased and there were scarce references to homeopathy, electroacupuncture, chiropractic, and osteopathy (Domingues et al. 2022).

These findings support a survey in Sweden by Sohlberg et al. (2021) who found the use of CAVM uncommon with newer graduates more likely to use it than older graduates and the most frequently used methods included massage, stretching, and acupressure. The authors of the study noted that whilst CAVM use is uncommon, there needs to be a scientific assessment of safety and effectiveness.

By comparison, a survey of German veterinary practitioners by Stanossek and Wehrend (2022) found that there was an increasing demand for naturopathy and complementary medicine over the past 5 years. Of the veterinarians, 57.9% stated there was an increasing demand and 28.5% stated a stable demand. It was also found that users of veterinary naturopathy and complementary medicine tend to be older, female, and self-employed. A majority of veterinarians polled (85.4%) used veterinary naturopathy and complementary treatment options in their practical work with homeopathy the most commonly used treatment.

The Animal Medicines Australia's Pets in Australia 2022 survey noted that Australian pet owners spent on average $65 on alternative healthcare treatments for dogs and $7 for cats in 2022, compared to 2019 where pet owners spent an average of $57 for dogs and $44 for cats. Certainly, no evidence of increased demand here.

According to a statement from Pet Industry News 2023 (petnews.com.au), 'people are demanding holistic alternatives to what traditional vets are prescribing to support the health and wellbeing of their animals'. They quote animal naturopath Ruth Hatten, who states that 'holistic therapies honour animals with reference to their evolutionary history, their natural state. They reduce and remove the negative effects of toxins and optimise health' and that vets 'have a heavy reliance on artificial products, drugs, pharmaceuticals and processed prescription foods, which for chronic health issues can do more harm than good'. 'Evidence is subjective', argues Hatten. 'Anecdotal evidence is science and there is plenty of that in natural medicine because ancient cultures have been using it for centuries and still stand by those medicines because they work'.

This is of course an excellent example of the thinking behind the use of complementary and alternative 'therapies' and whilst one could dismiss this as spoken by a non-veterinarian, veterinarians who practise CAVM are prone to make the same claims, especially in regard to 'ancient cultures'.

Veterinarians who engage in CAVM are easy to find in Australia, and there are ample educational opportunities. IVAS, the International Veterinary Acupuncture Society, is the leading international provider for acupuncture, and the College of Integrative Veterinary Therapies (CiVT) runs an IVAS certification in Veterinary Chinese medicine as well as offering a graduate diploma of veterinary acupuncture (civedu.org). In Western Australia there is a Veterinary Acupuncture College (vetacupcollege.com.au).

Australian Holistic Veterinarians (ahvets.com.au), at the time of writing, lists 48 veterinarians, with the vast majority acupuncturists and most with homeopathy as well. A few advertise 'therapies' I've never heard of such as 'intuitive counselling' and 'biomechanical medicine' and 'radionics', and run the full gamut of CAVM from osteopathy to Bach flowers and Bowen massage. Traditional Chinese Medicine (TCM) looms large and so does titre testing, of course. Australian holistic veterinarians stated aim is to foster the use of CAVM in a professional and caring manner in order to benefit the health of animals and to render a positive image of holistic care in the general community.

The Australian Veterinary Acupuncture Group (AVAG), a special interest group of the Australian Veterinary Association (AVA), at the time of writing, has a membership of 73 and lists 35 veterinarians Australia wide who carry out acupuncture. Some AVAG members undertake other alternative modalities such as homeopathy and chiropractic. The AVA also has an Integrative Veterinarians Australia (IVA) Special Interest Group with a membership of 48 at the time of writing and a stated aim to foster the use of integrative therapies in a professional manner in order to benefit the health of animals. Their list of integrative therapies include acupuncture, chiropractic, and traditional Chinese herbal medicine.

No doubt veterinarians who engage in CAVM belong to a number of these organisations, so the actual number of veterinarians engaged in CAVM in Australia is small considering there are around 15,000 practising veterinarians nationwide, of which only 5,400 belong to the AVA. Despite this CAVM practitioners appear to exert a disproportionate influence and manage to find spots at various veterinary conferences.

Presentations are, not surprisingly, predominantly attended by CAVM practitioners and one on moxibustion a few years ago raised eyebrows and concerns over the animal welfare impacts of 'burning' animals. IVA in 2024 had a webinar on TCM 'tongue diagnosis' in dogs. I found it difficult to visualise this method of diagnosis and assumed that it would depend on avoiding sharp teeth.

We may think that pet owners are disillusioned with everyday veterinary care and a lack of scientific literacy has propelled them into the 'warm embrace' of 'alternatives'. There's actually not a great deal of evidence, despite what CAVM practitioners state, that owners are seeking CAVM in increasing numbers. Rather, there is evidence that the demand is driven by veterinarians incorporating CAVM into their practices supported by and given credibility by professional veterinary associations, educational bodies, and veterinary pain guidelines and even, unfortunately, promoted to increase practice income.

14.3 WHERE IS THE EVIDENCE? WHAT IS THE POINT OF NEEDLESS NEEDLING?

According to AVAG, acupuncture is a branch of traditional Chinese medicine which 'has the ability to alter various physiological body functions' and is 'probably one of the oldest forms of human and veterinary medicine in the world' and 'has been used to treat horses, pigs and cows in China for well over 3000 years'. A claim, similar to that of the animal naturopath Ruth Hatten.

Further to this, the AVAG website states, 'Traditional Chinese Medicine aims to rebalance the whole body and promote healing and a sense of wellbeing throughout. It can relieve muscle tension, improve blood and lymphatic circulation, stimulate nerve regeneration, the immune systems and endocrine functions . . . it stimulates many pathways in the body always bringing the body back to a state of balance and homeostasis'. Furthermore, 'MRI studies have shown . . . most acupuncture points have a regulating effect on the amygdala thereby reducing the body's stress levels and reestablishing the normal diurnal rhythms of the body', and 'acupuncture points to treat eye problems will stimulate the optic section of the brain'. 'Many other conditions also respond to acupuncture e.g. diseases of the skin . . . and behavioural problems'.

This single MRI study which is mentioned but not referenced on the AVAG website makes big claims which practitioners of CAVM tend to do; however, the study is on humans, not animals, so it is quite irrelevant and even more so since it has recently been found that a placebo cream had a similar effect on brain MRI studies.

AVAG further states, 'Traditional Chinese Veterinary Medicine is another approach to understanding medicine. It has evolved over thousands of years from simple observations of nature and the patterns of disease to the current sophisticated and elegant paradigm for treating disease that it is today'.

Acupuncture has been variously described as a theatrical placebo (Colquhoun & Novella 2013), astrology with needles (Kavoussi 2009), and modern bloodletting (Novella 2010). Not just needles but other techniques such as bee venom acupuncture, ozone acupuncture, moxibustion, and others. These are presented to pet owners as accepted and established veterinary therapies, adversely affecting animal welfare, and posing a serious reputational risk to the profession.

Current evidence does not support that acupuncture, chiropractic, homeopathy, reiki, or aromatherapy are effective, yet people still use them even if it is pointed out that they are implausible and ineffective. This is for various reasons, but it seems that alternative therapies suit their interests in environmentalism and spirituality for example. They assume that the treatments are without risk and are 'natural', which is not true, of course, as the use of alternative therapies can increase the risk of death due to delays in proper treatments, and some of the so-called natural treatments can be toxic. Chiropractic manipulation may lead to unintended injuries.

In the human field, there are thousands of papers on acupuncture and an abundance of controversy, claims, and counterclaims. Since 2013 there have been 434 systematic reviews and a systematic review of systematic reviews (Allen et al. 2022). It was found that acupuncture 'rated only a minority of high or moderate certainty evidence, and most of these were about comparisons with sham treatment or had conclusions of no benefit of acupuncture. Conclusions with moderate or high-certainty evidence that acupuncture is superior to other active therapies were rare'.

Despite the 'humanisation' of pets, there is no doubt that the mind of the human is not that of the dog, and we know that cognitive behaviour therapy and the placebo effect can be powerful tools in treating chronic pain in humans. Not so for the family pet, and there is no evidence for the use of acupuncture in animals (Magalhães-Sant'Ana 2019), and the use of acupuncture for pain relief in animals could be considered not only unethical but cruel.

Furthermore, research studies mentioning acupuncture, electro-acupuncture, chiropractic, and homeopathy have been found to be relatively scarce and remained so for some time, supporting the assertion that there is not an increased interest and certainly no further scientific research to support claims of efficacy (Domingues et al. 2022).

14.4 CAVM AND ANIMAL HEALTH AND WELFARE

CAVM raises important legal and ethical issues for the veterinarian which are discussed in more detail in this book in the chapter 'Should complementary and alternative medicine be considered malpractice? An ethical reflection', by Manuel Magalhães Sant'Ana.

The use of ineffective therapies on animals is an ethical and animal welfare issue. Surely it is unethical to offer and charge for ineffective 'therapies' and poor animal welfare to subject an animal to a worthless 'therapy'. The human owner can look for other options if a 'treatment' doesn't work for themselves, not so the unwell, hapless pet at the hands of ill-informed owners and CAVM practitioners. Furthermore, there is a concern that the use of CAVM is associated with anti-vaccination sentiments and the raw feeding movement, both of which could negatively impact on animal health and welfare.

14.5 DONKEYS, BEARS & PANGOLINS

Veterinarians who have as their first priority the health and welfare of animals and who act as advocates for them should be the first professionals to shun, and certainly not embrace, any aspect of alternative medicine associated the use of animal parts and animal welfare concerns, from bear biling to the use of rhino horns, from the decimation of the pangolin and ejiao made out of donkey skins.

Demand for bear bile has outstripped supply since a paper in *Nature* noted that ursodeoxycholic acid (UDCA) derived from bear bile could have an important role in the management of COVID-19. Although UDCA can be synthesised from chemical ingredients, bear bile is still a major source.

According to an editorial (Nature 2017), new draft guidelines would do away with clinical testing requirements for TCMs made according to classical recipes. As the editorial points out the world needs more rigorous trials of herbal remedies and 'hundreds of years of use in clinics that don't standardise or analyse the clinical data are no match for blinded controlled studies'.

The global TCM market size was worth USD 247.22 billion in 2024 and projected to reach USD 449.69 by 2033 (Business Research Insights 2025).

Pleasingly, there are indications that there is a move away from the use of threatened species in TCM. Because of concerns around the use of animals in TCM, a number of concerned TCM practitioners launched the Coalition for Wildlife

Protection in TCM in April 2024 (Coalition for Wildlife Protection in TCM 2024) as a new initiative to preserve global biodiversity by abstaining from the use of endangered species in healing practices. This recognises the positive role that many influential TCM practitioners have played in protecting wildlife over the past 30 years.

Despite these efforts and newer laws, shops in various Asian countries continue to illegally sell pangolin scales, rhino horn and tiger bone, driven by the illegal trade and commercial interests. Pangolins, for example, continue to be at risk from illegal poaching and trafficking with at least 15 tonnes of pangolin seized globally in 2024, an increase from 2023 (Environmental Investigation Agency 2025).

TCM is one of the drivers for the illegal trade in wildlife, not just animals but plants as well with impacts on biodiversity (Mozer & Prost 2023).

In 2019 the WHO formally recognised TCM, and this created a backlash and a concern that the increased interest in TCM was responsible for the surge in illegal wildlife trafficking. The London based Environmental Investigation Agency (EIA) claims that the expansion of TCM in many African countries risks fuelling the illegal wildlife trade and threatens the future of some of the world's most endangered species. 'The growth of the TCM market coupled with the perception of Africa as a potential source of TCM ingredients is a prescription for disaster for some endangered animal species such as leopards, pangolins and rhinos'.

There has been a dramatic increase in the commercial interest in wildlife related products over the last 50 years including threatened and illegally traded species as evidenced by the above average growth of patent-filing. This suggests future unsustainable use of wildlife, such as pangolins and even the farming of rhinoceros. Of particular concern is the fact that no correlation was found between regulations that banned or restricted the wild animal trade and changes in patent-filing behaviour with CITES listing, bans and restrictions even leading to increased patenting rates (Hinsley et al. 2023).

To quote Taylor and Gough (2017), 'TCM relies on a non-scientific philosophy of ill health, promoted for political reasons by Mao. Its diagnostic methods are unsafe, its evidence base is poor, there are significant risks of toxins both from the medicines used and contaminants, and there are major ecological and welfare issues involved in the production of TCM'.

14.6 THE PET WELLNESS INDUSTRY

Whilst the extent of the use of CAVM can be difficult to define in Australia the pet supplement and pet 'wellness' market appears to be booming and supplement manufacturers are doing very nicely with more than half of Australian pet owners reporting that they give supplements to their pets. (Animal Medicines Australia survey 2022). This market has been steadily growing since 2018.

It is estimated that the global pet supplement market was worth a staggering AUD $2.8 billion in 2022 and estimated to grow to AUD $4.6 billion by 2030 with multivitamin chews, fish oil supplements, and products for soothing stress and anxiety. The Australian animal wellness industry also includes items such as pet-friendly yoga classes.

Post-COVID-19, supplements for stress reduction are anticipated to be a huge market as pets are left alone when their owners returned to work. Australia's multibillion-dollar pet supply industry was growing at around 4% annually pre-COVID-19 but doubled between 2020 and 2021. However, much of the demand comes from increasing pet ownership in the Asian market and not Australian cattle dogs named Bluey.

Products on the shelves in Australia only need to be safe and don't need to be proven efficacious and there is no regulation around pet supplements or pet food. I asked one of the prominent supplement makers to provide evidence of efficacy, which elicited a surprising response – an admission of no evidence but an assurance that research will be carried out in future. I doubt this will happen as there would be little point in proving efficacy for a product which is, in any case, already a best seller.

At a time when there is a concern around climate change and sustainability and the environmental impacts of pet ownership, the wasteful production of useless products to satisfy 'pet parents' must surely merit debate.

14.7 COUNTERACTING CAVM

Unfortunately, as I have found over many years, initiating change is difficult and those veterinarians who practise CAVM are not so easily going to change their spots. Hopefully, instead, especially for students and new veterinary graduates they can be steered towards the use of evidence-based medicine and importantly encouraged to question what they do from a scientific viewpoint and to develop a healthy scepticism.

It can be difficult to counteract the use of CAVM when the 2022 World Small Animal Veterinary Association (WSAVA) guidelines for the recognition, assessment, and treatment of pain endorse acupuncture, contrary to the stated WSAVA aim of 'medical and ethical duty to mitigate suffering from pain to the best of our ability'.

The WSAVA pain guidelines state for acupuncture that 'evidence is limited in veterinary medicine' whilst contradicting this by stating that 'studies generally indicate analgesic effects of acupuncture for the management of acute and chronic pain in dogs and cats i.e. ovariohysterectomy, OA, hemilaminectomy and other neurological and musculoskeletal diseases'. 'Acupuncture has been shown to reduce opioid requirements and is increasingly being suggested as an alternative to opioid based treatments in chronic pain'.

The suggestion of limited evidence is lost here and the reader may mistakenly believe that the WSAVA wholeheartedly endorses acupuncture for pain relief. It certainly does in a statement underneath an item on the WSAVA guidelines for neuropathic pain. 'Acupuncture and medical massage. These should be included in the analgesic regimen as soon as possible. Neuropathic pain is difficult to manage with pharmaceutical agents alone, therefore the use of acupuncture and other integrative techniques should be included as adjuncts to a multimodal pharmaceutical regimen'.

The guidelines also state that 'in human medicine acupuncture as a treatment for various forms of acute and chronic pain has risen in esteem', which perpetuates the idea of acupuncture as a valid therapy for humans as well as animals.

The challenge is for veterinarians to counteract pseudoscience and stop giving CAVM further credibility. We know that cognitive biases run deep and changing behaviours can be extremely difficult. As with any behaviour change, you need enablement and restrictions. What needs to happen is for the profession and regulators to make it more difficult for CAVM vets to operate and ensure there is no further promotion.

Whilst quackery and pseudoscience have been around for a long time it is clear that we are living at a time of a distrust of science where opinion-based medicine threatens to overwhelm evidence-based medicine. Anyone can tweet or do a podcast and of great concern to those of us on the frontline of preventative care of animals, social media advertising of anti-vaccine myths and uninformed people writing about 'overloading the immune system' doesn't help. I'm concerned that the promotion of titre testing by 'alternative' practitioners, for example, could lead to outbreaks of diseases such as distemper and parvovirus because pet owners fail to follow up vaccinations later, especially if costs become an issue.

Finally, as Taylor and Gough (2017) eloquently state 'CAVM is an unnecessary embellishment, a lucrative exercise in smoke and mirrors. While on occasion appearing to offer hope and consolation to owners, these are mere illusions; CAVM brings no benefit to the individual animal, its net effect is harmful, and it has no place in the treatment of animals'.

REFERENCES

Allen J, Mak S, Begashaw M, et al. Use of acupuncture for adult health conditions, 2013 to 2021: a systematic review. *JAMA Netw Open*. 2022;5(11). Available at: https://pubmed.ncbi.nim.gov/3646820/.

Business Research Insights. Traditional Chinese Medicine (TCM) Market Size, Share, Growth, and Industry Analysis by Type (Acupuncture, Chinese Herbal Medicine, Cupping, Tui Na, Others), by Application (Healthcare, Treatment), Regional Insights and Forecast From 2025 To 2033. Last Updated: 31 March 2025. Base Year: 2024. Available from: https://www.businessresearchinsights.com/market-reports/traditional-chinese-medicine-tcm-market-109110.

Coalition for Wildlife Protection in TCM. April 2024. Available from: https://www.wildlife-protectionintcm.com/pressrelease2024/.

Colquhoun D, Novella SP. Acupuncture is theatrical placebo. *Anesth Analg*. 2013;116(6):1360. Available from: https://doi.org/10.1213/ANE.0b013e31828f2d5e.

Domingues K, Franco NH, Rodrigues I, et al. Bibliometric trend analysis of non-conventional (alternative) therapies in veterinary research. *Vet Q*. 2022;42(1):192–198.

Environmental Investigation Agency. 2025. Available from: https://eia.org/blog/highlighting-eias-illegal-trade-concerns-for-wildlife-and-trees-at-cites-standing-committee/

Hinsley A, Challender D, Masters S, et al. Early-warning of trends in commercial wildlife trade through novel machine-learning analysis of patent filing. *Natureportfolio* 2023 Sept 26;15.

Kavoussi B. Acupuncture is astrology with needles. *Science-Based Medicine* [Internet]. 2009 Aug 3. Available from: https://sciencebasedmedicine.org/astrology-with-needles/.

Magalhães-Sant'Ana M. The emperor's new clothes: an epistemological critique of traditional Chinese veterinary acupuncture. *Animals*. 2019;9:168. Available from: https://doi.org/10.3390/ani9040168.

McKenzie B. *Placebos for pets? The truth about alternative medicine in animals*. Ockham Publishing; 2019.

Mozer A & Prost S. *An introduction to illegal wildlife trade and its effects on biodiversity and society, Forensic Science International: Animals and Environments*, Volume 3, 2023. Available from: https://www.sciencedirect.com/science/article/pii/S2666937423000021.

Nature, Editorial. *Traditional Chinese medicine needs proper scrutiny* [Internet]. 2017 Nov 29. Available from: https://www.nature.com/articles/d41586-017-07650-6.

Novella SP. Acupuncture and modern bloodletting. *Science-Based Medicine* [Internet]. 2010 Jul 7. Available from: https://sciencebasedmedicine.org/acupuncture-and-modern-bloodletting/.

Ramey DW, Rollin BE. *Complementary and alternative veterinary medicine considered*. Wiley and Sons; 2005.

Sohlberg L, Bergh A, Sternberg-Lewerin S. A questionaire study on the use of complementary and alternative veterinary medicine for dogs in Sweden. *Vet Sci*. 2021 Dec 8;12:331.

Stanossek I, Wehrend A. Application of veterinary naturopathy and complementary medicine in small animal medicine: a survey among German veterinary practitioners. *PLoS One*. 2022;17(2):e0264022. https://doi.org/10.1371/journal.pone.0264022.

Stephens T. What is the point of veterinary acupuncture? *Australasian Science*. 2018 May–Jun.

Taylor N, Gough A. *No way to treat a friend: lifting the lid on complementary and alternative veterinary medicine*. 1st ed. Portland: 5M Publishing; 2017.

15 Should Complementary and Alternative Veterinary Medicine be Considered Malpractice?
An Ethical–Legal Analysis

*Manuel Magalhães Sant'Ana
and Alexandre Azevedo*

15.1 BACKGROUND

In 2018, I (MM-S) was involved in a debate on the use of traditional Chinese medicine (TCM) with a so-called 'integrative' veterinary practitioner. This veterinarian claimed publicly that animal acupuncture was a thousand-year-old practice, and that hip dysplasia was caused by Jing deficiency. Faced with such claims, I presented an evidence-based view of TCM in a series of press articles and on social media, aiming to steer away from folklore. Later, during a veterinary conference, I used analogical reasoning to argue that acupuncture and TCM were based on similar principles as humoral medicine (Magalhães-Sant'Ana 2019) and were not proven more valid than homeopathy, Bach flower remedies, reiki, or predestination. This stance didn't sit well with the alternative vets in the audience. Instead of triggering debate focusing on scientific evidence, I was accused of defaming traditional Chinese veterinary therapists and things escalated quickly. The situation became so tense that I had to be escorted out of the room. Subsequently, those accusations materialised into a defamation claim – a strategy frequently used by alternative therapists to silence their critics (Jarry 2019) – of which I was acquitted (Loeb 2020).

This story illustrates how the field of complementary and alternative medicines (CAM) is rife with legal and ethical issues. This time, the defendant was the conventional vet, but should veterinarians employing ineffective or potentially harmful therapies be held accountable? Shouldn't CAM be held to the same standards as conventional therapies to be safely administered, prescribed, or referred? More specifically, should the use, prescription, or referral of unproven or ineffective veterinary therapies be considered malpractice? In this chapter we will delve into the legal and ethical dimensions of complementary and alternative veterinary medicines (CAVM), including recommendations for the future.

15.2 ALTERNATIVE MEDICINE – WHAT'S IN A NAME?

Several hurdles arise when dealing with CAM – or in the words of Edzar Ernst, SCAM, the so-called alternative medicines (Ernst 2018), particularly in the veterinary field, namely, the lack of clear definitions and lack of harmonisation in terms of regulation. The term 'alternative medicine' is 'broadly used in the Western world to refer to a group of therapeutic systems and interventions that exist largely outside of the established, conventional healthcare system' (Chatfield 2015). In humans, CAM have been categorised into distinct domains based on their underlying principles and therapeutic approaches, namely, biologically based practices, energy therapies, manipulative and body-based methods, and mind-body medicine (Chow et al. 2023). It is not possible to make an exhaustive list of all CAM used in animals, but these include homeopathy, acupuncture, chiropractic, herbal medicine, aromatherapy, low-level laser therapy, prolotherapy, and orthomolecular therapy, to name but a few (McKenzie 2019).

In Table 15.1, we categorize complementary and alternative veterinary medicines (CAVM) into four domains: energy therapies (which aim to achieve healing

TABLE 15.1
Four Domains of Complementary and Alternative Veterinary Medicines

Energy therapies	Natural therapies	Manual and physical therapies	Post-modern therapies
Reiki and energy healing	Herbal medicine	Osteopathy	Ozone therapy
Pranic healing	Cannabinoids	Chiropractic	Prolotherapy
Magnetic field therapy	Nutritional therapy	Massage	Orthomolecular medicine
Bach flower remedies	Naturopathy	Reflexology	Low-level laser therapy
Homeopathy	Aromatherapy	Tai-chi-xuan	Homotoxicology
Acupuncture and acupressure	Traditional Chinese medicine	Yoga	Pulsed electromagnetic field therapy

Note: The four domains of CAVM are energy therapies (healing is achieved by regulating the flow of a vital energy or force), natural therapies (healing is based on ingredients found in nature), manual and physical therapies (healing through exercise and manipulative interventions), and post-modern therapies (novel therapies based on the combination and reshaping of concepts or references from the past).

by regulating the flow of a vital energy or force), natural therapies (where healing is based on ingredients found in nature), manual and physical therapies (which use exercise and manipulative interventions), and post-modern therapies (which integrate and reinterpret past concepts into novel approaches). While not an exhaustive classification, this division serves to illustrate the broad diversity within CAVM practices.

The main problem with the suggested classification is that it does not account for the fact that therapies within the same domain may have very little in common and can be based on different (and even opposing) philosophical foundations. In effect, CA(V)M are more easily defined for what they are not than for what they are (Ernst et al. 2004), and others have preferred to use the term non-conventional therapies (NCTs) to refer to therapies based on unscientific principles and/or lacking reliable scientific evidence of effectiveness (Domingues et al. 2022). A non-conventional therapy is considered complementary or alternative, provided it is used together or in place of conventional medicine, respectively.

As with every complex topic, there are grey areas in these definitions. Acupuncture, for example, can be divided into the so-called Western acupuncture, arguably based on modern scientific principles, and traditional acupuncture, based on the principles of traditional Chinese medicine. Is the former as much of an alternative therapy as the latter? And consider what is one of the most popular alternative therapies of the moment: cannabinoids. As their pharmacokinetic mechanism is unravelled, clinical research points towards their usefulness in some pathologies, despite the low quality evidence (Morrow & Belshaw 2022). Does this mean that cannabinoids are conventional after all? Finally, some therapies are deemed conventional because they are based on plausible pathophysiological mechanisms but have been used for decades despite little to no evidence of effect. That is arguably the case of alpha-amylase to treat oedema, chondroprotectors to control osteoarthritis, or antihistamines to treat symptoms of allergic diseases. Should they be considered alternative therapies or at least judged in the same way as these?

15.3 REGULATORY APPROACHES TO CAVM

David Ramey (2003) identifies three challenges emerging from the regulation of CAVM: defining what constitutes acceptable standard of care, whether non-veterinarians should be allowed to apply them, and the view that CAVM are not acts of veterinary medicine and therefore should not be regulated. The lack of clear definitions constitutes an additional challenge to establishing consistent regulations of CAVM. In Europe, for example, there is no harmonised regulatory framework for CAVM and veterinarians in different countries seem to rely more upon certain alternative therapies for cultural and geographic reasons rather than scientific reasons. In the UK, the debate regarding alternative therapies in veterinary practice has been mostly dominated by homeopathy (Limb & Waters 2018; Waters 2018; Loeb 2018), whereas in Portugal the use of homeopathy seems marginal and traditional Chinese medicine takes the main stage with acupuncture in particular being viewed by a large proportion of the veterinary community as a respected practice,[1] as if it was conceptually, historically, and scientifically validated (Magalhães-Sant'Ana 2019).

The fundamental regulatory dilemma concerns the conflict between the necessity to consider CAVM as acts of veterinary medicine in order to exercise control over their use, and the danger of, in doing so, legitimising procedures that have no scientific validity (Schommer 2012). Finding a balance between encouraging innovation and protecting animals from ineffective, or even fraudulent, practices becomes a delicate ethical conundrum. As shown in Figure 15.1, veterinary therapies (either conventional or non-conventional) can be arranged in an evidence-based continuum, ranging from those for which no evidence is available and are based on belief and tradition to those for which effectiveness has been demonstrated by systematic reviews and meta-analyses. Restrictive regulations of CAVM may limit the availability of prospective therapies, denying animals access to practices that may have a therapeutic effect, whereas a more lenient regulatory approach may expose animals and their owners to unproven or potentially harmful practices. The challenge lies in determining where to draw the line between what should be considered an acceptable or unacceptable standard of care.

Regulatory bodies in various jurisdictions have approached the regulation of CAVM differently, and their positions have evolved over time (Ramey 2003). For example, in their 2009 Position Statement, the College of Veterinarians of Ontario (CVO) decided to integrate complementary and alternative therapies into mainstream veterinary practice, considering that they could only be performed by veterinarians or under their supervision or delegation (CVO 2009). This position, however, was recently changed to a more permissive approach, and the CVO no longer considers what they now call non-conventional therapies as acts of veterinary medicine based on the demand of the public for such therapies and their inability to retain control over their practice (CVO 2021). The opposite position was taken by the Portuguese Order of Veterinary Surgeons (Ordem dos Médicos Veterinários) in 2019, when they attempted to include acupuncture in the Veterinary Act, which was at the time submitted to the Portuguese Parliament. The Parliament passed a preliminary version of the legislation, but the final version of the Veterinary Act was never enacted.

At least two arguments can be drawn against the inclusion of CAM as veterinary acts, namely, corporatism and consumerism. When restricting CAM to veterinary professionals, veterinary regulatory bodies can be accused of corporatism

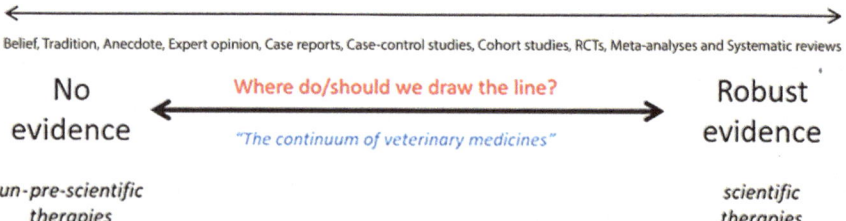

FIGURE 15.1 The continuum of veterinary medicines in terms of evidence and the challenge of where to draw the line between what is deemed acceptable standard of care.

Complementary and Alternative Veterinary Medicine 141

for restricting their use to members of the veterinary profession while failing to demonstrate that public health and animal welfare are protected by having non-veterinarians prevented from practising such therapies. That is arguably the case for therapies that involve minimal risk, such as massage or acupressure. Moreover, the prevalence of CAM is notably higher in affluent societies, thus suggesting that their inclusion in veterinary care is driven by consumerism rather than necessity (Ernst et al. 2004). This reflects the increasing commodification of veterinary services, especially the pet care industry, fuelled by consumer demand for therapies marketed as natural and holistic, none of which necessarily align with evidence-based veterinary medicine. Schommer (2012) describes how the futile attempt of the American Veterinary Medical Association (AVMA) to retain control over the use of CAVM led to the inclusion of 'animal communication' as a veterinary act and how AVMA failed to secure *Aesculapian authority* (Rollin 2002) in the process.

15.4 CAVM AND PROFESSIONAL MALPRACTICE

Should CAVM be considered malpractice? And is there a duty for the veterinary profession to protect animals and the public from CAVM? These questions require an ethical reflection, drawing on examples from both human and veterinary medicine. In human medicine, CAM have been considered harmful for at least three reasons: for causing direct harm to patients (Leon-Sanchez et al. 2007), for working like a placebo and having no real therapeutic effect (Beedie et al. 2018), and for delaying or replacing the use of more effective conventional therapies (Johnson et al. 2018). Weighing the harm of CAVM is challenging because adverse effects in veterinary practice are underreported (De Briyne et al. 2017), and there is no indication whether alternative veterinary therapists are any more likely to be prosecuted than conventional practitioners.

In the UK, the Royal College of Veterinary Surgeons Disciplinary Committee had one case in October 2016 of a veterinary surgeon considered guilty of disgraceful conduct for promoting on his professional website misleading therapeutic claims regarding such therapies as Aerobic Oxygen ('supports brain and nerve function including memory, headaches, Alzheimer's, senile dementia, Parkinson's'), Quinton Marine Plasma ('excellent for allergies and sinusitis'), Russian Healing Blanket ('enables the body to correct the overall homeostasis of the organism'), and e-Lybra Bio-Resonance Technology ('reveals weaknesses in the immune system and strengthens it to increase resistance to disease'). The hearing was adjourned indefinitely after the defendant took measures to amend the information on his website in compliance with professional standards (Woodmansey 2016).

In Portugal, the Order of Veterinary Surgeons has convicted three alternative veterinary therapists of disciplinary offenses within the last six years (2018–2023): one in 2022 for practising pranic healing as an act of veterinary medicine and two in 2018 for publicly defending anti-vaccination policies (and consequently putting at risk public health and bringing the veterinary profession into disrepute). The first defendant was sentenced to pay a fine of three Social Support Index (the equivalent to two minimum wages), whereas regarding the *anti-vax* vets, one was sentenced to pay a fine of one Social Support Index, and the other was reprimanded (Magalhães-Sant'Ana, personal communication). These represent a fraction (2.4%) of the total 127 convicted veterinarians within that time frame. Since the number of veterinarians practising alternative therapies is unknown, the prevalence of convictions among alternative vets cannot be computed or compared with prevalences in conventional practitioners.

At the heart of the ethical dilemma of CAVM lies a tension between the need to safeguard animal health and welfare and the recognition of the autonomy of pet owners seeking alternative therapies for their animals. Furthermore, the demand for alternative therapies for animals raises questions about informed consent. Should pet owners be free to explore alternative treatments for their animals, even if the scientific community remains sceptical about their efficacy? CAM are often portrayed as being natural, holistic, and non-invasive, with none of the side effects of the corresponding conventional therapies, which can convey a message of trust, efficacy, and non-maleficence. These assertions do not stem from scientific evidence, thus hindering autonomous choices and precluding genuine informed consent (Ernst et al. 2004).

While the autonomy of the client to choose any therapeutic option for his or her animal should be respected, even if ineffective, several circumstances can deem situations when a veterinarian might administer, prescribe, or refer CAM unethical (although a non-veterinary practitioner might not be liable in any of these circumstances). The first is when CAM are not clearly differentiated from acts of veterinary medicine and are conferred unfounded credibility by being proposed by a veterinarian, who (as in the misconduct cases described earlier) is expected by society to provide a suitable standard of care. The second is when clients are not made fully aware of the uncertainty regarding the efficacy of CAM, or when CAM are presented as scientifically proven, in which cases the consent of the client is not informed. Interestingly, it is easy to find veterinary clinics touting the benefits of acupuncture in treating just about everything, including cancer, without regulators condemning this information as being misleading, in the same way as aerobic oxygen or pranic healing. The third is when CAM are unsafe, present more risks than benefits, or will reduce the likelihood of using more effective therapies. That is arguably the case of chiropractic, particularly when associated with anti-scientific claims (McKenzie 2019).

The use of CAM raises an additional concern of malpractice liability when patients are referred to these therapies by a licensed medical or veterinary practitioner (Studdert et al. 1998). Cohen and Eisenberg (2002) explore this concern in the case of human medicine, which is founded on the referral to a therapy that is below the standards of care for the medical profession, in terms of efficacy and safety. However, when being applied by a non-medical or non-veterinary practitioner, no reference standards of care exist, which leads to the pressing need to either establish such standards for specific CAM (Raposo 2019) or include them in regulations defining standards of care for conventional therapies. Ideally, to be prescribed by veterinarians, CAM need to be held to the same standards as any other conventional therapy, in terms of evidence of efficacy and safety, to avoid conferring undue credibility. However, this is arguably unrealistic for most alternative therapies, as a series of systematic reviews have shown (cf. Bergh et al. 2021). Taking acupuncture as a case example, researchers from China Agricultural University have disputed my claims that there is no historical support for animal acupuncture, in an attempt to perpetuate the myth of the antiquity of veterinary acupuncture (Hu & Liu 2020), but no attempt was made to challenge the claims that animal acupuncture is clinically ineffective or that it works as a placebo (Magalhães-Sant'Ana 2020).

In the current paradigm, or in the absence of specific regulations, any veterinarian administering, prescribing, or referring CAVM must exercise absolute transparency to clients. As veterinarians, we have a professional obligation to refrain from portraying CAVM as veterinary acts, or as proven and effective therapies unless reasonable scientific evidence is available. Erroneously portraying CAVM as scientifically proven or effective is unethical, violates informed consent, and should be considered malpractice.

15.5 RECOMMENDATIONS

The field of complementary and alternative veterinary medicines (CAVM) is rife with legal and ethical issues. At the heart of these issues lies a tension between the need to safeguard animal welfare and the recognition of the autonomy of pet owners seeking alternative therapies for their animals. Stricter regulations may limit the availability of future therapies, denying animals access to practices that may have a therapeutic effect, whereas a more lenient regulatory approach may expose animals and their owners to unscrupulous practitioners. Veterinarians are both ethically and legally bound to society by rules of professional conduct to provide the best possible standard of care, considering current scientific knowledge. While individual veterinarians cannot be prevented from prescribing, applying, or referring CAVM, they are required to exercise transparency regarding the scientific evidence of efficacy of CAVM and their risks and side effects, and refrain from referring to these therapies as acts of veterinary medicine. A regulatory framework is needed that acknowledges the heterogenicity of alternative therapies, respects the autonomy of owners, and fulfils the duty to protect the welfare of animals under veterinary care.

15.6 DISCLOSURE STATEMENT

At the time of writing, MM-S was a member of the Disciplinary Council of the Portuguese Order of Veterinary Surgeons and was directly involved in the disciplinary hearings concerning alternative veterinary therapists. MM-S would like to thank Fundação para a Ciência e a Tecnologia (FCT), I. P., Portugal, for funding the research projects *VETHICS 2022 – A structured approach to describing and addressing the ethical challenges of the veterinary profession in Portugal* (grant number: SFRH/BPD/117693/2016), co-funded by the European Social Fund (ESF), and *EviEdVet – Promoting education and training for evidence-based veterinary medicine* (ref: PTDC/CEDEDG/0187/2020), funded by national funds.

NOTE

1 These differences are reflected in the fact that in the UK we can find the British Association of Homeopathic Veterinary Surgeons (www.bahvs.com), whereas in Portugal there is no such organisation. Both countries have veterinary acupuncture organisations (the Association of British Veterinary Acupuncturists, www.abva.co.uk, and the Associação Portuguesa de Acupuntura Médico-Veterinária, www.apamv-assoc.pt).

REFERENCES

Beedie C, Whyte G, Lane AM, et al. 'Caution, this treatment is a placebo. It might work, but it might not': why emerging mechanistic evidence for placebo effects does not legitimise complementary and alternative medicines in sport. *Br J Sports Med.* 2018;52(13):817–818.

Bergh A, Lund I, Boström A, et al. A systematic review of complementary and alternative veterinary medicine: 'miscellaneous therapies'. *Animals (Basel).* 2021;11(12):3356.

Chatfield K. Alternative medicine. In: ten Have H, editor. *Encyclopedia of global bioethics.* Berlin: Springer International Publishing; 2015. p. 1–14.

Chow SL, Bozkurt B, Baker WL, et al. Complementary and alternative medicines in the management of heart failure: a scientific statement from the American Heart Association. *Circulation.* 2023;147(2):e4–e30.

Cohen MH, Eisenberg DM. Potential physician malpractice liability associated with complementary and integrative medical therapies. *Ann Intern Med.* 2002;136(8):596–603.

College of Veterinarians of Ontario (CVO). Position statement: the practice of complementary and alternative veterinary medicine. *Docplayer* [Internet]. 2009 Jun. Available from: https://docplayer.net/59540713-The-practice-of-complementary-and-alternative-veterinary-medicine.html.

College of Veterinarians of Ontario (CVO). Position statement on the use of non-conventional therapies in the practice of veterinary medicine. *CVO Standards* [Internet]. 2021 Jul. Available from: https://www.cvo.org/standards/use-of-non-conventional-therapies-in-the-practice-of-veterinary-medicine.

De Briyne N, Gopal R, Diesel G, et al. Veterinary pharmacovigilance in Europe: a survey of veterinary practitioners. *Vet Rec Open.* 2017;4(1):e000224.

Domingues K, Franco NH, Rodrigues I, et al. Bibliometric trend analysis of non-conventional (alternative) therapies in veterinary research. *Vet Q.* 2022;42(1):192–198.

Ernst E. *SCAM: so-called alternative medicine.* 1st ed. Exeter: Imprint Academic, Ltd.; 2018.

Ernst E, Cohen MH, Stone J. Ethical problems arising in evidence based complementary and alternative medicine. *J Med Ethics.* 2004;30(2):156–159.

Hu Y, Liu Z. 2020. Historical facts of acupuncture and traditional Chinese veterinary medicine – a letter to the editor re: Magalhães-Sant'Ana, M. *Animals* 2019;9:168. *Animals (Basel).* 2020;10(7):1196.

Jarry J. Censoring science communication by screaming defamation. *McGill Office for Science and Society Separating Sense from Nonsense* [Internet]. 2019 May 10. Available from: https://mcgill.ca/oss/article/general-science/censoring-science-communication-screaming-defamation.

Johnson SB, Park HS, Gross CP, et al. Use of alternative medicine for cancer and its impact on survival. *JNCI J Natl Cancer Inst.* 2018;110(1):121–124.

Leon-Sanchez A, Cuetter A, Ferrer G. Cervical spine manipulation: an alternative medical procedure with potentially fatal complications. *South Med J.* 2007;100(2):201–203.

Limb M, Waters A. Heating up: homeopathy debate turns 'nasty'. *Vet Rec.* 2018; 182(17):470–471.

Loeb J. Changing tack on complementary medicines. *Vet Rec.* 2018;183(4):110–111.

Loeb J. Veterinary ethicist sued by acupuncturist. *Vet Rec.* 2020;187(9):336–337.

Magalhães-Sant'Ana M. The emperor's new clothes – an epistemological critique of traditional Chinese veterinary acupuncture. *Animals (Basel).* 2019;9(4):168.

Magalhães-Sant'Ana M. Reply to the comment re: Magalhães-Sant'Ana, M. *Animals.* 2019;9:168. *Animals (Basel).* 2020;10(7):1197.

McKenzie B. *Placebos for pets? The truth about alternative medicine in animals.* 1st ed. Aberdeenshire: Ockham Publishing; 2019.

Morrow L, Belshaw Z. Is cannabidiol an effective supplementary treatment for reducing pain in dogs with osteoarthritis? *Vet Rec.* 2022;191(10):420–421.

Ramey DW. Regulatory aspects of complementary and alternative veterinary medicine. *J Am Vet Med Assoc.* 2003;222(12):1679–1682.

Raposo VL. Complementary and alternative medicine, medical liability and the proper standard of care. *Complement Ther Clin Pract.* 2019 May;35:183–188.

Rollin BE. The use and abuse of Aesculapian authority in veterinary medicine. *J Am Vet Med Assoc.* 2002;220(8):1144–1149.

Schommer M. Opening the door: non-veterinarians and the practice of complementary and alternative veterinary medicine. *J Animal Ethics.* 2012;2(1):43–52.

Studdert DM, Eisenberg DM, Miller FH, et al. Medical malpractice implications of alternative medicine. *JAMA.* 1998;280(18):1610–1615.

Waters A. Homeopathy – need it get so personal? *Vet Rec.* 2018;182(17):469.

Woodmansey D. Misleading website DC hearing adjourned. *Vet Times* [Internet]. 2016 Oct 24. Available from: https://www.vettimes.co.uk/news/misleading-website-dc-hearing-adjourned/.

16 Pointless Supplements and 'Therapeutic' Pet Foods

Andrea Tarr

16.1 WHAT ARE SUPPLEMENTS?

There is a lot of interest in supplements nowadays. Humans use supplements for themselves and increasingly seem to want to buy them for the animals in their care. But defining the term 'supplement' is not as easy as you might think. The term clearly started out as short hand for 'food supplement', and that is how you will often find it defined. But 'supplement' now represents a huge array of products sold for people to give to their pets. Some supplements, like individual vitamins or fish oil, are normal components of food. Some, like garlic or ground turmeric root, are traditional ingredients that humans add to food. Other supplements, for instance, cannabidiol (CBD), are not normal food components or accompaniments but are better described as plant-based drugs.

In regulatory terms, supplements are not medicines in that they do not contain ingredients with a medicinal function (in other words, a pharmacological effect) and cannot be promoted for medicinal uses. However, there is not always agreement between regulators about whether a substance is a supplement or a medicine: for instance, in the UK, the veterinary medicines regulator has decided that veterinary products containing CBD are veterinary medicines on the basis that CBD is medicinal by function (Veterinary Medicines Directorate 2018), whereas CBD products for humans are considered to be food supplements (Food Standards Agency 2023) unless the product is marketed for a medicinal use.

Some pet supplements look like medicines because they come as tablets or capsules; some are presented in the form of treats, and others as a product for adding to the feed or already included in feed. All are promoted, or used, for some sort of benefit to health, such as support for joint health or immune function or helping with stress or anxiety. The range of substances and products covered by the term supplement includes, but is not limited to the following:

- Vitamins and minerals
- Herbs and herbal extracts (e.g. curcumin, hemp, turmeric, valerian)
- Probiotics and prebiotics

Pointless Supplements and 'Therapeutic' Pet Foods 147

- Extracts from animals or animal products (such as green-lipped mussel, salmon oil, cod liver oil, and other sources of omega-3 fatty acids; alpha-casozepine and other milk proteins; and glucosamine and chondroitin from shellfish)
- antioxidants
- amino acids, peptides, and proteins
- hyaluronic acid.

What is clear is that supplements are big business. The global veterinary dietary supplements market was valued at USD 1.6 billion in 2020 and is expected to continue growing, with an estimated annual growth rate of 8.2% by 2028 (Grand View Research n.d.).

16.2 DO PETS NEED SUPPLEMENTS?

In theory, a balanced diet should provide all the nutritional requirements to maintain the health of a pet. Most simply and logically, a supplement is a nutritional component added to the feed, or administered separately, when an essential item is missing from, or insufficient in, the diet or is poorly absorbed. For instance, vitamin B12, an essential dietary vitamin naturally present in animal products, is usually consumed in the diet of a dog. Vitamin B12 deficiency can lead to ill health and even death in severe cases; such deficient dogs require vitamin B12 supplements (Kather et al. 2020). This example shows that some supplements are essential for life and wellbeing.

Other than this, why does a pet need a supplement? Treating or preventing a disease in an animal that is not due to a nutritional deficiency might involve the use of a medicinal substance. Put simply, such use of an intervention should always be based on evidence that the likely benefit outweighs any potential harm. This is the principle underlying the use of veterinary medicines and veterinary medicines regulation. There must be certainty about the quality of the substance being given to the animal and a reasonable degree of certainty about its efficacy and safety. In other words, pets do not need unnecessary and unproven supplements.

16.3 SO WHY DO PET OWNERS BUY SUPPLEMENTS?

A person might want to try a supplement to solve a problem (e.g. a behavioural issue), to make something better (e.g. managing body weight), for enhancement (e.g. a shinier coat), or to prevent something from going wrong in the future (e.g. preserving joint health). The culture of 'a pill for every ill' means that the promise of a remedy in a product that is accessible and easy to use, and that seems safe and not too expensive, is attractive. Pets are increasingly 'humanised' and seen as members of the family. It follows that owners who use supplements in the pursuit of a 'healthier lifestyle' might seek the same for their pets. Or maybe someone has told them that a product will solve or prevent a problem or make something better. A supplement is a marketer's dream: identify a problem – offer an easy solution.

> **BOX 16.1 THE TALE OF A PET OWNER
> WHO BOUGHT A SUPPLEMENT**
>
> My story is about the time I went into a pet shop to buy a new leash for my dog and came out with a herbal supplement. I didn't plan to buy the supplement. The visit was a pleasant experience for me and my dog because the woman in the store was very helpful and seemed knowledgeable about dog nutrition and behaviour. She was particularly kind and understanding when I told her about the difficulty I had coping with my dog's reactivity towards other dogs. She suggested the dog was anxious and recommended that I try a supplement containing valerian to help reduce his anxiety while out walking. So I bought it. Did the valerian work? I've no idea. I doubt it. I used it a few times. One time my dog seemed a bit calmer or more focused, but that might have been due to a change in my own behaviour. Who knows?

Of course, the woman stood to make a sale through her recommendation, but I have no doubt that she believed in the supplement's efficacy. I did not expect that someone in her role would be trained in science and understand evidence hierarchy. In contrast I have been immersed in the theory and practice of evidence-based therapy for decades and my rational mind told me not to rely on personal anecdote because it is subject to major bias. But I left the shop having bought a bottle of valerian extract. Why? I think this experience illustrates the powerful effect of personal anecdote, particularly on someone who is desperately seeking a solution to a difficult problem. I believe I was persuaded by the woman's personal enthusiasm and confidence about the product's efficacy, and this was reinforced by the trust that I felt in relation to the other advice she was giving, and a gratitude for the empathy she showed. So, imagine the effect if an unproven supplement is recommended by a veterinarian?

16.4 GIVING AN IMPRESSION OF EFFICACY

Supplement companies cannot legally claim that their products treat or prevent diseases, but they can legally make general health-benefit claims, such as 'helps support natural kidney function' or 'maintains and supports joint health'. However, companies sometimes find ways to convey a more 'medicinal' or scientific impression, for example, through the use of phrases such as 'recommended by vets' and 'clinically proven'. Or they might sell supplement products only through veterinary practices or make them available only on veterinary prescription even though this is not a legal requirement. Advertisements for supplements might allude to trials conducted by reputable institutions, giving enough information to create the impression of supporting scientific evidence but not enough for the advert to contravene veterinary medicines regulations. Promotion of supplements typically relies on the use of powerful personal anecdotes – only positive ones of course!

16.5 WHY IS EVIDENCE OF EFFICACY NEEDED FOR SUPPLEMENTS?

There is usually a rational theoretical basis for using a supplement, but often robust scientific evidence of benefit is lacking. However, it is not enough to base the use of an intervention on theory alone – on hope or expectation that it might work. There are many examples in human medicine where an intervention has been used because it was thought to be a good idea, only later to be proven to do no good or to be harmful. One example is placing babies to sleep on their fronts (Hauck & Tanabe 2009). A more recent example is the use of ivermectin in the treatment of COVID-19 infection (Naggie et al. 2022). This means that we should have a high level of confidence that an intervention is useful and that the likely benefits outweigh the potential harm.

The accepted way to find out if an intervention works is to test it in a randomised controlled trial. This is considered to be the most reliable method because it aims to rule out bias and the effects of factors other than the intervention itself. Most medicines have only a modest effect, and relatively large and well-designed trials are needed to show convincing effects, particularly in chronic conditions like joint disease in which signs wax and wane and there is a large caregiver placebo effect (Conzemius & Evans 2012).

To find out if a supplement has a noticeable beneficial effect, it should be subject to the same standards as medicines. But there is no requirement for any proof of the effects of a supplement, so it is not surprising that companies do not go to the trouble and expense of conducting trials that would give a convincing result.

A supplement should not be recommended without examining all the evidence. However, supplement trials are usually small and difficult to interpret because they use various doses, frequencies, and durations of administration and different formulations and because of the lack of standardisation of products. Research reports often present insufficient information about study design, such as randomisation or research blindness. Also, the use of subjective measures often assessed by owners and non-validated measurement tools may be susceptible to bias and a placebo effect. In Veterinary Prescriber's review of the evidence on green-lipped mussel supplements, fundamental design problems made it impossible to reach a confident conclusion about whether green-lipped mussel has beneficial effects in dogs with osteoarthritis (Veterinary Prescriber 2020). There is also a possibility of publication bias in that trials showing a benefit may be more likely to be published and to be publicised than those showing a lack of effect.

The effects of a supplement, if any, are likely to be subtle, and so it is inevitable that it will be difficult to demonstrate a convincing effect in a small trial. The reality is that a continuing state of uncertainty is in the interests of companies that market supplements. When there is uncertainty, people will look for hope, something marketers are good at selling.

16.6 THEY CAN'T DO ANY HARM CAN THEY?

Supplements have a reputation for being innocuous. People often associate 'natural' with safe. But supplements are not safer alternatives to pharmaceutical drugs. All need to be treated with the same caution. Just because something is a supplement, not a medicine, does not make it safe.

Even if a food or plant has been used with apparent safety for a long time, when it starts to be used in a different way, as an extract or a concentrate, or in a high dose, or in a different species, we cannot be sure that it is safe. For instance, garlic extract has a potential to cause haemolytic anaemia in dogs (Lee et al. 2000). The use of CBD in dogs has been associated with raised liver enzymes and the potential to interact with other medications (Gamble et al. 2018; Mejia et al. 2021). In March 2023, an omega-3 supplement product for cats and dogs was recalled because of possible raised levels of vitamin A and a potential risk of vitamin A toxicity (US Food and Drug Administration 2023). Unlike medicines, the side effects of supplements are not routinely monitored.

Even if unproven supplements are not harmful in terms of directly causing adverse effects in the animal, they can harm in other ways:

- Supplements can be expensive, especially if they are used regularly and for long periods. The marketing strategy of some supplement companies is to encourage people to sign up to a subscription to capture loyalty and long-term sales.
- Supplements may distract from proven therapies, including lifestyle measures and medicines. A supplement can never match the beneficial effects of weight reduction in an overweight animal.
- There may also be negative environmental effects as a result of the use of supplements, some of which involve the harvesting of natural resources. There is also a carbon footprint associated with the manufacture and transport of supplements, as well as packaging waste. It is probably difficult or impossible for the pet owner or veterinarian to check the eco credentials of supplements. Undoubtedly, the greenest unproven supplement is the one that is not used.

16.7 PET OWNERS NEED HELP TO MAKE BETTER CHOICES

The veterinary supplements industry is large but does not have to provide evidence of the efficacy of supplements to market them. Yet companies use persuasive marketing techniques to sell supplements for pet owners to administer to animals. There is a wide variety of substances in supplements in various formulations that are not of a standard quality. Little is usually known about safety particularly with long-term use. A supplement might be needed if an essential dietary component is missing but supplements do not replace food or medical treatments.

A supplement will consume financial and other resources and possibly divert pet owners away from effective interventions. It is not acceptable to give unproven supplements the benefit of the doubt. Veterinarians should help pet owners to know that different standards apply to supplements compared to medicines, and help them to understand the uncertainties about the benefits and harms of interventions.

REFERENCES

Conzemius MG, Evans RB. Caregiver placebo effect for dogs with lameness from osteoarthritis. *J Am Vet Med Assoc*. 2012;241(10):1314–1319.

Food Standards Agency. Cannabidiol (CBD). *Food Standards Agency Safety and Hygiene* [Internet]. 2023 Oct 12. Available from: https://www.food.gov.uk/safety-hygiene/cannabidiol-cbd.

Gamble L-J, Boesch JM, Frye CW, et al. Pharmacokinetics, safety, and clinical efficacy of cannabidiol treatment in osteoarthritic dogs. *Front Vet Sci*. 2018;5:165.

Grand View Research (GVR). Veterinary dietary supplements market size, share & trends analysis report by animal type (livestock, companion), by application, by type, by dosage form, by distribution channel, by region, and segment forecasts, 2021 – 2028. *Grandview Research Industry Analysis* [Internet]. n.d. [cited 2024 May 10]. Available from: https://www.grandviewresearch.com/industry-analysis/veterinary-dietary-supplements-market-report.

Hauck FR, Tanabe KO. Sids. *BMJ Clin Evid*. 2009 Jun 5;2009:0315.

Kather S, Grützner N, Kook PH, et al. Review of cobalamin status and disorders of cobalamin metabolism in dogs. *J Vet Intern Med*. 2020;34(1):13–28.

Lee K-W, Yamato O, Tajima M, et al. Hematologic changes associated with the appearance of eccentrocytes after intragastric administration of garlic extract to dogs. *Am J Vet Res*. 2000;61(11):1446–1450.

Mejia S, Duerr FM, Griffenhagen G, et al. Evaluation of the effect of cannabidiol on naturally-occurring osteoarthritis-associated pain – a pilot study in dogs. *J Am Anim Hosp Assoc*. 2021;57(2):81–90.

Naggie S, Boulware DR, Lindsell CJ, et al. Effect of ivermectin vs placebo on time to sustained recovery in outpatients with mild to moderate COVID-19. A randomized clinical trial. *J Am Med Assoc*. 2022;328(16):1595–1603.

US Food and Drug Administration (FDA). Stratford Care USA, Inc recalls omega-3 supplements for cats and dogs because of possible elevated levels of vitamin A. *FDA Recalls, Market Withdrawals, & Safety Alerts* [Internet]. 2023 Mar 10. Available from: https://www.fda.gov/safety/recalls-market-withdrawals-safety-alerts/stratford-care-usa-inc-recalls-omega-3-supplements-cats-and-dogs-because-possible-elevated-levels#recall-announcement.

Veterinary Medicines Directorate (VMD). VMD statement on veterinary medicinal products containing cannabidiol. *GOV.UK* [Internet]. 2018 Sept 14. Available from: https://www.gov.uk/government/news/vmd-statement-on-veterinary-medicinal-products-containing-cannabidiol.

Veterinary Prescriber. Green-lipped mussel – is it effective in canine OA? *VETRx CPD Modules* [Internet]. 2020 [cited 2024 May 10]. Available from: https://members.veterinaryprescriber.org/app/cpd/module/green-lipped-mussel-is-it-effective-in-canine-oa.

Part IID Exotic Animal Medicine

17 Zoo Vet Dilemmas – A Personal Perspective

Andrew Routh

Though zoos have a role to play in endangered species' conservation, the vast majority of specimens held in zoological collections come from a relatively small number of non-conservation species. Moreover, for a zoo to function, specimens need to be exhibited to the public and maintained as managed captive populations over generations.

Legislation and licensing should ensure minimum standards of health and welfare. However, through their professional oath it falls, ultimately, to veterinary surgeons to uphold both the health and the welfare of the animals in the zoo. To achieve this requires the recognition and resolution of numerous ethical quandaries.

17.1 INTRODUCTION

Like many, it was an interest in wildlife and conservation from an early age that set me off on a career as a veterinary surgeon. Pre-university influences included conservationist Peter Scott, David Attenborough, and Gerald Durrell (who wrote in one of his books that vets and architects were the biggest dangers to zoo animals). As an undergraduate, I channelled my pre-clinical and clinical extramural studies towards zoo work. I joined the British Veterinary Zoological Society. After graduating the only work I found was in mixed veterinary practice (whilst volunteering with wildlife work). A handful of veterinary colleagues worked in the non-domestic field. It was thirteen years before I moved full-time into zoo and wildlife medicine. Thirty years later there is much for reflection.

17.2 WHAT IS A ZOO?

Before considering the role of the zoo vet, it is essential to consider the role of the modern zoo and broader perceptions within society. The UK Zoo Licensing Act (1981), with a few caveats, defines a zoo as 'an establishment where wild animals (as defined by section 21) are kept for exhibition to the public'.

Though a number of zoos are run as business concerns, most zoos are charities. (This ratio varies around the world.) There are some zoos run directly by government departments (national or local). Whether a zoo is openly commercial or run as a not-for-profit organisation, there is a need for income to at least match year on year running costs. Age and size of organisation does not offer immunity, with the Zoological Society of London having several financial close calls in the late 20th and early 21st centuries.

Sources of income other than gate receipts are available, most frequently from donors, sponsorship, individual memberships, and grants. These often arise through using the zoo as a 'shop window' to maintain the organisation's profile. Conservation programme species will only make up a small proportion of collection species, with the zoo promoting the organisation's work through the exhibition of the charismatic species. However, there are conflicting arguments with one camp saying that without the crowd pullers, there would be no money for conservation and the other camp railing against the 'Disneyfication' of zoos, arguing for a purity of focus on endangered species. Taken to extremes, there are collections which exhibit e.g. white tigers. These are phenotypic abnormalities resulting from intentional inbreeding and contrary to, for example, a British and Irish Association of Zoos and Aquaria (BIAZA) position statement on the intentional breeding for the expression of rare recessive alleles (BIAZA 2022).

Zoos undertake other roles beyond that of simply exhibiting wild animals to the public. Varying proportions of their work go on away from direct public gaze. To degrees, they act to prevent species' extinctions through keeping endangered species in captivity and breeding them, a role analogous to a safety net (Conway 2011). For this to be successful, the ambition must be to return specimens to the wild through reintroductions. The greatest successes are achieved through in-country programmes and the training of in-country colleagues (veterinarians, educators, and conservationists). Many projects must run over years or decades to achieve success. Training, transfer of skills, and capacity-building to achieve project self-sufficiency are essential for success.

Only a small percentage of the species that would benefit from conservation action end up in zoological collections. This is backed up where data has been scrutinised, e.g. with endangered amphibians (Jacken et al. 2020) and turtles and tortoises (Ahmed et al. 2024). Thus, the zoo vet must anticipate that the bulk of their work will be on the non-endangered but frequently encountered zoo species rather than Gerald Durrell's beloved, endangered, and often overlooked 'little brown jobs'.

Worldwide, visitors (normally after paying an entrance fee) come to zoos to see 'wild' animals exhibited. Zoos aspire for that visit to be an educational experience, but it could also be argued that a visitor expectation is to be entertained. These expectations underpin the veterinary care of zoo animals, providing their own unique challenges.

17.3 WHAT IS A ZOO VET?

The levels of veterinary services provided to zoological collections vary. Generally, zoos either employ an in-house veterinary team or have an external vet-client relationship (with routine visits and emergency call-out). For the latter the veterinary surgeons may have zoo work as part of a general practice workload or may be employed in a practice working full-time to provide veterinary cover to numerous zoological collections.

These differing terms of engagement provide a contrast in working circumstances.

A salaried zoo vet has better oversight of husbandry, health, and sickness in a collection. Daily presence on-site should mean greater case continuity. They are in a better position to determine standard operating procedures e.g. on quarantines and biosecure management, plus should be given the opportunities to actively contribute to the organisation's policies on e.g. welfare and ethics. However, they will sit within the zoo's organisational structure and will likely have non-veterinary line management. They will have to negotiate and establish case treatment plans with colleagues (as opposed to with clients). As part of an organisation, they will be subject to overall intra-organisational management and discipline, which may be a challenge if their professional opinion differs from that of non-veterinary colleagues and management.

Conversely, the visiting clinician works within a conventional client-vet relationship. They may have no involvement with a case or its management from when they leave the zoo until their next visit.

All zoo staff have responsibility for disease prevention, control, and exclusion. Similarly, 'notifiable diseases' must be reported to the authorities even if only suspected. This is not a veterinary responsibility, though an animal holder may seek clarification from their veterinary surgeon before reporting.

Overall disease management and control must be a veterinary responsibility, especially with reference to statutory pre- or post-export quarantines. Quarantine and testing are integral to animal moves, national and international. Export health certificates will require official veterinarian (OV) sign-off. This is currently permitted to be done by an OV who can be an employee of the exporting zoological collection, but the OV's ultimate accountability is to the statutory authorities and the RCVS and not their employer.

Irrespective of the working arrangement, any zoo vet must make sure that, above all, their constant endeavour ensures the health and welfare of animals committed to their care.

17.4 REGULATION, LEGISLATION, AND ZOO ETHICS

Zoos, as entities, are subject to legislation. In the UK the baseline legislation is the Zoo Licensing Act (ZLA) (1981). Through a system administered by the local authority, zoos are inspected at intervals and issued a licence. The inspection team's judgments are underpinned by central government's secretary of state's Standards of Modern Zoo Practice (SSSMZP), but decisions on licence conditions or revocation are determined locally.

In addition, UK zoos also must comply with the overarching Animal Welfare (Sentience) Act (2022).

Zoos can, themselves, become members of self-regulated industry bodies, e.g. British and Irish Association of Zoos and Aquaria (BIAZA) and the EAZA. Membership requires certain standards to be met and member zoos are subject to inspection. The aims of these organisations are similar. EAZA, for example, describes its aim as furthering 'professional quality in keeping animals and presenting them for the education of the public, and of contributing to scientific research and to the conservation of global biodiversity'. It also looks to promote and coordinate research to support these objectives, provide resources to its members, to inform and to influence relevant legislation.

The baseline for any veterinary surgeon providing services to a zoological collection is that they must be appropriately registered (in the UK registered with the Royal College of Veterinary Surgeons). (This also holds true when dealing with wildlife.) Post-graduate qualifications, ranging from university-run MSc courses to diplomas, are available globally. There is an increasing number of resources available, including peer-reviewed journals, books, courses, and conferences plus online material, offering the opportunity for a veterinary surgeon to keep up to date. Membership of organisations, e.g. British Veterinary Zoological Society (BVZS) and the European Association of Zoo and Wildlife Veterinarians (EAZWV), is beneficial. Their aims broadly align with e.g. EAZA in looking to advance knowledge, to provide resources, and to inform statutory bodies regarding legislation.

Research is an oft-cited objective for zoological collections. There is a legal and an ethical aspect to any research.

In the UK there is the Animal (Scientific Procedures) Act (1986). There is no exemption in this act for zoo animals (nor for wildlife). Any proposed research must undergo thorough scrutiny. If likely to pass the thresholds set by the act, then Home Office advice should be sought before proceeding. (Any research to be undertaken overseas must comply with local law. Best practice would be to have a documented review of the proposed work undertaken by the relevant ethics committee.)

Ethics committees are required under the ZLA, mandating 'a written policy and process for dealing with ethical issues that is credible, transparent, and effective'. The remit for the committee is broad as it requires review 'of all ethical issues related to the operation of a zoo, both human and animal'. It suggests that a rotating membership, including a veterinary surgeon, will aid in dealing with all these diverse considerations. Included in its list and of most direct relevance to the zoo vet are as follows:

- Animal experiences
- On-site events that may impact upon animal behaviours
- Husbandry practices
- Painful interventions
- Treatment of abnormal behaviours
- Animal training activities, including purpose and intent

- Hand-rearing of animals
- Shows and performances involving animals, including purpose and intent
- Euthanasia of animals (except those euthanised on veterinary advice)
- Isolation of individuals of social species
- Population management, including breeding and culling policy
- Research projects involving animals or human participants (in and ex situ)

17.5 THE PATIENTS

With the exception of some individuals from some species (primarily conservation programme specimens and aquatic specimens), almost all zoo animals have been captive born.

Pre-move screening and quarantine act as barriers to disease ingress, but within a collection, there are often few barriers to pathogen transference. However, with the increased risk of avian influenza from wild birds and the potential culling of collection birds, the concept of managed 'epidemiological units' is becoming more widely accepted.

Conservation programme species may be held in strict isolation, technically never entering the collection, to minimise the risk of acquired infections being transferred to the wild on reintroduction. In the field of infectious diseases, the Rumsfeldian 'unknown unknowns' abound. In the 1980s the Mallorcan midwife toad (*Alytes muletensis*) was endangered in the wild and a captive population established in a zoo. Some were released into the wild in 1991 infected with zoo-acquired chytrid fungus *Batrachochytrium dendrobatidis* (Bd). Deaths occurred and it was not until 2015 that the wild population recovered through active management of the disease. Measures to screen the health of the toads in 1991 did not pick up the fungus because at the time it was not known to science (Walker et al. 2008).

Though the disease status of multigenerational captive-bred specimens may be better known there are other concerns. Genetic management should be a priority, with planned programmes and studbooks for the higher profile species. However, options may be limited, especially if the numbers of founder specimens for the captive population was low and/or founders were closely related. Diseases are seen with presumed genetic or familial components. Detection of diaphragmatic defects in golden lion tamarins (*Leontopithecus rosalia rosalia*) was made early in the programme. This required extensive diagnostic work and breeding management to reduce its severity (Bush et al. 1996). Eyelid coloboma in snow leopards (*Panthera uncia*) is well-recognised and frequently seen (Georoff & Marlar 2007). The defect can be rectified surgically but, with a presumptive inheritable component, should these specimens be used for future breeding? In addition, in the same study, some cubs had concurrent congenital, developmental, or potentially heritable conditions (hip dysplasia, swimmer's syndrome, stifle osteochondrosis, cardiac anomaly, and/or hydrocephalus). Future management of this species in captivity and its welfare will be a challenge; something recognised in other species.

Inadvertent selective breeding occurs even in the best managed programme. The ability of individuals to successfully breed is well recognised; the concept of certain lines becoming over-represented in studbooks is known. However, the individuals that breed are likely to be more tolerant of captive conditions and tractable to manage. The net effect can be domestication over generations, giving a population well-adapted to captivity but becoming less likely to adapt to the wild on release.

17.6 DETECTING ILLNESS

The veterinary surgeon will need to have an overview of 'zoo health' and that of species within the collection. For licensing and regulatory requirements, including the sign-off of export health certificates, documented monitoring programmes and routine health surveillance are required. This includes post mortem examination of dead specimens.

There are some species-specific, prescribed, health-check schedules. In Europe these are generally mandated by the EEP (variously, the EAZA Ex-situ Programme or the European Endangered Species Programme). Some zoos carry out structured elective health checks at fixed intervals, the frequency of which increase as a specimen ages (Barrows et al. 2017; Kershaw et al. 2020).

Otherwise, the zoo vet is reliant on day-to-day observations from the keepers of individual specimens in their care. For many species the daily duration of observation on which to make assessments is short. These observations often coincide with elements of positive reinforcement, i.e. when food is presented or, more simply, keeper presence; this can lift the specimen's behaviour. A more rounded appraisal, potentially through 24 hours, can now be achieved using remote cameras or cameras with a memory card. Nocturnal species provide additional challenges, even when on reverse day-night cycles, but again technology and cameras can help.

Decisions to intervene are often based solely on observations. Some species will hide clinical signs and the progression of disease can be rapid in some. Catch-up and intervention will always carry inherent risks, as will not intervening. Observation and review has its merits but is not a safe, neutral action.

17.7 HOW TO TREAT A PATIENT

One examines, one diagnoses, and now one needs to treat.

There are almost no drugs licensed for use in the species one encounters in zoos. If one knows where to look there are numerous resources. Many zoos use a recording system called ZIMS. This can be searched, both at local and global level, to obtain drug doses used in the same or in allied species. Much can be extrapolated from documented use in domestic and non-conventional pet species. For primates one can look at what is used in humans. Peer-reviewed papers are published, conference presentations given and there is a network of ever-helpful colleagues. Ideally one then makes a decision at a personal level and carries out science-based medication. In principle, selection of medication for non-domestic species should go through the 'cascade'. If antimicrobials are to be used then choice for each case should be scrutinised and backed-up, where possible, with laboratory analysis. Prevention of transfer of antimicrobial resistance requires responsible use. However, the only antimicrobial licensed in non-domestic species is a fluoroquinolone: a category of antimicrobials on the restricted-use list.

Science-based medicine does not equate to evidence-based medicine. The zoo vet should not despair; they are not on their own. When published data on clinical management for domestic species is reviewed (for example, in periodic 'Evaluating the Evidence' articles in the *Veterinary Record*), there is often a lack of robust evidence to underpin one's treatment choices. One can only do one's conscientious best.

For surgical management, extrapolating from domestic species and reviewing the literature, the options are more proven. Anatomy, restraint, and anaesthesia will differ. More importantly, post-surgical case management can differ markedly.

What a zoo vet must accept is that they are a generalist, working across many taxa and diseases but in a discrete, speciality niche. There are other colleagues who are better, through specialisation, in their own field and can bring skill sets that readily transfer to the treatment of zoo animals. Do not overlook diagnostic specialists who can be used from the start to provide key information to inform the treatment plan and ultimate prognosis.

No one likes to fail. Reporting unsuccessful case outcomes is challenging but should be encouraged. The use of non-validated tests and non-licensed medications and management of difficult species will all conspire against the veterinary team (Bouts et al. 2009). Not reporting when things do not go to plan risks others repeating your misfortune.

17.8 WHEN NOT TO TREAT A PATIENT

Before embarking on any veterinary intervention and treatments, a realistic appraisal of intended outcomes must be made. Not all cases will have a 100% successful outcome. What level of sub-optimal outcome would be acceptable for all, in particular for the animal? It is best to discuss and plan from as early on as possible.

The easiest cases to plan for are those where a rapid (and successful) outcome is anticipated; a case with minimal disruption to the specimen and any social group in which it is held.

More complex cases need greater circumspection. Mitigating factors will include whether a specimen will require frequent interventions for e.g. medication or dressing changes. Will this then require the specimen to be separated from its social group with a poor chance of returning to that group? Is full rehabilitation expected? If treatment is partially successful what will be the specimen's subsequent welfare status?

Though a specialist may be fully capable of treating or of operating on a 'like for like' condition in a domestic animal, would that be appropriate for the zoo animal? These decisions need to be made with the zoo vet being pragmatic, whilst factoring in that zoo management may have a more utilitarian view of the specimen's worth. Solitary specimens may have compromised welfare, old specimens may not have a future role to play in the social group or breeding programmes, and surplus males may never be reintegrated. Thus, euthanasia must be considered where poor welfare is likely to be the outcome.

17.9 OVERALL WELFARE

Welfare in a zoo, which sits squarely in the professional oath, is always a challenge to quantify and to optimise. A captive environment is not the wild environment but, whilst some perceived freedoms may be reduced, the expectation is of a life with a consistent food supply, reduced diseases, and absence of predators. It should be no surprise, therefore, that many zoo specimens exceed their life expectancy in the wild. Consequential geriatric conditions and degenerative disease, with allied pain, must be appropriately managed by veterinary surgeons and the animal staff.

The Zoo Licensing Act originally structured itself around the Five Freedoms found in farm animal welfare, but these evolved into the Five Domains and have been subsequently taken further with scoring systems and the Animal Welfare Assessment Grid (Justice et al. 2017; Barrows et al. 2017). Welfare assessments are seen as a gauge of animals in health but, especially in ageing zoo populations, later life assessments are directed more towards quality of life (Föllmi et al. 2007; Vogelnest & Talbot 2019). These systems often generate a score and thresholds for action. In the first instance they may offer routes to improve quality of life but, ultimately, will inform decisions on elective euthanasia.

The mental health of zoo animals is often raised as a concern. This should be flagged up via the welfare assessments and may be manifest by e.g. stereotypic behaviour or a social animal not integrating into a group and then held alone. Though overall nutrition can be good in zoological collections, the food given can be calorie dense when compared with food consumed in the wild. Foraging time, often hard-wired in, is reduced and can lead to aberrant behaviours. Overcompensating by providing additional food results in obesity.

Exhibit design can be modified and enrichment provided, with these actions informed by behavioural studies supported by measurements of faecal cortisol metabolites (Clark et al. 2012). There are psychoactive drugs that could be used in an attempt to address behavioural issues. However, these should be used prudently and in conjunction with pre- and post-administration behaviour studies to determine their efficacy.

17.10 HUSBANDRY AND MANAGING THE CAPTIVE POPULATION

Flight restraint in birds is a procedure in which a veterinary surgeon may be involved and must be involved if it is a surgical procedure, often referred to as pinioning. Pinioning involves the removal of the distal tip of one wing soon after hatching. The birds can then be exhibited in large open bodies of water without the risk of escape. This procedure has always been controversial and may occur less frequently as more exhibits are netted over to prevent contact with wild birds due to avian influenza.

Training is a double-edged sword. Many zoos have animal shows as part of their programme for visitors. Animals carry out behaviours, with varying degrees of naturalism to them, whilst one of the show team will provide commentary highlighting e.g. the behaviour, the traits of the species and threats to the species in the wild. These should have prior ethical review and should fit within the educational remit of the zoo licence but are also indicative of the degrees of domestication that are now seen in zoo specimens. Hand-reared specimens may be used.

Conversely, training, using positive reinforcement and protected contact, can be a huge asset to the veterinary management of animals. Blood samples can be taken and blood pressure checked, readings taken from indwelling cardiac monitors, and eyes and teeth examined all without the need for general anaesthesia. If general anaesthesia is needed then induction by hand injection, safer and less stressful for all, is easily achieved. Medications can be administered and post-operative care provided.

There is veterinary involvement in both aspects of breeding programmes.

On the one hand there are efforts to manage and augment populations of endangered species. At the most simplistic level, there is veterinary involvement in the movement of key animals, often internationally, as part of breeding programmes. Less common, and thus needing prior ethical review, are techniques of assisted breeding, harvesting of gametes, artificial insemination, cloning, and utilisation of previously bio-banked material to resurrect lost genetic material.

On the other hand, there are excess numbers of some species in captivity. Population control is required. This is most problematic in mammals. Stopping breeding can be carried out by contraception. EAZA runs a Reproductive Management Group that offers guidance and shared experiences. Some techniques, e.g. implants, are considered temporary with the potential that animals can rejoin the programme. Others, such as castration, are irreversible.

As the norm in the wild is for repeated breeding, there is a school of thought that contraception is physiologically detrimental and that the captive situation should mimic the wild. This is the 'breed and cull' approach, which reached a high public profile in 2014 with the euthanasia of a surplus male giraffe in Denmark. There are vocal proponents and opponents of this policy. EAZA published a policy statement on management euthanasia/culling in 2023 which supports all courses of actions if criteria are met. As a veterinary surgeon, the zoo vet would likely be involved in ethical discussions and, probably, be required to perform euthanasia on young, healthy (and possibly globally rare) specimens. Keepers, who are frequently emotionally invested in their animals, often attempt to distance themselves from 'culls' by referring to them as KBO (killed by order).

17.11 THE GOAL

One would imagine that the role of a zoo vet is to return the rare species with which they work to their range country and into a wild where threats have been removed. That does occur but not very often.

One step down is their involvement in breeding programmes ensuring optimal health and genetic viability with releases on the horizon but not in the immediate future. Conservationists work tirelessly to provide safe habitats in the wild, but (and more so with climate change coming into play) they are not always successful.

Realistically, the bulk of the day-to-day work of the zoo vet is upholding the health and the welfare of the animals in the zoo, some rare and many not yet, most destined to be in zoos as ambassadors educating the public for generations to come.

17.12 CONCLUSION

The job of a zoo vet should be described as challenging but rewarding. An article in the *Veterinary Record* (Agathou et al. 2022) looked at stereotypes in areas of veterinary work as perceived by their colleagues in the profession. Zoo and wildlife vets, whilst scoring almost no adverse characteristics, were seen to be 'adventurous, interesting, cool, and lucky'. Fair enough, but it would be good if sight were not lost of attributes ascribed to other sectors of the profession, including 'caring, intelligent, and thoughtful'.

REFERENCES

Agathou A, Stratis A, Routh J, et al. Professional stereotypes among specialties and fields of work within the veterinary community. *Vet Rec*. 2022;191(8):e1486.

Ahmed K, Tapley B, Michaels CJ. Global and regional patterns in distribution and threat status of zoo collections of turtles and tortoises. *Herpetol J*. 2024 Jan;34:1–10.

Barrows M, Killick R, Saunders R, et al. Retrospective analysis of elective health examinations as preventative medicine interventions at a zoological collection. *J Zoo Aquar Res*. 2017;5(1):25–32.

BIAZA. https://biaza.org.uk/policies-guidelines/BIAZA Rare Alleles Policy. 2022 (Accessed March 2025

Bouts T, Vordermeier M, Flach E, et al. Positive skin and serologic test results of diagnostic assays for bovine tuberculosis and subsequent isolation of *Mycobacterium interjectum* in a pygmy hippopotamus (*Hexaprotodon liberiensis*). *J Zoo Wildl Med*. 2009;40(3):536–542.

Bush M, Beck BB, Dietz J, et al. Radiographic evaluation of diaphragmatic defects in golden lion tamarins (*Leontopithecus rosalia rosalia*): implications for reintroduction. *J Zoo Wildl Med*. 1996;27(3):346–357.

Clark FE, Fitzpatrick M, Hartley A, et al. Relationship between behavior, adrenal activity, and environment in zoo-housed western lowland gorillas (*Gorilla gorilla gorilla*). *Zoo Biol*. 2012;31(3):306–321.

Conway WG. Buying time for wild animals with zoos. *Zoo Biol*. 2011;30:1–8.

Föllmi J, Steiger A, Walzer C, et al. A scoring system to evaluate physical condition and quality of life in geriatric zoo mammals. *Animal Welfare*. 2007;16(3):309–318.

Georoff TA, Marlar AB. Retrospective review of eyelid coloboma in snow leopards (*Panthera uncia*) housed under managed care in North America: 49 cases (2000–2020). *J Am Vet Med Assoc*. 2007;261(12):1–8.

Jacken A, Rödder D, Ziegler T. Amphibians in zoos: a global approach on distribution patterns of threatened amphibians in zoological collections. *Int Zoo Yearbook*. 2020;54(1):146–164.

Justice WSM, O'Brien MF, Szyszka O, et al. Adaptation of the animal welfare assessment grid (AWAG) for monitoring animal welfare in zoological collections. *Vet Rec*. 2017;181(6):143–143.

Kershaw T, Hall EJ, Dobbs P, et al. An exploration of the value of elective health checks in UK zoo-housed gibbons animals. *Animals (Basel)*. 2020;10:2307.

Vogelnest L, Talbot JJ. Quality of life assessment and end of life planning for geriatric zoo animals. In: Miller RE, Lamberski N, Calle PP, editors. *Fowler's zoo and wild animal medicine current therapy*. St. Louis: Elsevier; 2019. p. 83–91.

Walker SF, Bosch J, James TY, et al. Invasive pathogens threaten species recovery programs *Curr Biol*. 2008;18(18):R853–R854.

FURTHER READING

Rose P, Riley L. Five ways to wellbeing at the zoo: improving human health and connection to nature. *Front Psychol*. 2023;14:1258667.

18 The Value of Mice

R. Eddie Clutton and Amanda Novak

18.1 INTRODUCTION

Animals have been an integral part of human existence for millennia and continue to play diverse and changing roles in human societies. In these roles, each animal has an intrinsic (inherent or implicit) value as a sentient entity living within a diverse biological system. It also has an extrinsic (explicit or instrumental) value for meeting human requirements alone. The sum of an animal's intrinsic and extrinsic values determines how society and individuals, including veterinarians, regard them. This is useful because humans naturally rank animals in terms of worth. For example, what makes the use of primates in biomedical research less defensible than the use of sheep? The Nuffield Council on Bioethics (2005) suggest sentience, cognitive capacity, the capacity to flourish, sociability, and the possession of a life, are the five criteria for making such decisions. This chapter examines the factors affecting an animal's worth and circumvents problems with inter-species differences by focusing on one: *Mus musculus*. It then examines how this value affects the welfare and the quality of veterinary treatment that mice with a similar common disease, e.g. tumours, are likely to receive. The intent of this is to provoke thought as to what makes some animals 'more important' than others – at least in the public eye, and in turn, that of the veterinary profession itself, thereby revealing the apparent arbitrariness with which veterinary treatment is sometimes dispensed. The chapter also aims to (i) promote interest in *Mus musculus*, (ii) provoke a more thoughtful approach to the veterinary treatment of small mammals in general, and (iii) reveal the benefits of being a laboratory animal in the United Kingdom (UK).

18.2 THE IMPLICIT AND EXPLICIT VALUES OF ANIMALS

Animals are implicitly valued because they are sentient, i.e. capable of experiencing positive and negative feelings, e.g. pleasure, joy, pain, suffering, and distress, that matter to them as individuals. Intrinsic values are self-ascribed, i.e. arise from within the animal itself and identify the value it places on its own existence. Intrinsic values are not easily measured but nevertheless reveal the moral responsibilities humans have towards animals, including ascribing them rights and treating them with respect and compassion. Recognising their capacity to suffer mandates a moral responsibility to protect them from unnecessary harm while accepting their intrinsic worth also means their interests are not automatically subordinated to human interests. More recently, it has become accepted that animals have an intrinsic value in maintaining ecological balance and biodiversity.

Extrinsic values are conferred on animals by humans and are based primarily on the economic contributions animals make to agriculture (as labour, food, or fibre providers), tourism, entertainment, and the ecosystem. As such, they are usually measurable econometrically. However, more nuanced is their value as sources of emotional, recreational, aesthetic, or spiritual gratification, which can have secondary therapeutic benefits for humans. An animal's extrinsic value varies according to cultural, economic, and individual factors but in most cases is defined by their economic contribution. Where animals reduce commercial gain, e.g. mice in a grain shed, they incur a net negative value and are categorised as pests or vermin. The ethical considerations surrounding the use of animals for economic gain are important in a humane market economy. These things said, there are at least four other forms of explicit value beyond hard economics.

For example, an animal's value in scientific and medical research goes beyond Big Pharma's profits: laboratory animals provide greater, though more abstract, benefits in the form of new knowledge and understanding or hope for more effective treatments of human and animal disease. The ethical debate related to animal experimentation and the pursuit of alternatives is important: while both extremes of view recognise the intrinsic worth of the laboratory mouse, scientific debate is increasingly focused on their instrumental value as reliable models of human biology.

Third, many animals – particularly pets – are emotionally valuable to humans and, by providing companionship, can act as emotional support. This has therapeutic value and health benefits in numerous settings, e.g.˙ assistance. For reasons explored later, mice make excellent pets.

Fourth, animals may have an abstract symbolic worth, deeply rooted in cultural and historical contexts. Cultural perceptions can influence the treatment and conservation of different species. Some societies hold specific species in regard and consider them sacred, while others may view them as resources for exploitation. These perspectives influence how animals are treated and protected. Laboratory mice play a significantly greater symbolic role than their troublesome free-ranging conspecifics.

Fifth, conservation efforts to protect endangered species tend to be greatest amongst the rarest because the rarer a thing, the greater its value. Conservation attempts, however, are influenced by cultural factors, with people preferring to save charismatic megafauna like pandas rather than insects. Being neither rare nor mega, mice are seldom the focus of conservation efforts, although from a moral viewpoint, conservation efforts on behalf of any species are always justified because all animals have worth beyond (immediate) human requirements in their contribution to ecosystem health and biodiversity. Conservation is also a moral imperative: as William Beebe proposes, *'When the last individual of a race of living beings breathes no more, another heaven and another earth must pass before such a one can be again'*.

Pragmatically, an animals' overall worth is reflected in the ethical and legal frameworks that society establishes and determines how they are treated: laws and regulations provide explicit protections for animals, recognising their intrinsic worth and setting standards for their care and welfare. Ethical theories and principles, such as animal rights and animal welfare, explicitly address the moral standing of animals.

There are five readily identifiable mouse populations in the UK: wild, free-ranging animals; those kept as pets; those used in laboratories; and fancy mice, i.e. those bred for their physical characteristics and exhibition. There are also mice which are bred for feeding other animals, such as snakes and birds of prey. This chapter will focus on the different values of wild, pet, and laboratory mice and consider how this affects the veterinary options available when mice from these populations develop tumours.

18.3 WILD MICE: HISTORY AND INTRINSIC VALUE

Genomic studies indicate the modern feral mouse (see Figure 18.1) arose from an ancestral form in the Indian subcontinent some 700,000 years ago. By 13,000 BC they were infesting the Mediterranean and by 1000 BC had reached Northern Europe. Mice accompanied the conquistadors in the 16th-century colonisation of South and Central America and were probably responsible for the domestication of *Felis muricidalis*. Murine success can be attributed to their prolificacy: in theory and under optimal conditions, a single breeding mouse pair may generate up to 5,082 mice in one year (Milchevskaya et al. 2023). This high reproductive rate and their adaptability in varied environments make them a potential threat to human resources. However, individual wild mice usually live less than one year because of high predation levels, exposure to harsh environments, and possibly too much sex.

On the basis of sentience, the intrinsic value of wild mice does not differ from that of laboratory or pet animals. However, unlike their housed conspecifics,

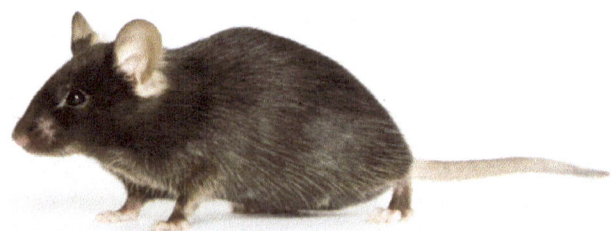

FIGURE 18.1 A wild mouse.

wild mice play a major role in ecosystem dynamics, providing food for muricidal animal and bird species, while dispersing fruit and other seeds throughout the environment.

18.4 WILD MICE: EXTRINSIC VALUE

Wild mice and other rodents are of major economic importance through their effects on food production. In Asia it is estimated the rice lost every year to rodents could feed about 200 million people. In Australia's southeastern grain belt, mice breed so successfully that they achieve densities of 1000 animals per hectare and cause losses to agriculture worth A$36 million annually (Brown & Henry 2022).

Wild mice populations have scientific value: by exhibiting significant genetic diversity, they provide an opportunity to study the effects of natural genetic variation on traits, behaviour, and disease susceptibility. The study of wild mice has also contributed to ecological research by providing insights into population dynamics, adaptation to different environments, and the effect of environmental changes on genetic diversity.

Wild mice have little emotional value: the stress it would cause the animals involved, and the wide availability of pets bred selectively for human companionship mean the domestication of wild mice cannot be advocated.

Despite their pestilential potential, the wild mouse holds considerable symbolic value amongst those not economically affected by them. In 1785, Robert Burns wrote 'To a Mouse', an apologetic reflection 'on turning her up in her nest wi the plough'. More recently, Hannah & Barbera's *Tom and Jerry* – an American animated film series – awards Jerry (a wild mouse) the attributes of heroism, fortitude, and inventiveness. In response to the cat's (Tom's) repeated assassination attempts, Jerry cuts Tom's head off, saws him in half, and binds him to a giant sky-rocket before lighting the fuse. Robert (Mousey) Thompson (1876–1955), an oak furniture manufacturer from North Yorkshire, UK, incorporated a carved mouse on almost every piece he made in recognition of the impoverishment of *Mus ecclesiasticus*.

18.5 WILD MICE: LEGAL AND ETHICAL CONSIDERATIONS

In the UK, the Wildlife and Countryside Act (1981) and the Animal Welfare Act (2006) define the legal framework for pest control in the UK. The former protects wildlife species, including mice, from certain activities that may cause harm, disturbance, or unnecessary suffering. The Act emphasises the need for humane and ethical treatment of wildlife, even in the context of pest control. Section 11(1) of the Act makes it an offence to use certain killing methods considered to be cruel or inhumane, e.g. self-locking snares and poisons. Licensed pest control companies ensure that the mice are dealt with legally and use methods that prioritise human and animal safety, including the targeted use of approved rodenticides. Beyond legality, the ethical analysis of pest control must consider any suffering of the target species, the risk of harm to non-target species, and the environmental effects of control measures. In the UK, the hazel dormouse, the water vole, and the fat dormouse are legally protected under Schedule 5 of the Wildlife and Countryside Act 1981.

18.6 WILD MICE AND VETERINARY CARE

A wild mouse with a large ulcerating tumour is going to die a slow and unpleasant death unless a predator destroys it first. If such a mouse can be caught by hand, then it is probably severely debilitated, has suffered enough, and will have no prospects of a life worth living. Such animals should be killed immediately using any method causing instant death, e.g. cervical dislocation or concussion. People making the case that an animal's 'wild' status shouldn't preclude it from veterinary care might reflect on the major stresses likely to be experienced by animals undergoing major surgery and subsequent 'nursing' whilst being entirely unaccustomed to humans.

18.7 PET MICE: HISTORY AND INTRINSIC VALUE

The earliest written references to pet or fancy mice originated in China, ca 1100 BC, where coat-colour mutations have been recorded ever since. Many domesticated (pet) mice varieties were imported from China, Japan, and India by 18th-century Europeans and led to the foundation of the National Mouse Club (of England) in 1895 (Rozenbaum 2022). Since then, the value of mice as pets for individuals with limited space, funds, and time, i.e. children, has become well-established (see Figure 18.2). Their size allows for easy accommodation, and in general, they are low-maintenance: their minimal daily care routine includes feeding, fresh water provision, and periodical cage cleaning. Their low maintenance nature also contributes to the reduced stress levels recorded in most pet owners. Captured wild

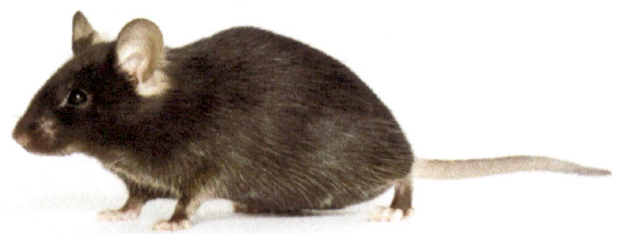

FIGURE 18.2 A pet mouse.

mice should not be 'used' as pets; it is recommended that pet mice be purchased from reputable dealers or preferably rehomed from charities, e.g. the RSPCA. Some licensed establishments now allow the rehoming of ex-laboratory wild-type mice.

Pet mice have the same self-ascribed intrinsic value as laboratory mice and, being withheld from the natural breeding pool, are unlikely to make a significant contribution to biodiversity, beneficial or otherwise.

18.8 PET MICE: EXTRINSIC VALUE

Pet mouse ownership generates little, if any economic gain for the owner. In contrast, breeders, pet shop owners, feed, bedding, and accessory manufacturers, pet insurance companies, and veterinarians stand much to gain. That said, the therapeutic benefits of pet mouse ownership may reduce the owner's medical bills!

The pet mouse is of little scientific value beyond stimulating an interest in zoology in young owners – or medicine, when the pet inevitably sickens. However, they have enormous educational value, especially amongst urban children who, unlike their farm-reared counterparts, are likely to be less acquainted with the processes of sex, birth, lactation, growth, and death. Pet mice have the potential to provide at least three learning objectives. First, caring for them may instil a sense of responsibility. Feeding, grooming, bedding, and providing for the animal's needs demand consistency and routine. Collectively, these are valuable life skills and help youngsters develop a sense of accountability. Second, interacting with pet mice may promote empathy and compassion. Recognising and satisfying an animal's basic needs cultivates a sense of consideration and care for the feelings of other animals and humans. Finally, the brief life expectancy of pet mice (about three years) provides young owners with several important life lessons – including the inevitably of death. Ritual attempts to cope with grief at the death of a small pet by laying it in a bedding-filled shoe box and burying it in the garden under some form of marker are probably a useful preparation for coping with the future loss of a loved human relative.

Irrespective of a pet's capacity to offer unconditional love and loyalty, the belief that they do is sufficient to imbue young owners with a sense of companionship and security that may reduce feelings of loneliness. Importantly, emotional interactions with small mammals have therapeutic benefits: petting and playing with animals can trigger oxytocin release, which is associated with bonding and stress reduction (Marshall-Pescini et al. 2019). In some situations, pet mice may be of immense emotional value.

Pet mice *per se* do not figure prominently in the pantheon of distinguished non-human animals, although the murder and subsequent resurrection of Mr Jingles in the film adaptation of Stephen King's *The Green Mile* (see: The Best of The Mouse On The Mile (Mr. Jingles) | The Green Mile (1999) | Screen Bites [SUPPLIER DMO ROTORUA 2a YT 16x9 15s (youtube.com)]) received 7.8K "likes" (and no "dislikes") as of March 12th 2024.

18.9 PET MICE: LEGAL AND ETHICAL CONSIDERATIONS

In the UK, the Pet Animals Act 1951 (Amendment) Act 1983 (Gov.UK 1951) protects the welfare of mice sold as pets. It requires those who sell pets to be licensed by the local authority (council). In granting a licence, the council must be satisfied that the animals have suitable and clean accommodation, are supplied with food and drink, and are protected from disease. Licensed premises may be inspected at reasonable times and the licence withdrawn if unsatisfactory conditions found or if the terms of the licence are not being complied with.

As pets, mice (and other animals) are also protected under AWA 2006. The Act places a legal duty of care on pet owners, i.e. providing a suitable environment, a proper diet, the ability to exhibit normal behaviour, housing with or apart from other animals, and protection from pain, suffering, injury, and disease. The Act grants enforcement powers to the police and local authorities, to prosecute cases of cruelty or neglect. Penalties for offences include fines, imprisonment, and disqualification from owning animals. Authorities are allowed to inspect premises where animals are kept and can remove animals, if welfare standards are not met. The Act holds those in charge of animals responsible for their welfare, whether they are the owners or temporary caretakers.

18.10 PET MICE AND VETERINARY CARE

Despite protective legislation, the benefits of being a pet mouse ultimately depend on the care afforded by the owner. The attention pets require may become inadequate when children – and their parents – lose interest, and the animal is ignored but perhaps not released. Under these conditions, a growing tumour may go unnoticed. The AWA 2006 requires that a pet's health problems must be addressed, and so the discovery of a large, ulcerated tumour obliges the owners to have the animal humanely killed or receive veterinary treatment, e.g. surgical excision (at least) with or without chemotherapy.

The thought of providing such veterinary treatment to pet mice would at one time have been ridiculed given the animal's primary role in educating urban children. This may no longer be the case: the animal has value so is entitled to treatment, the client demands that it be treated, the vet has never done this before and is excited by the challenge, the fee for attempted treatment is greater than that for euthanasia, etc. However, the tendency for murine tumours to metastasise to the lungs indicates the need for pre-operative thoracic imaging for the purpose of prognostication. Despite justification, this measure is likely to be considered too expensive for a child's pet with a limited lifespan. Whatever the decision, the animal retains its educational value for young owners by demonstrating that veterinary treatment does not always prevent death, that vet bills can be eye-wateringly large, and that pet insurance might be considered should future pets be acquired.

18.11 LABORATORY MICE: HISTORY AND INTRINSIC VALUE

In 1903, William Castle of Harvard University published work on murine coat colour genetics which his student, Clarence Little, used to create the first inbred strain of mice. The collaboration of Castle and Little with Abbie Lathrop, a fancy mouse breeder, saw the onset of an exponential growth in the breeding and production of laboratory mice in the early 20th century (Rozenbaum 2022). Thereafter, mice rapidly superseded rabbits, guinea pigs, and dogs as the most popular vertebrate laboratory species because of their genetic similarity to humans, ease of keeping, a brief generation time, and high fecundity. Their availability, size, low cost, and ease of handling were also important. Depending on context, mice are now considered to be the optimum model of hereditary human disease, as they share 95% of their 30,000 genes with humans (see Figure 18.3). Developments in genetic engineering technology mean that genetically modified mice can now be created as required. In future, 'humanised' rodents that carry human genes, cells, tissues, or organs may lead to improved and refined models for developing therapeutics for human disease (Bryda 2013; Rozenbaum 2022).

In 2022, some 900,000 experimental procedures were conducted on mice in the UK. In addition, over 1 million genetically modified animals were created. In the United States (US) the numbers of rats and mice used are not reported because they were explicitly excluded from the US Animal Welfare Act of 1966 as the legislation does not regard them as 'animals' (Department of Agriculture Animal and Plant Health Inspection Service 2016).

Well-maintained specific-pathogen-free animals can live 26 to 30 months, although different strains develop life-limiting conditions which skew this statistic. In the UK, the regulatory authorities tend to request that mice are euthanatised before geriatric health conditions develop (at an approximate age of 15 months). In the UK, most laboratory mice are euthanatised at the end of study (as re-use is

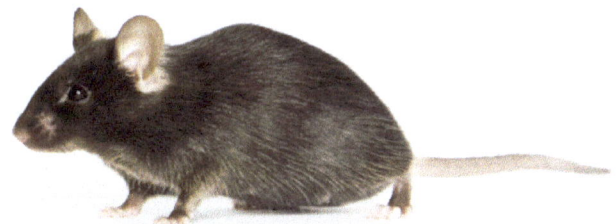

FIGURE 18.3 A laboratory mouse.

discouraged) although the rehoming of suitable animals is increasing throughout the UK, Europe, and the US.

Laboratory mice are unlikely to possess any greater or lesser intrinsic value than their conspecifics living in small cages or under floorboards. Escaped rehomed intact wild-type laboratory mice are unlikely to affect biodiversity should they consort with the natives as they only carry selected traits that are already within the wild mouse population. The ecological effects of GM mice escaping into the wild population is a potentially greater and less frivolous matter; hence, their rehoming is forbidden.

18.12 LABORATORY MICE: EXTRINSIC VALUE

The enormous worldwide economic value of laboratory mice arises from their breeding and sale and the supply of equipment and commodities to provide their basic requirements. The global mouse model market was estimated to be worth $1.5 billion in 2024 and is set to reach $2.2 billion by 2029 (Markets and Markets 2024). Furthermore, laboratory mouse housing manufacture and supply was valued at USD 0.45 billion in 2022 and is predicted to reach USD 1.9 billion by 2030 (Verified Market Research 2024). The value of individual laboratory mice varies considerably and depends on numerous factors. Specific mouse lines are usually preserved as frozen embryos and cost up to $3500 to be recovered and to produce at least two carriers of the desired alleles. One common modified line, the CD21-KO inbred mouse, currently costs approximately $30.

Mice have made a major contribution to biomedical research. Of the 114 Nobel Prizes in Physiology and Medicine between 1901 and 2023, 101 used animals, and of these, the modal species (40) were mice (animalresearch.info 2020). Initially, inbred mice were used to study the biological effects of genetic mutations or environmental influences, e.g. diet, because such effects are obvious in genetically identical animals. Natural mutants from inbred strains emerged which conferred proclivity to obesity, cancer, or immune defects. For example, discovery of the mutation causing severe combined immune deficiency (SCID) in 1983 provided an unprecedented opportunity to examine the immune response. Throughout the 1980s, developments in gene-modifying techniques culminated in 'knockout' mice, which allowed the study of the role of sequenced genes whose functions were unknown. These and related techniques have produced invaluable models of human illnesses ranging from heart disease to cystic fibrosis, Alzheimer's disease, and Parkinson's disease. In addition to providing a better understanding of certain forms of deafness, psychiatric conditions, e.g. depression, vaccination responses to diseases including TB, and the immunological aspects of malaria, mice have provided (non-genetic) diagnostic tools and treatments, e.g. humanised monoclonal antibodies, which are now available as therapies for breast cancer, leukaemia, and arthritis (Medical Research Council 2000).

Strong emotional bonds can develop between laboratory mice and their carers, which accounts for the moral stress (arising from doing tasks which one believes should not be done) and/or emotional dissonance (behaving according to rules or conventions that run counter to what one feels) that affect personnel who simultaneously care for animals whilst recognising the necessity for facilitating scientific outcomes, e.g. killing animals for post-mortem examination (LaFollette et al. 2020). The large-scale euthanasia of laboratory mice as occurs with surplus animals arising from the generation of GM lines or, more significantly, when massive animal depopulation is necessary – as was the case with lockdown during the COVID-19 outbreak – can have major adverse psychological effects on animal care staff (King & Zohny 2022).

The symbolism of mice as laboratory animal representatives is greater amongst the scientific community and bodies supporting animal research, e.g. Understanding Animal Research, than those opposed to it. For example, entering 'Cruelty Free International' into the Google search engine for images reveals that amongst the first 50 images, mice only feature in two, while rabbits appear 53 times. The same exercise using the search term 'laboratory animals' yields 37 mice (and 14 rats). Until recently, the logo of the British Laboratory Animal Veterinary Association showed a set of scales upon which a small laboratory mouse outweighed a human figure (Figure 18.4). The greatest token of appreciation of mice in research is found in the Novosibirsk Institute of Cytology and Genetics of the Russian Academy of Sciences, where a 70 cm bronze statue depicting an elderly female laboratory mouse wearing a pince-nez and knitting a double helix of DNA may be found. The monument commemorates 'the sacrifice of mice in genetic research used to understand biological and physiological mechanisms for developing new drugs and curing diseases'. The statue, pedestal, and surrounding garden cost $50,000 revealing something about the animals' perceived value (Panko 2017).

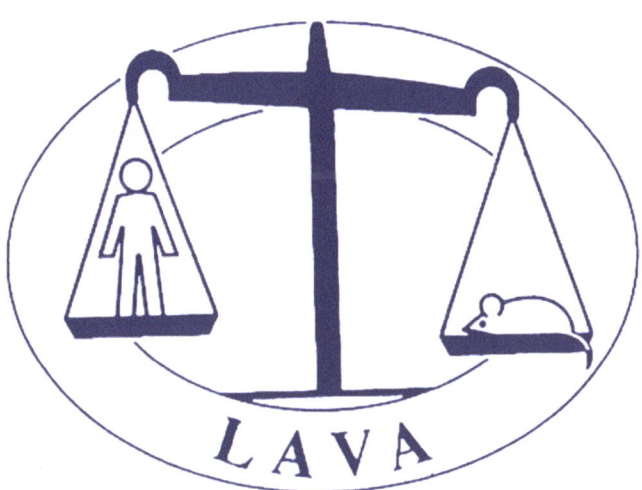

FIGURE 18.4 The former logo of the Laboratory Animals Veterinary Association (used with permission).

Laboratory mice have no conservational importance, while isolation within laboratories, and the non-rehoming policy of GM animals minimises the risks of escapees exerting any ecological effects.

18.13 LABORATORY MICE: LEGAL AND ETHICAL CONSIDERATIONS

The ethical defence of animal use in research rests on the 3Rs principles espoused in 'Principles of Humane Experimental Technique' (Russell & Burch 1959). The Rs refer to replacement, reduction, and refinement, and their combined objective can, in brief, be taken to mean that when scientific goals cannot be achieved using non-animal alternatives (replacement), the fewest number (reduction) of the least sentient animals which are living a life of maximum welfare and minimum suffering (refinement) should be used. The 3Rs principle is globally recognised and adherence to it mandated throughout the scientific process that begins with the application for research funding through ethical study approval and licensing to study prosecution and report publication.

In the UK, animals in research are protected by the Animals (Scientific Procedures) Act 1986 (ASPA 1986). In brief, procedures (defined as scientific interventions that would cause a similar or greater level of pain, suffering, distress, or lasting harm to the animal as the superficial introduction of a hypodermic needle) can only be performed by Home Office (HO)–licensed individuals (with proven competency in the procedures involved) working on HO-licensed projects in a HO licensed laboratory. Project licences are only granted if the study's benefits to people, animals, or the environment are likely to exceed the harms experienced by the animals involved and where alternatives don't exist. This harm-benefit ratio is established by a mandatory ethical and scientific review process undertaken by an institutional animal welfare and ethical review board (AWERB). For each study, AWERBs approve established humane endpoints (HEPs) which are clear criteria that trigger the termination of a procedure before an animal experiences harm that is not authorised or scientifically justified. The welfare of laboratory mice is the prescribed and legal responsibility of all licence holders but, within the laboratory, is assured on a day-to-day basis by designated named animal care and welfare officers (NACWOs). The overall health and welfare of all mice within a given establishment is the responsibility of the named veterinary surgeon (NVS).

18.14 LABORATORY MICE AND VETERINARY CARE

The anticipated harms of any study must be specified on the project licence application which requires approval before the study can proceed. Once animals are on study, any expected harms exceeding HEPs, or unexpected complications, will trigger the animal's immediate and humane termination. Each mouse scheduled to go on study will have a custom care plan, monitoring sheet, and humane endpoint agreed beforehand, while a full health check, including body condition scoring, will be carried out on all animals to ensure they meet the study's inclusion criteria.

Testing substances for tumourigenicity is commonly performed on NUDE mice, a mildly immunocompromised strain. Therefore, their diet will be irradiated, and their water will be treated to remove bacteria and fungi. Initially, their daily assessment (as required by the HO) will include food and water intake levels. Typically, mice will be bedded on chipped aspen or corn cob. All cages will contain nesting material (typically cotton pads, paper-based products, or some combination) for thermoregulation and to meet the murine obsession with nest-building.

The study itself will involve a small volume of test compound being injected under the flank skin. Thereafter, the mouse will be body condition scored and undergo general health assessment weekly. Assessment findings will be scored objectively, and the results recorded on a health record. The absolute score and trend will determine the proximity of HEPs. During examination, mice will be restrained using cupped hands or tunnels because picking up mice by the tail induces aversion and high anxiety so is now condemned (Gouveia & Hurst 2019).

As the tumour grows, the mouse will receive support to ease discomfort, e.g. analgesics, additional softer bedding, and soft palatable food within easy access. Once the lesion is clearly apparent, assessment frequency will increase. If the tumour location affects ambulation or the tumour begins to show surface abrasion, the animal will be terminated using methods prescribed in Schedule 1 of ASPA (1986). The method chosen will be carried out by someone who has been assessed as competent to use the prescribed technique on mice. The decision to kill the mouse will be taken by the animal care staff in conjunction with a NACWO or an NVS. When a mouse is to be humanely killed, it is first moved to a separate room to avoid stressing remaining pen-mates (NC3Rs 2017).

18.15 CONCLUSION

In the UK, the AWA 2006 recognises the equivalent intrinsic value of laboratory, pet, and wild mice and protects them all equally, although this is of little practical significance in veterinary medical terms. The ASPA (1986) affords considerably more protection to laboratory mice, whose welfare is optimised, irrespective of experimental conditions, by NACWOs and NVSs with extensive experience in murine matters, including pain recognition and treatment. Once tumours develop in laboratory mice, they will be detected promptly, and the animal terminated once HEPs are reached. For the rest of their brief lives, laboratory mice will receive veterinary care whenever it is needed, and in the UK, most will be killed before diseases of advanced age become apparent. In contrast, a pet mouse with large tumours is unlikely to receive similar standards of care, although much depends on the vagaries of the owner and whether veterinary treatment is sought. If referred, vets with varying degrees of mouse experience may elect to surgically remove the lesions, but given the animal's low extrinsic value, the pet mouse is unlikely to receive the same suite of care, i.e. imaging, surgery, and follow-up chemotherapy, that a dog or cat with similar lesions might receive. While ethically challengeable, this option is probably in the animal's interests because a strong case can be made for tumorous mice (and many dogs and cats) to forego treatment and live a relatively peaceful life until the tumour's growth adversely affects their welfare and demands euthanasia. Free-ranging mice? Alas, unless killed beforehand by predators, those with terminal metastatic disease are likely to die slow and painful deaths. Yet despite this unpleasant certainty, the intrinsic value of the wild mouse remains recognised, clear, and incontestable – immortalised in Burn's second verse:

I'm truly sorry Man's dominion
Has broken Nature's social union,
An' justifies that ill opinion,
Which makes thee startle,
At me, thy poor, earth-born companion,
An' fellow-mortal!

REFERENCES

Animal Welfare Act 2006. *The National Archives* [Internet]. Up to date 2024 Sept 10. Available from: https://www.legislation.gov.uk/ukpga/2006/45/contents.

animalresearch.info. Nobel prizes. *animalresearch.info Medical Advances* [Internet]. 2020 Oct 1. Available from: https://www.animalresearch.info/en/medical-advances/nobel-prizes/.

Animals (Scientific Procedures) Act 1986. *The National Archives* [Internet]. Up to date 2024 Sept 10. Available from: https://www.legislation.gov.uk/ukpga/1986/14/contents.

Brown PR, Henry S. Impacts of house mice on sustainable fodder storage in Australia. *Agronomy*. 2022;12(2):254.

Bryda EC. The mighty mouse: the impact of rodents on advances in biomedical research. *Mo Med*. 2013;110(3):207–211.

Department of Agriculture Animal and Plant Health Inspection Service. Thresholds for de minimus activity and exemptions from licensing under the Animal Welfare Act. *Federal Register* [Internet]. 2016 Aug 4. Available from: https://www.federalregister.gov/documents/2016/08/04/2016-18452/thresholds-for-de-minimis-activity-and-exemptions-from-licensing-under-the-animal-welfare-act.

Gouveia K, Hurst JL. Improving the practicality of using non-aversive handling methods to reduce background stress and anxiety in laboratory mice. *Sci Rep*. 2019;9(1):20305.

King M, Zohny H. Animal researchers shoulder a psychological burden that animal ethics committees ought to address. *J Med Ethics*. 2022;48(5):299–303.

Laboratory mouse housing cage market size and forecast. *Verified Market Research* [Internet]. 2024 Feb. Available from: https://www.verifiedmarketresearch.com/product/laboratory-mouse-housing-cage-market/#:~:text=What%20is%20the%20projected%20market,4.8%25%20from%202023%20to%202030.

LaFollette MR, Riley MC, Cloutier S, et al. Laboratory animal welfare meets human welfare: a cross-sectional study of professional quality of life, including compassion fatigue in laboratory animal personnel. *Front Vet Sci*. 2020;7:114.

Marshall-Pescini S, Schaebs FS, Gaugg A, et al. The role of oxytocin in the dog-owner relationship. *Animals (Basel)*. 2019;9(10):792.

Medical Research Council. Mice and medicine: animal experiments, medical advances and the MRC. *UK Research and Innovation* [Internet]. 2000 Jul. Available from: https://www.ukri.org/wp-content/uploads/2021/08/MRC-0208212-Mice-and-Medicine.pdf.

Mice Model Market. *Markets and Markets* [Internet]. 2024 Feb. Available from: https://www.marketsandmarkets.com/Market-Reports/mice-model-market-1308.html#:~:text=The%20global%20mice%20model%20market,trend%20analysis%20of%20the%20market.

Milchevskaya V, Bugnon P, ten Buren EBJ, et al. Group size planning for breedings of gene-modified mice and other organisms following Mendelian inheritance. *Lab Animal*. 2023;52(8):183–188.

NC3Rs. Euthanasia. *NC3Rs Resource Library* [Internet]. 2017 Apr 1. Available from: https://nc3rs.org.uk/3rs-resources/euthanasia.

Nuffield Council on Bioethics. The ethics of research involving animals. *Nuffield Council on Bioethics* [Internet]. 2005 May. Available from: https://www.nuffieldbioethics.org/assets/pdfs/The-ethics-of-research-involving-animals-full-report.pdf.

Panko B. This Russian monument honors the humble lab mouse. *Smithsonian Magazine* [Internet]. 2017 Aug 2017. Available from: https://www.smithsonianmag.com/smart-news/russian-statue-honoring-laboratory-mice-gains-renewed-popularity-180964570/.

Pet Animals Act 1951 (Amendment) Act 1983. *The National Archives* [Internet]. Undated [cited 2024 Apr 23]. Available from: https://www.legislation.gov.uk/ukpga/1983/26/contents.

Rozenbaum M. A history of mice in scientific research. *Understanding Animal Research* [Internet]. 2022 Jul 7. Available from: https://www.understandinganimalresearch.org.uk/news/a-history-of-mice-in-scientific-research.

Russell WMS, Burch RL. *The principles of humane experimental technique*. London: Methuen & Co. Ltd; 1959.

Wildlife and Countryside Act 1981. *The National Archives* [Internet]. Up to date 2024 Sept 10. Available from: https://www.legislation.gov.uk/ukpga/1981/69.

Part III

Why Are These Controversies Arising Through Changes at Numerous Levels of the Veterinary–Client–Patient Relationship?

The Animal Population

19 Problems with Pedigrees

Righteous Rage and the Need for Nuance

Alison Skipper

19.1 INTRODUCTION

When veterinary professionals discuss pedigree dog breeding together, they seldom seem to say anything positive. It's easy to see why. Those toiling at the coalface of clinical practice encounter a seemingly endless succession of patients with painful, debilitating diseases that are directly linked to their body shapes and which could therefore have been entirely avoided with a different set of aesthetic priorities. The breeder is too often a shadowed bogey in the consulting room, invoked by puppy buyers to justify adherence to a bizarre diet or inaccurate medical advice. Many campaigners dismiss the various national kennel clubs that regulate pedigree dog breeding, such as the Royal Kennel Club (RKC) in the UK (recently given 'Royal' status to mark its 150th anniversary), as arcane and reactionary self-serving institutions that ignore modern science. And dog shows – which drove the original creation of the pedigree dog – are a niche activity nowadays, largely invisible to outsiders, except when a social media storm follows a noteworthy incident at a high-profile event such as the RKC's Crufts, the largest dog show in the world. No wonder, then, that, insofar as overworked veterinary staff even think about pedigree dog breeding, they tend to view it with bemusement, distaste, or outright contempt.

19.2 BACKGROUND

What is a pedigree dog, anyway? Strictly speaking, a pedigree is just the written record of an individual's ancestry: write that down, and it's a dog with a pedigree. But the term now usually describes dogs that are registered with an official organisation such as the RKC. Each kennel club defines every breed in two ways: through its physical appearance, as described in an official breed standard, and by a breed register. This lists all dogs of each breed and is generally restricted to those whose parents were also registered (a 'closed registry' system). However, both breed standards and closed breed registries are potential causes of ill health. Isolating each breed as a separate gene pool inevitably reduces genetic diversity and can increase the risk of inherited disease. These problems can be exacerbated when breeders use 'popular sires' or deliberately breed from closely related dogs, which happens quite often. And while many breed standards are unproblematic, some traditionally call for physical features, such as short legs, flat faces, excess skin, or heavy coat, which can be so exaggerated through selective breeding that they affect welfare. These attributes may be rewarded in the show ring, despite increasing evidence that dogs with extreme conformation often have serious associated health issues and sometimes shortened lives.

19.3 THE CONTROVERSY

From this perspective, it's unsurprising that many critics of pedigree dog breeding are deeply frustrated by the ongoing perpetuation of what they see as a blindingly obvious and easily avoidable set of problems. They neither know nor care about the arcane practices of the dog show world, which are so dear to its aficionados. Campaigners' arguments range through a spectrum: that health should be prioritised above looks, that breeding regulations should be changed, that certain breeds should be banned, that dog shows should be abolished, that pedigree breeding should be banned, or even that there should be no human control of canine reproduction or canine lives at all. Dan O'Neill (my former boss, incidentally), a leader of the International Collaborative on Extreme Conformations in Dogs (ICECDogs) initiative to promote the breeding of dogs with good 'innate health' (ICECDogs 2024) – bodies that don't impair the quality of their lives – recently suggested that, if dogs were not selectively bred within different breed populations, future generations would all revert back to a generic street-dog-like appearance with no physical exaggeration – a 'Goldilocks' dog (because it's 'just right') (Chadwick 2024). To opponents of pedigree dog breeding, this might be nirvana: to its proponents, it's anathema.

Nevertheless, there's no denying the toxic paradox that human preferences have driven the production of many dogs whose welfare is directly compromised by the design of their own bodies. Moreover, critics have been denouncing these practices for a very long time. 'The tendency in every fancy is to develop certain points and peculiarities to excess, and we have our reward in weak constitutions, and tendencies to some sort of specific disease', wrote one journalist of the early show scene, in 1889 (Dalziel 1889, 423). It is both surprising and depressing to discover that some Victorian dogs were already suffering from breed-related diseases and that the underlying human causes of these biological problems were recognised even then. If the issue is obvious and the solution clearly under human control – just stop breeding unhealthy dogs – then why has this been continuing for well over a century? It's not for lack of awareness: this essay's title comes from a 1980 veterinary editorial (Anon 1980), one of many interventionist campaigns over the last 60 years, all seeking to solve these issues (Skipper 2021). The answer, of course, is that this problem is so difficult to address precisely *because* it's ultimately a human problem, not a canine one. Canine bodies are simply the battlefield where this conflict between aesthetics and functionality takes place. This is a 'wicked problem', where complex multiple factors drive the views and opinions of different stakeholders with incompatible perspectives (Rittel & Webber 1973). It remains intractable for that reason, despite the plethora of recent research, campaigning and legislation intended to deal with this issue.

19.4 PATHWAYS TO PROGRESS?

Faced with this frustrating tangle, it's easy to take a reductive approach, arguing that 'crossbreds are healthier'. Of course, it is sadly true that some pedigree dogs – especially some of the brachycephalics – experience poor health and reduced lifespans (O'Neill et al. 2020). But breeds vary in their longevity and health, influenced by other confounding factors, such as body size and inbreeding. Some breeds have longer lifespans than crossbreeds; others, shorter (McMillan et al. 2024). Moreover, assumptions can be misplaced. For instance, pedigree breeders tend to condemn designer crossbreeds as less healthy than their pedigree parent breeds, while veterinarians might assume the reverse – yet, fascinatingly, a recent study did not identify any meaningful overall difference in health between these groups (Bryson et al. 2024). How many of our expectations about canine health are similarly shaped by prejudice rather than evidence? Lumping all pedigree dogs together as 'unhealthy' is too simplistic. Highlighting specific points of concern – this breed is too exaggerated, or those breeders are ignoring a major health problem – draws attention to troubling practices without alienating other breeders who aren't involved and who may indeed agree. And a targeted criticism is harder to refute.

Similarly, campaigners for better dog breeding often direct wholesale criticism at national kennel clubs, arguing that their customs perpetuate breed-related disease and that they don't do enough to drive change. Most kennel clubs certainly could be more proactive. However, I have always felt that it's more productive to support existing governance in pedigree dog health to improve than to bypass it. These organisations have significant potential power to improve breeding practices – for example, the RKC registers about one-third of the dogs bred in the UK. Kennel clubs in various countries already revise breed standards, fund health research, develop health testing schemes, control permitted breeding, and maintain health-testing databases. They can introduce controls to reduce inbreeding. They can apply pressure to reduce extreme conformation through internal initiatives. Some forward-thinking organisations are even rethinking closed breed registries: for example, the Norwegian Kennel Club has led an outcrossing programme for the genetically vulnerable Norwegian Lundehund (Melis et al. 2022), and similar projects are likely elsewhere. I've been involved in various aspects of RKC health work, from committees to vetting at Crufts, for over a decade, and have observed significant progress during that time: change does happen, albeit sometimes slowly. Yet some activists almost seem disappointed when the pedigree sector introduces a new health initiative, as if reluctant to admit that the 'enemy' could ever do anything positive.

Dog shows are frequently depicted as a negative influence on pedigree dogs, and it's certainly true that closed breed registers and show ring preferences have historically been a major driver of the breed-related diseases that we see today. But it's not a simple story. Human nature being what it is, public commentary tends to skew negative: exhibitors of healthy dogs with moderate body shapes tend to get on with it under the radar. For good reason, critics focus instead on the breeds with the most extreme conformation, with frequent calls to change the wording of their breed standards. Undoubtedly, this was originally much needed. For example, the first (English) Bulldog breed standard called for a 'strikingly massive' head ('the larger the better'), an 'extremely short' face, and 'much loose, thick and wrinkled skin' (Dalziel 1889, 88–89). These features would clearly predispose to respiratory difficulty and dystocia, as late Victorian Bulldog breeders already realised.

However, the RKC and many other international kennel clubs have significantly revised this and many other breed standards over recent decades so that the current wording heavily emphasises moderation. Some campaigners seem to be unaware of this shift, which is counterproductive, because a rallying call that focuses primarily on breed standards is misdirected if they are no longer the most pressing problem. If show ring judges ignore revised breed standards, then further change to standards won't help: it's the judges who need to change instead. But it can be tricky to police judging decisions effectively. Therefore, the RKC introduced show veterinary checks in certain breeds (for clinical signs of conformation-related disease), which in some breeds has encouraged judges to change their priorities, successfully driving a cultural shift away from the most extreme conformation. These improvements can quickly vanish if restrictions are eased, so there's no room for complacency, but it does suggest that shows can act as a positive lever for change. In the UK, the most extreme Bulldogs are now seen not in the show ring but on social media platforms – a world where breed standards are irrelevant anyway.

Inevitably, this progress is too limited for many frustrated campaigners, who in several European countries have worked to implement new legislation intended to ban or drastically alter various breeds affected by conformation-related disease. But most legislation is only effective with stringent enforcement; otherwise, only the law-abiding comply. Issue-specific legislation may become outdated as science and society move on: conversely, legislation that is vaguely worded will have little impact. And, all too often, legislation that is intended to tackle wicked problems turns out to drive unexpected and often unwelcome consequences as well as intended outcomes. For all these reasons, I don't think that breed-specific legislation is an easy answer to the problems of pedigree dog health, although I understand its appeal.

19.5 BOTHERSOME BREEDERS

Recently, at least in the UK, stakeholders in pedigree dog health have begun to explore human behavioural change interventions, recognising that this is essentially a human problem. Almost nobody deliberately breeds dogs with the intention of causing them misery, but many people are reluctant to accept that their breeding aims might need revision to improve canine welfare. Why are people so attached to such breeding practices, despite the external criticism they trigger and the considerable evidence of the problems they too often cause? Fundamentally, this is because many people in the pedigree dog world have their own worldview. As with any special interest groups, be they political parties or online fandoms, breed communities can provide their members with friendship, a sense of purpose, a shared value system, and a body of knowledge which take years to master and is impenetrable to outsiders. These powerful social paradigms act as significant barriers to change. Moreover, breed communities can also be surprisingly insular, with those involved in one breed sometimes having little awareness of health problems in others. Group identities can have positive or negative impacts on engagement with canine health and welfare because breed community cultures vary enormously in their willingness to engage with breed-related disease, in their transparency around health testing, and even in acknowledging whether exaggeration that they consider a noteworthy feature or 'normal for the breed' could have any adverse consequences.

Nevertheless, it's important to remember that it's breeders who actually breed the dogs and who therefore choose the next generation. Those of us who talk about better breeding instead of doing it will only make a difference if we alter the behaviour of those who breed, either directly or by influencing puppy buyers. Breed clubs and communities may not always welcome change, but they are networks through which conversations can be started. The history of this conflict clearly shows that past progress in pedigree dog health – for example, the introduction of screening for hip dysplasia and inherited eye diseases, or the recently introduced Kennel Club/University of Cambridge respiratory function grading scheme (RFGS) for brachycephalic obstructive airway syndrome (BOAS) (Ladlow 2021) – has always involved discussion and collaboration between veterinary or scientific experts and breed communities. Through acquiring knowledge, breeders have gradually shifted their views and adopted new practices. A breed community with strong leadership and a supportive culture can make enormous collaborative efforts to engage with health problems once convinced of the need to address them, and can identify and overcome key barriers to intervention, thus further accelerating progress, sometimes with transformative results.

Yet, ironically, constructive dialogue about pedigree dog health is often hampered by partisanship and prejudice, which entrenches and exacerbates the divisions between stakeholders. We live in a polarised society. Thirty years ago, early adopters of the Internet were so few that those of us who shared a niche interest were inevitably brought together on a single discussion list or board, making connections across national and factional boundaries, and often reaching new understandings of contentious issues in the process. But those times have gone. Today, social media algorithms funnel us into echo chambers with our own kind – a particular problem when the issue is controversial or political because online affirmation too often encourages a sort of blinkered self-righteousness that impedes effective engagement with the very people we want to influence.

Consequently, online veterinary groups frequently default to an indiscriminate condescension towards the pedigree dog world, which is generally unhelpful and sometimes entirely undeserved. Participants deride the breeder as inherently ignorant and stupid. But people who breed pedigree dogs span the whole of society, ranging from hardened criminals to the late Queen Elizabeth II. Some recalcitrant or dishonest breeders can be nightmares to deal with; others bring the vet cake. Critics often claim that 'they're all in it for the money', but this clearly isn't true; while there obviously are many commercial breeders, some of whom are undoubtedly problematic, there are also many people who breed dogs entirely as a loss-making hobby. Some breeders couldn't care less what a dog looks like; for others, appearance is everything. There are highly responsible people (including some veterinary professionals) who put huge amounts of effort into breeding healthy dogs, there are many who pay lip service to health matters, and there are others who neither know nor care about any health considerations whatsoever. Yet blanket judgemental statements about breeders lump all these people together rather than thinking critically about whether they are actually a homogenous group.

19.6 VETERINARY RE-EVALUATION?

Thinking in stereotypes is tempting but lazy. It's inevitable that many busy veterinary professionals at the coalface of general practice simply don't know, or want to know, much about the technicalities of pedigree dog breeding. Consequently, however, an experienced breeder has probably seen more normal whelpings than the clinician and may well know more about the specific health problems of their own breed. Veterinary authority is not threatened by acknowledging that some breeders are also knowledgeable. Yet the veterinary pendulum has currently swung so far towards criticism and contempt of all things breeder-related that some veterinarians seem automatically to approach all breeders in a spirit of antagonistic superiority. Unsurprisingly, breeders – being human – are (like vets!) generally reluctant to engage with people who are overtly hostile or who belittle their expertise, and so these encounters often end badly for both the people and the animals involved. This is a real pity, because where individual vets and breeders overcome their mutual suspicion and build a good working relationship, both sides can benefit. It's a loss for animal welfare that current attitudes and working practices often make this so difficult.

As a veterinarian with longstanding involvement in pedigree dog health, I think of myself as a communicator working in the liminal space between the veterinary and pedigree dog communities, trying to promote dialogue and understanding between them. In the current climate, this position can be lonely. I respect hardline campaigners for their passion for animal welfare. Robust criticism of breeding practices is often justified, and hard-hitting campaigns to increase awareness of issues such as brachycephalic disease undoubtedly have great value. But I find it very troubling when veterinary professionals become so committed to an ethical agenda that they prioritise ideology over individuals. For example, many veterinary campaigners believe that dogs with brachycephaly should not exist. Some consequently argue that veterinary involvement with these dogs should be confined to the relief of suffering, so it's acceptable to carry out an emergency caesarean or to surgically relieve respiratory distress, but unacceptable to perform an elective section or respiratory health testing. While I obviously deplore conformation that predisposes to dystocia or dyspnoea, I'm concerned that such attitudes override the contextualised care appropriate to each patient: does a pregnant bitch suffer unnecessarily if she is then transported much further to see a vet? Similarly, I understand why some veterinarians feel that engaging with health initiatives such as respiratory function testing legitimises brachycephalic breeding. But I disagree. These dogs exist, and BOAS has a major impact on their welfare. The RKC/University of Cambridge RFGS provides breeders with a practical way to identify breeding dogs that are less severely affected. As this tool has become more widely used by UK show breeders, their views have changed. Little by little, through hundreds of conversations at respiratory checks and with their friends, these breeders are increasingly regarding noisy breathing as unacceptable, rather than as an inevitable side effect of brachycephalic life. This sort of cultural shift takes time, but it progressively makes a real difference to actual dogs. How can anyone who cares about canine welfare think that's a bad thing, no matter how much they disapprove of brachycephalic breeding?

These issues have such complicated ramifications. Indisputably, exploitative breeding that compromises animal welfare is ethically wrong. But, given that there is always going to be a demand for companion dogs that cannot, for various reasons, be met from rescue alone, a substantial puppy trade of some sort is inevitable. Anti-pedigree campaigning has encouraged a shift towards 'designer' crossbreds, whose owners often choose them precisely because they think they will be healthier than a pedigree dog. But, with little regulatory oversight and a high commercial demand, such dogs are often bred in low-welfare facilities: many purchasers would be horrified to see the supply chain behind their fluffy doodle puppy. Other people, following the mantra of 'adopt, don't shop', increasingly end up negotiating the murky waters of international rescue. Although some dogs reach happy homes through these channels, low-welfare breeding for the rescue market, rehoming of street dogs unsuited to household life, problematic transportation and the importation of serious zoonotic diseases are all well-documented issues with this growing sector. So the alternatives to the pedigree dog trade have their own problems, as experts in the field are increasingly realising. We somehow need to find a way of supporting a supply of ethically bred dogs to satisfy the evident demand. Simply attacking the pedigree dog sector because of what it does badly, no matter how justified, does not solve this problem.

19.7 CONCLUSION

The word 'eugenics' is a verbal missile that's often deployed in the pedigree dog breeding debate, reflecting the strength of feeling on all sides. When animal rights activists denounce pedigree dog breeding as 'canine eugenics', they mean that people are deliberately breeding unhealthy or deformed animals. Intentionally emotive, this terminology is unhelpfully confusing, because it's describing the exact opposite of what human eugenics was intended to achieve. The concept of eugenics was created by the British Victorian, Francis Galton (Gillham 2001). It was disseminated and enacted around the world in the early 20th century, at all levels from newspaper columns to genocide, by people who thought that manipulating the reproduction of human populations (both by encouraging the 'good' and by preventing the 'bad') to 'improve' future generations was a worthwhile thing to do that would advance the interests of humanity. Of course, we now consider human eugenics abhorrent, both because of its racist and ableist perceptions of what constitute 'better people' and because we believe that manipulating human reproduction is morally wrong anyway (other than to help individual couples, with informed consent, who are trying to conceive a healthy child). But animals are not people. Most of us don't think that deliberately trying to breed healthier dogs is bad; that's exactly what we think should happen. Campaigners for healthier pedigree dogs are therefore actually advocating *for* canine eugenics, if you think about it.

I end with this rather sensationalist point to emphasise that so much of the debate around pedigree dog health is shaped by understandable emotion rather than by critical thinking. Consider all the pedigree dogs that we don't talk about, because there's nothing wrong with them: when breeds aren't a problem, what's the problem? If pedigree breeding practices were altered to holistically prioritise health and welfare, then any ongoing objection to them would be rooted in prejudice, not evidence. What's wrong with breeding dogs that you consider beautiful, or that suit your lifestyle, as long as they are also bred to be healthy? While the average dog owner may not care about the fine details of their pet's lineage, most people surely like to have a rough idea of the eventual size, temperament, and physical characteristics they can expect from their new family member. At its best, this is exactly what the pedigree dog world can offer, providing carefully reared puppies with predictable characteristics and experienced post-sales mentorship to support new owners, optimising both animal welfare and human satisfaction. There will always be disagreement about what 'good breeding' entails, and of course, this is to some extent a utopian dream. But there are already some breed communities which absolutely do prioritise health. They deserve support and encouragement. Condemning a whole sector without critical appraisal and nuanced analysis feeds entrenched division and hostility; it doesn't promote meaningful engagement that leads to change. We can do better than that, and we should.

REFERENCES

Anon. Problems with pedigrees. *Vet Rec.* 1980;107:1.
Bryson GT, O'Neill DG, Brand CL, et al. The doodle dilemma: how the physical health of 'designer-crossbreed' Cockapoo, Labradoodle and Cavapoo dogs' compares to their purebred progenitor breeds. *PLoS One.* 2024;19(8):e0306350.

Chadwick J. Meet Goldilocks, the breedless dog of the future. *Daily Mail Online* [Internet]. 2024 Apr 6. Available from: https://www.dailymail.co.uk/sciencetech/article-13268285/breedless-dog-merge-humans.html.

Dalziel H. *British dogs: describing the history, characteristics, breeding, management and exhibition of the various breeds of dogs established in Great Britain.* Vol. 2. London: L. Upcott Gill, 1889.

Gillham NW. Sir Francis Galton and the birth of eugenics. *Annu Rev Genet.* 2001;35(1):83–101.

International Collaborative on Extreme Conformations in Dogs (ICECDogs). First ever international agreement on what are naturally healthy bodyshapes for dogs. *ICECDogs Press Releases* [Internet]. 2024 Apr 9. Available from: https://www.icecdogs.com/home/press-releases.

Ladlow J. Brachycephalic obstructive airway syndrome: guide to the respiratory functional grading scheme. *In Pract.* 2021;43(10):548–555.

McMillan KM, Bielby J, Williams CL, et al. Longevity of companion dog breeds: those at risk from early death. *Sci Rep.* 2024;14(1):531.

Melis C, Pertoldi C, Ludington WB, et al. Genetic rescue of the highly inbred Norwegian Lundehund. *Genes (Basel).* 2022;13(1):163.

O'Neill DG, Pegram C, Crocker P, et al. Unravelling the health status of brachycephalic dogs in the UK using multivariable analysis. *Sci Rep.* 2020;10(1):17251.

Rittel HWJ, Webber MM. Dilemmas in a general theory of planning. *Policy Sci.* 1973;4(2):155–169.

Skipper A. A historical perspective on brachycephalic breed health and the role of the veterinary profession. In: Packer RMA, O'Neill DG, editors. *Health and welfare of brachycephalic (flat-faced) companion animals.* Abingdon: CRC Press Taylor & Francis Group; 2021. p. 7–24.

20 Ageing Pets and Physical Rehabilitation

Mary Ellen Goldberg, Sheilah Robertson, and Polly Taylor

20.1 INTRODUCTION

Jack was a German shepherd crossbreed who lived with his owner from the age of nine months. He had enjoyed a long and active life, but as he grew old, he developed a variety of age-related conditions, and by the time he was 18 years old he had osteoarthritis, lipomas, cataracts and was almost deaf. He had not lost weight; his appetite was good and he could still navigate around his home including the stairs. However, he developed urinary incontinence, necessitating sheets to be placed around the house. Yoga mats were put in the kitchen and on other slippery surfaces to provide better traction so he could still navigate the home without falling over. Soon, both his mobility and his appetite deteriorated. When he would no longer eat home cooked food and could not get up without assistance, his owner opted for euthanasia at home: a happy life and a peaceful, stress-free end.

Since the early part of the 20th century, human life expectancy has increased dramatically and the same now applies to companion animals. This is generally considered to be due to improvements in hygiene, nutrition, and medical care. The consequences of a longer life are that an ever-increasing proportion of both the human and pet population are geriatric (McKenzie et al. 2022). There are numerous unpleasant health conditions associated with ageing, and these must be managed appropriately to ensure a good quality of life (QOL).

20.2 PHYSIOLOGY OF AGEING

In spite of medical progress, the ageing process is accompanied by characteristics, diseases and conditions which adversely affect daily life – the process of becoming geriatric. The term 'geriatric' is a statement of health status rather than chronological age (McKenzie et al. 2022). It includes physical and behavioural changes as well as increased caregiver burden. The main clinical characteristics of this process are the physical effects of muscle atrophy, degenerative joint disease and decreased proprioception, along with systemic problems, including reduced exercise tolerance, obesity, loss of sensory acuity, and neoplasia (Bellows et al. 2015, 2016).

Impaired cardiac contractility and decreased functional reserve, along with a number of specific cardiac abnormalities may contribute to poor cardiac function. Ageing impairs pulmonary function and, coupled with the cardiovascular changes, reduces the desire for exercise. For dogs in particular, this may seriously affect their QOL. What is life to an old Labrador who cannot swim or fetch their ball?

Intestinal malabsorption, altered drug metabolism and elimination, reduced ability to combat infection (immunosenescence), resistant urinary tract infections, decubital ulcers, blindness and deafness often accompany the ageing process. It is not uncommon for geriatric dogs to have cataracts causing blindness.

Many old cats have chronic kidney disease (Marino et al. 2014). Intact male dogs may have prostatic enlargement and urinary incontinence is common in spayed females (VetCompass 2019). Decreased renal glomerular filtration rate and tubular function may lead to electrolyte imbalances, increased urination and altered drug excretion. Urinary incontinence has a range of consequences – for both animal and owner. Keeping an incontinent dog or cat leads to problems of cleanliness, excoriated skin, and worse still, the potential for animal-owner/animal-carer relationships to break down: the pet may be distressed with soiling itself or its bed and the owner frustrated with the constant need for cleaning.

Changes in liver function may influence drug pharmacokinetics. This may affect analgesic dosing for chronic pain, and altered pharmacodynamics may necessitate revising the dose and the dosing intervals to provide effective treatment without adverse side effects. Non-pharmacological strategies, such as modifications to the living environment, may provide additional management of pain and poor mobility (Monteiro et al. 2023).

A number of neurological changes contribute to a geriatric state. Loss of fine motor control, decreased proprioception, poor balance and coordination, alteration and slowing of the gait, and decreased reaction times all develop in old age. The brain shrinks, with decreased blood flow, neuronal connections and neurotransmitter production, leading to decreased adaptability. Sensory perception and thermal regulation may be impaired. Geriatric dogs and cats commonly have a degree of cognitive dysfunction.

Muscle mass and strength decrease with old age (sarcopenia), leading to stiffness, loss of function and change in gait. Cats may lose the ability to retract their claws. Old dog and cat skin loses its elasticity making it easily damaged, and wound healing is slower. Calluses, skin tumours and ulceration may develop. The term 'frailty' has been used in relation to age-related deterioration in the musculoskeletal system and appears to be a risk factor for death in dogs (Hua et al. 2016). Frailty is a multisystem impairment associated with increased vulnerability to stressors and describes individuals that are at increased risk of poor health, comorbidity, disability and death.

Overall, the geriatric changes that occur with old age impair the QOL of the ageing dog and cat. Physical rehabilitation (rehab) has often been proposed to improve the QOL of such pets (Pease 2024), and a number of texts are available describing a range of methods and programs which can be applied to old animals

(Goldberg & Tomlinson 2024). Any program, for instance, to improve muscle strength, must in itself improve QOL – not simply produce a purely physical benefit sometime in the future. A rehab program must be pleasant for the animal as well as being physically beneficial in the longer term. Fortunately, many older animals appear to enjoy rehab; however, this is not always the case, and a dog (or cat) cannot understand that there may be future benefit from a current experience it is finding unpleasant. Imposing subjective human perception onto animals is a common human failure.

20.3   QUALITY OF LIFE

Most diseases associated with ageing are not pleasant and cause substantial decline in the QOL. However, old animals deserve a good life just as much as younger pets. As veterinary surgeons and animal carers, it is our duty to make that life worth living. From a caregiver perspective, the question whether that life is worth living hinges around perceived QOL, mobility, pain, faecal and urinary incontinence, appetite and maintenance of the animals' interaction in the household.

QOL does not have a universally consistent or accepted definition. The World Health Organization defines QOL as the perception of an individual's position in life in the context of the culture and value systems in which they live and in relation to their goals, expectations, standards, and concerns (Wiseman-Orr 2006). The International Association of Animal Hospice and Palliative Care (IAAHPC) defines QOL as 'how well or poorly an animal is doing, considering the totality of an animal's feelings, experiences, and preferences, as demonstrated by the animal' (IAAHPC 2022). QOL is far more important than longevity (Belshaw et al. 2015).

Assessment of QOL is potentially entirely subjective, and it is essential to use tools to keep track of a slow decline and to set a point beyond which QOL is inadequate for that life to be worth living. There are many QOL tools available, and disease-specific versions are particularly valuable for animals with certain diseases, such as diabetes, cardiac disease, hyperthyroidism, osteoarthritis, or Cushing's syndrome.

All means of assessing QOL are involved in the process of deciding that the animal's life is not worth living and euthanasia is now the best option for the pet. The owner's ability to care for their pet inevitably has a considerable effect on this decision. The four caregiver budgets (finances, emotional, physical, and time) come into play. For instance, a very busy family or an owner who works long hours away from home may not have the time to devote to supplying the ageing pet's increased needs; a geriatric or disabled owner may not have the strength to lift a large pet.

20.4   PHYSICAL REHABILITATION FOR AGEING ANIMALS

Physical rehabilitation is widely believed to contribute substantially to maintaining a good QOL – a 'life worth living' – in the pet faced with the numerous unpleasant effects of old age. Most experience of this is in dogs, although universal evidence of benefit is hard to establish. Such rehabilitation is based around three aspects: managing pain, improving mobility and adjusting the home environment to enable the pet to carry out the activities of daily living (Goldberg & Tomlinson 2024).

Evidence from human geriatric care has shown that regular physical training, and particularly multicomponent training (MCT) has many health benefits. MCT includes endurance training, muscle strengthening, balance exercises, stretching (flexibility training) and coordination training. Reduced mobility is an independent risk factor for morbidity, hospitalisation, disability, and mortality. Health benefits of rehabilitation include better oxygen transport and oxygen capacity, reduction in osteoporosis, lower blood pressure, improved respiratory capacity, improved joint mobility, less anxiety and enriched social interaction. How much this human experience relates to dogs, cats, and horses is largely unknown. However, programs based on tools used in human physiotherapy are applied to dogs. For instance, functional mobility assessment, evaluating posture, attitude and function, is used to provide a foundation for canine exercise or other treatment programs.

20.4.1 Pain Management

Chronic pain is often a feature of the geriatric pet and is most commonly a result of osteoarthritis (OA). It is best monitored using a validated pain scale (Gruen et al. 2022; Monteiro et al. 2023).

Nonsteroidal anti-inflammatory drugs (NSAIDs) are the mainstay for pain management of osteoarthritis in all species, including humans; they are usually well tolerated. This applies even in geriatric dogs and cats with decreased renal function as long as they are monitored to allow bespoke dosing. Less conventional analgesics such as amitriptyline, gabapentin, pregabalin, amantadine, cannabidiol (CBD), ketamine and tramadol are also used, although the evidence for their effectiveness is limited (Gruen et al. 2022). Therapies involving new classes of drugs and species-specific monoclonal antibodies are now coming into use for osteoarthritis: a piprant-class drug and anti-nerve growth factor monoclonal antibody are available but the long-term benefits or harms in old animals are yet to be elucidated.

Enriched therapeutic diets and nutraceuticals are widely recommended to relieve pain related to osteoarthritis in dogs and cats. However, a recent meta-analysis showed no benefit for chondroitin-glucosamine nutraceuticals but did reveal a clinical benefit of omega-3-enriched diets or omega-3 supplements (Barbeau-Grégoire et al. 2022). Pye et al. (2024) reviewed non-pharmaceutical or surgical treatment for OA in dogs and came to a similar conclusion. Feeding marine-based omega-3 is, however, environmentally suspect.

Excessive weight exerts additional mechanical load on the joints, therefore maintaining normal lean body weight is critical in preventing osteoarthritic pain. In addition, adipose tissue secretes proinflammatory cytokines which exacerbate osteoarthritis.

Acupuncture has long been advocated as a means of providing analgesia and improving comfort for chronic pain (Monteiro et al. 2023). However, these WSAVA guidelines are contradictory as, whilst advocating for use of acupuncture, they also point out a lack of evidence of effectiveness. Regardless of considerable controversy as to whether acupuncture is beneficial in old animals, suffice it to say that some, but not all, appear to find it a pleasant experience.

20.4.2 Physical Therapy

Manual treatment, such as massage, muscle stretches, myofascial release and passive joint mobilisation, are well recognised in management of human OA pain and have been employed in dogs and cats. Likewise, electrotherapy, including therapeutic ultrasound, shockwave therapy, pulsed electromagnetic field therapy and neuromuscular electrical stimulation, have also been employed in geriatric humans and pets. The benefits or otherwise of these processes have not been clearly demonstrated, and it is tempting to suggest that the flashier (and more expensive) the process, the more popular its use – even though the benefits may be negligible. Hydrotherapy, in the form of an underwater treadmill or swimming is well recognised in human physiotherapy, and there are some reports of its value in dogs. Water support reduces concussive forces on the joints and allows compromised mobility patients to stand, and steady paced walking is achieved against water resistance. Many dogs appear to enjoy hydrotherapy, but the evidence for true benefits in pain relief is still limited.

A therapeutic exercise program aims at balance, strength, endurance and flexibility' and focuses on activities of daily living to train the muscles in the way they will be used. Geriatric pets have limited reserves, and exercises must allow rest periods and should not cause distress. Impaired cardiovascular or respiratory function must be considered, as excessive exercise may be stressful and even cause collapse. Old dogs with limited sight can still participate in therapeutic exercises but must be made aware of obstacles and be given time to gauge their location. Animals with urinary incontinence need space and time for urination – especially during hydrotherapy sessions.

Assistive devices may be useful to enable extremely weak pets to start muscle strengthening exercises. Such assistive devices are not a permanent way of life but aid in therapy. Particularly when a patient is large, assistive devices such as slings, physiotherapy rolls, mobility carts, wheelchairs, or lifts may be helpful to maintain a standing position. Smaller patients can be supported manually. The pet should never be left unsupervised in an assistive device; the support is a means to strengthen muscle, not a crutch to be used for life.

Sarcopenia will respond to strength training by improving gait and proprioception (Freeman 2012). The concept of frailty as applied to humans appears adaptable to dogs (Lemaréchal et al. 2023). For instance, food-motivated gait speed off leash proved to be an effective indicator of age-related deterioration and cognitive decline. It is a relatively easy variable to measure in a clinical setting and more useful than gait speed on leash (Mondino et al. 2023). Rehabilitation including exercise, socialisation, training, and manual therapy can be extremely effective in preserving cognitive function. Old dogs and cats can learn new tricks! This is undoubtedly beneficial although it probably takes longer than in younger animals (Frye et al. 2022; Sordo & Gunn-Moore 2021).

Pye et al. (2024) provide a thorough review of non-pharmaceutical or surgical treatment of OA in dogs. The overall conclusion is that physical therapies, such as hydrotherapy and acupuncture, have little evidence of benefit, but the jury is still out on the true benefits of most of the electrical therapies.

20.4.3 Environmental Adjustments

Home reorganisation is often the most logical and simple way to improve the QOL of an old pet. Obvious requirements are providing suitable (e.g. soft) bedding and maintaining cleanliness, orthopaedic beds, raised food bowls, carpeted stairs, non-slip surfaces such as yoga mats to provide adequate traction on the floor, and ramps for easier access to raised areas. Cat litter boxes with a low entrance facilitate access for cats with OA. Other modifications include obstacle-free spaces to move around. Keeping furniture in one place and not changing room layout will aid an animal who is becoming blind.

20.5 LIFE CANNOT BE PROLONGED FOREVER

Human obsession with immortality has been fuelled by advances in medical technology and skills to the point where the inevitability of death is often no longer even acknowledged. This has led to many cases of prolonged lives with terrible quality both for the human patient concerned and for their caregivers. A quotation from a comment in a newspaper article (Gorman 2020) about the US's Dog Aging Project sums it up: 'Mother nature doesn't do old age. This is something that humans have dragged themselves into, and now we're going to drag our pets along with us. We are the people that are struggling to warehouse ancient humans who are immobile, demented, fearful, and in pain simply because "well, she seems to enjoy ice cream"' (Anthes 2023).

What are the projects aiming to prolong canine life such as Loyal's Helping dogs live longer, healthier lives (https://loyalfordogs.com/) and the Dog Aging Project (DAP) (https://dogagingproject.org/) going to achieve? They appear to care deeply about the health and happiness of dogs, implying that it is not simply about prolonging life but for that prolonged life to be healthy and happy – a life worth living. This is reassuring, as the human world is not good at differentiating the benefits of QOL from quantity. Surely there is no benefit to anyone from a prolonged but miserable life of pain and disease.

Loyal states, 'We're helping dogs . . . live longer and stay healthier as they age. Our products focus on preventive care, addressing the underlying causes of a range of age-associated diseases to delay their onset and reduce their impact'. The DAP (which has recently lost much of its funding from the National Institute on Aging) 'conducts rigorous scientific research designed to define, explain and ameliorate the effects of ageing'. The project aims to study ageing *per se*, primarily for its relevance to humans. 'Studying ageing in humans is challenging and expensive', but although dogs age more rapidly than humans, they experience some of the same diseases of ageing and share the human environment. It is hoped that studying dogs can contribute to knowledge of the ageing process in humans.

Are these investigations of benefit to dogs? Loyal is assessing correcting for an overexpression of insulin-like growth factor-1 (IGF-1), which is the principal mediator of growth hormone in large and giant breed mature dogs that is believed to lead to early mortality. Their STAY project is a double-blinded, placebo-controlled study recruiting 1,000 senior dogs in partnership with veterinary clinics across the United States (https://loyal.com/clinical-trials). This is an effectiveness study for their LOY-002 drug which has recently received Food and Drug Administration (FDA) preliminary efficacy acceptance.

The TRIAD (Test of Rapamycin in Aging Dogs) clinical trial is looking at rapamycin (https://dogagingproject.org/triad), an mTOR inhibitor already licensed for a number of other indications and shown to increase lifespan and delay or reverse many age-related disorders in mice (Selvarani et al. 2021). The TRIAD is a multicentre, multidisciplinary, double-blind, placebo-controlled clinical trial. Healthy dogs, at least 7 years old and at least 20 kg, are enrolled to receive rapamycin or placebo and provide a range of biological samples for the rest of their life. Currently, only dogs are included; there are no equivalent feline projects.

In such investigations, healthy animals, who cannot themselves give informed consent, are subjected to non-therapeutic administration of a drug or placebo, and lifelong supply of biological data, for a largely unknown outcome. A pet is not able to understand that this might prolong their life; even if they could, would they want it? These treatments are heralded as a benefit to the dogs themselves – although, in reality, the research is to understand human ageing. It could be argued that using dogs is simply an economical way to conduct a preclinical trial for humans. A preclinical trial using pet dogs is not in itself unethical, but flagging the project as a benefit to your pet dog is potentially misleading, even if it is unlikely to do more harm than subjecting them to repeat injections and biological sampling. The supposed benefit of an intervention to prolong life, although not everyone would wish it, can be understood by a human in a way that a dog cannot. Only time will tell if there is a real benefit in improved health during any prolongation of life.

Should we not just accept that a dog or cat has a shorter life span than a human and make that life as good as possible – from an animals' perspective?

20.6 CONCLUSION

Ageing pets can be helped to maintain a high QOL and remain comfortable. They can interact with their family and other pets in their home. Physical rehabilitation is an integral part of keeping these pets active long into their 'golden years'. However, if physical rehabilitation is not helping and particularly if it is harming QOL it should be stopped. The goal is not to make them live forever, only as long as their life is worth living. The balance between prolonging life and maintaining good quality is precarious. Dogs and cats do not live as long as humans and must be cared for according to the needs of their species, not those of *Homo sapiens*. Veterinarians are privileged to be able to provide euthanasia to end suffering. The story of Jack at the start of this chapter serves to remind us how this can result in a life that was worth living, peacefully ended.

REFERENCES

Anthes E. Could a drug give your pet more dog years? *New York Times* [Internet]. 2023 Nov 28. Available from: https://www.nytimes.com/2023/11/28/science/longevity-drugs-dogs.html.

Barbeau-Grégoire M, Otis C, Cournoyer A, et al. A 2022 systematic review and meta-analysis of enriched therapeutic diets and nutraceuticals in canine and feline osteoarthritis. *Int J Mol Sci*. 2022;23(18):10384.

Bellows J, Center S, Daristotle L, et al. Aging in cats: common physical and functional changes. *J Feline Med Surg*. 2016;18(7):533–550.

Bellows J, Colitz CM, Daristotle L, et al. Defining healthy aging in older dogs and differentiating healthy aging from disease. *J Am Vet Med Assoc*. 2015;246(1):77–89.

Belshaw Z, Asher L, Harvey ND, et al. Quality of life assessment in domestic dogs: an evidence-based rapid review. *Vet J*. 2015;206(2):203–212.

Freeman LM. Cachexia and sarcopenia: emerging syndromes of importance in dogs and cats. *J Vet Intern Med*. 2012;26(1):3–17.

Frye C, Carr BJ, Lenfest M, et al. Canine geriatric rehabilitation: considerations and strategies for assessment, functional scoring, and follow up. *Front Vet Sci*. 2022;9:842458.

Goldberg ME, Tomlinson JE. *Physical rehabilitation for veterinary technicians and nurses*. 2nd ed. Hoboken: Wiley Blackwell; 2024.

Gorman J. Old dogs, new research and the secrets of aging. *New York Times* [Internet]. 2020 Nov 9. Available from: https://www.nytimes.com/2020/11/09/science/dogs-aging-behavior.html.

Gruen ME, Lascelles BDX, Colleran E, et al. 2022 AAHA pain management guidelines for dogs and cats. *J Am Anim Hosp Assoc*. 2022;58(2):55–76.

Hua J, Hoummady S, Muller C, et al. Assessment of frailty in aged dogs. *Am J Vet Res*. 2016;77(12):1357–1365.

International Association for Animal Hospice and Palliative Care (IAAHPC). Animal hospice and palliative care guidelines. *IAAHPC General Practice Guidelines* [Internet]. 2022 [cited 2024 Aug 31]. Available from: https://iaahpc.org/wp-content/uploads/2024/04/IAAHPC-Guidelines-2022.pdf.

Lemaréchal R, Hoummady S, Barthélémy I, et al. Canine model of human frailty: adaptation of a frailty phenotype in older dogs. *J Gerontol A Biol Sci Med Sci*. 2023;78(8):1355–1363.

Marino CL, Lascelles BD, Vaden SL, et al. Prevalence and classification of chronic kidney disease in cats randomly selected from four age groups and in cats recruited for degenerative joint disease studies. *J Feline Med Surg*. 2014;16(6):465–472.

McKenzie BA, Chen FL, Gruen ME, et al. Canine geriatric syndrome: a framework for advancing research in veterinary geroscience. *Front Vet Sci*. 2022;9:853743.

Mondino A, Khan M, Case B, et al. Winning the race with aging: age-related changes in gait speed and its association with cognitive performance in dogs. *Front Vet Sci.* 2023;10:1150590.

Monteiro BP, Lascelles BDX, Murrell J, et al. 2022 WSAVA guidelines for the recognition, assessment and treatment of pain. *J Small Anim Pract.* 2023;64(4):177–254. Available from: https://doi.org/10.1111/jsap.13566.

Pease M. Physical therapy for senior dogs. *The Grey Muzzle Organization Health and Well-Being Blog* [Internet]. Undated [cited 2024 Aug 31]. Available from: https://greymuzzle.org/resources/health-and-well-being-common-health-issues-care-mobility/physical-therapy-senior-dogs.

Pye C, Clark N, Bruniges N, et al. Current evidence for non-pharmaceutical, non-surgical treatments of canine osteoarthritis. *J Small Anim Pract.* 2024;65(1):3–23.

Selvarani R, Mohammed S, Richardson A. Effect of rapamycin on aging and age-related diseases – past and future. *GeroScience.* 2021;43(3):1135–1158.

Sordo L, Gunn-Moore DA. Cognitive dysfunction in cats: update on neuropathological and behavioural changes plus clinical management. *Vet Rec.* 2021;188(1):e3.

VetCompass. Early neutering of bitches increases incontinence risk, study finds. Royal Veterinary College *VetCompass News* [Internet]. 2019 Oct 7. Available from: https://www.rvc.ac.uk/vetcompass/news/early-neutering-of-bitches-increases-incontinence-risk-study-finds.

Wiseman-Orr ML, Scott EM, Reid J, et al. Validation of a structured questionnaire as an instrument to measure chronic pain in dogs on the basis of effects on health-related quality of life. *Am J Vet Res.* 2006;67(11):1826–1836.

Part IIIB The Veterinary Profession

21 Veterinary Education and the Changing Profession

Sarah Wolfensohn

If you think that veterinary medicine hasn't changed much since the days of James Herriott, you might be in for a rude awakening next time you visit a veterinary surgery. Gone are the days when a kindly, experienced veterinary surgeon who is a well-known and respected figure in the local community will examine your pet and send you both on your way, either with some reassuring advice or maybe a packet of pills, for a small charge which doesn't involve having to have an awkward conversation with the bank!

So how did this new generation of vets arise? Surely veterinary education has maintained the same objectives? Education? No, nowadays vets are trained; they have to follow the SOPs and tick the relevant boxes. Does this teaching prepare them for the challenges of general practice or push them down the route of narrow specialisation? How does the current education system develop the skills for achieving wider influence on the range of policies that could improve the welfare of animals, humans, and the environment?

21.1 DIFFERENT APPROACHES TO TREATMENT

Let's say you have just taken your dog, Ben, a Labrador, out for a walk and he's run through a barbed wire fence. Yes, we all know maybe he should have stayed on the lead but you happened to bump into Mrs Talksmoor and, while she was wittering on about the price of chocolate and how it's gone up since we left the EU, your pooch took it into his head to go exploring and cut his shoulder. He's got a one-and-a-half-inch cut on the shoulder, and by the time you get to the surgery with him, it has fortunately stopped bleeding, and he's keen to go in and see why all these other dogs are in this funny smelling building!

You've been there quite a few times before, but a young lady who you don't know comes out and before saying anything reaches out to Ben, which, slightly startled, takes a couple of steps back and woofs loudly. Having got over being introduced, you then take Ben into the 'consult' room while wondering what the hell happened to the word 'consultation'. A brief examination follows and ends with the recommendation that the wound should be 'thoroughly cleansed, debrided, and sutured' or, in plain English, stitched. Because Ben is now 8 years old, it is also recommended that pre-op blood samples should be taken, and, of course, he will need some antibiotics as the wound is probably contaminated. And, of course, as he is clearly not very friendly, he may need sedation to take the blood sample first. That all sounds fair enough, so you politely ask what it is going to cost and are given an estimate for about £175 for the blood sample plus £300 for the surgical repair but are told 'there isn't really much choice as it's quite a large wound and it could be very dangerous to anaesthetise Ben without checking his biochemistry and making sure he's not anaemic'.

You mutter something about having to check his pet insurance (which you know perfectly well he doesn't have because it was going to cost £35 a month and didn't seem to cover much) and hand over £52 for the 'consult' fee. You then go down the road to the surgery that you always used to go to before you started to think that maybe they were getting a bit expensive and you see an older bloke who gives Ben a treat, has a glance at the wound and says 'I wouldn't bother stitching that – it should heal fairly quickly and we've always got the option of trimming it up and stitching it in a few days if it's not healing OK. Better have some antibiotics for it though if he cut it on the wire round that field. Ted had some really grubby bullocks in there for the last few weeks'.

So why the difference? Is it just a perfectly legitimate difference of clinical opinion as to how a wound like this should be treated, with the addition of a difference in personality and ways of handling patients, together with a difference in approach to the risks of anaesthesia? Is the older bloke unreasonably blasé or even negligent in his recommendation or maybe just can't be bothered and in 'professional decline', while the younger vet is simply still keen and maybe also more risk averse? Or maybe this shows a lack of willingness to take responsibility resulting in 'Oh we need another test before I can treat this animal'. Does this demonstrate the decline of professional clinical judgement necessitating increasing dependence on laboratory tests and to what extent does undergraduate education affect the development of clinical judgement?

21.2 THE EFFECT OF BUSINESS OWNERSHIP AND PET HEALTH INSURANCE

Or might it have something to do with the ownership of the practice and related factors? Before we get on to that, let's just start by looking at pet health insurance. In the United States (US), where veterinary medicine has generally been 10 to 20 years ahead of Britain in terms of its approach to the business of veterinary medicine and to a similar extent in clinical practice, the pet health insurance market collapsed. That happened because claims became so expensive as a result of the extravagantly inflated fees that were being charged. There was also a suspicion that a significant percentage of procedures were actually unnecessary – but, of course, profitable! In Britain, the insurance market has worked quite well since

Patsy Bloom set up the first specialist insurance company to provide the cover way back in 1976. However, for many pet owners now, cover has become relatively unaffordable while the cover provided has become less comprehensive, and as a result, many pets are not now insured. In the States, that, combined with ever increasing fees in veterinary practice, has meant that a relatively high percentage of pets never go anywhere near a veterinary surgery. At the same time, the 'fortunate' few whose owners are insured or willing to pay regardless are treated as family members, and the owners will pay huge sums to save a pet – and at the same time, there are children starving all over our planet! That is, of course, an individual decision which owners are entitled to make, but for some of those animals, that results in significant welfare issues.

In veterinary companion animal practice, the health of the animal patient, and its best interests must be the main focus to follow the Royal College of Veterinary Surgeons (RCVS) Code of Professional Conduct (RCVS 2012). This code of conduct is becoming increasingly important as it has been recognised that there are increasing pressures in some circumstances that may override the patient's interest in decision-making. Other possible motivations to carry out interventions can include professional advancement for the clinician, financial gain for the practice, a training opportunity for less experienced clinicians, and the potentially unrealistic expectations of the client (with no positive prospect for the animal) (Grimm et al. 2018).

Obviously different professionals may quite reasonably choose different ways of treating the same problem, particularly as veterinary medicine does not have the same level of evidence-led treatment as in the human field. However, there are now several corporate groups who own a significant proportion of veterinary practices, and some give the veterinary staff protocols for treatment as well as targets for sales of medicines. The owners of these corporates are mostly companies, not veterinary surgeons, and are very profit-driven or obsessed with turnover, meaning that the veterinary surgeons working for these organisations are under pressure to charge, charge, charge. It would be unfair to suggest that employees of these corporate owners are deliberately doing unnecessary work, but in the example of poor old Ben's wound, which is a common real-life situation, there were clearly choices to be made with very different outcomes for the owner's bank balance.

Let's just look at a common procedure – pre-operative blood sampling. For sick animals where there are alternatives which need to be decided upon, it may be necessary to get some blood results before, for example, deciding on the risks involved in anaesthetising the patient. And of course, blood samples may be needed for diagnosis, which is a different matter entirely. It is also perfectly true that a very, very small number of young animals may have significant abnormalities but have no clinical signs, which would affect the safety of anaesthesia for routine procedures, such as neutering. Does that risk justify taking blood samples from every young patient undergoing routine surgery? Almost certainly not, but it's a procedure with a high profit margin and expected by a number of corporate practices.

21.3 VETERINARY SPECIALISATION

The role of specialisation is changing how vet students are taught and what their aspirations are. It has always been the case that much teaching – especially in the clinical years – is done by residents who are specialising in their particular subject, and so they teach that everything they are learning is relevant to the undergraduate vet student too. The result of this seems to be denigration of the role of the general vet practitioner, who actually has the more challenging (and interesting) job, and encourages them all to want to become specialists and consider that a GP is second class. Surely this is something affected by how we educate our students?

21.4 ENSURING GOOD ANIMAL WELFARE

There can be no question that the standard of care in veterinary medicine and the outcome for most of our patients is much better than in Herriott's day. At the same time, animal ownership, including horses and livestock, has become much more expensive, and we may be on the cusp of seeing it becoming unaffordable for many. Is that in any way desirable, and will we see a significant increase in welfare problems as a result? Advances in veterinary medicine mean prolongation of life is more easily achievable than in the past and have coincided with the companion animal's transition to family member status, encouraged by the development of cuteness. We may think that an animal is too cute to kill, but we must not leave them to suffer. The critical question about animals, as Jeremy Bentham (1748–1832) asked in 1789, is 'not, can they reason? nor, can they talk? but, can they suffer?' Then we must alleviate that suffering, and euthanasia may be the best and a perfectly acceptable option if we cannot improve quality of life.

Welfare concerns the quality of an animal's life rather than how long that life lasts (the quantity). Once an animal is dead, welfare is no longer a concern for that individual, but how an animal dies is a welfare concern, and high mortality rates are often indicative of poor welfare. There may be an effect on dependent offspring and conspecifics, and social groupings may be disrupted which need to be taken into account and managed. When considering an animal's quality of life, many people will also consider the value of that animal's life (Sandøe & Christiansen 2013). However, should we consider the value to itself, or to science, or to food production, or as a pet/companion, or to its peer group? How is its value affected by economics, culture, politics, emotion, religion, or its cuteness? Does it actually have no value? Does it only have value because it is here for man's use, or does it have inherent value simply by being sentient and having rational consciousness?

In modern veterinary medicine, there are numerous treatment options (Grimm et al. 2018), many of which lack evidence-based practices (Vandeweerd et al. 2012). As a result of this, there is increasing concern that these options are encouraging overtreatment and whether these modern and innovative potential treatments consider the best interests of the animal (Sandøe et al. 2016). Veterinary surgeons encounter many difficult decisions and regularly face ethical dilemmas (Bartram & Baldwin 2010; Yeates & Main 2011). Stress ratings are highest when there is conflict between the welfare of the animal and the interests of the client (Batchelor & McKeegan 2012). The vet's role has now moved beyond the short-term medical care of the animal to include long-term management of the emotional wellbeing of the attached human carer (Hutton 2019), who may prolong the animal's suffering by refusing to consider euthanasia as they come to terms with guilt and anticipatory grief. This delay as the vet waits for the client to psychologically accept the pending loss of the animal puts the vet into a pivotal, if not conflicted, position (Fox 2020), and leads to moral stress in veterinary practice with calls for improved decision-making tools (Persson et al. 2020). Veterinary surgeons, unlike doctors, are very privileged to have euthanasia as a treatment option for their patients in order to reduce potential suffering, but it is often perceived as indication of failure to make the animal better. Every animal will die at some point, and expert management of a timely and stress-free death is part of the veterinary surgeon's role. How that is perceived by owners can have a significant impact on the veterinary surgeon's mental wellbeing. They must learn to make well-reasoned, ethically justified decisions, reducing the influence of the animal's cuteness, thus promoting positive clinical experience and assurance for owners, which is of critical importance in veterinary practice. Specifically, including this in veterinary education will enhance the quality of decision-making and decisional conflict will be reduced, thereby improving the mental health of veterinary surgeons. The use of the AWAG (Wolfensohn 2020) can assist with client management because it provides a clear visual illustration of quality of life and thus supports the vet's decision-making and helps owners to understand the reasons for the vet's advice.

The ideal welfare law applies to all sentient animals, is clearly written, includes failing to meet an animal's needs among the offences, is easy to amend in line with new scientific knowledge and ethics, has high legal status which allows for prosecutions, has a clear enforcement responsibility, involves an enforcement body with sufficient power and funds, and includes education of the public and industry. Animal welfare is a complex concept and requires more than a token mention in the veterinary curriculum. Understanding it requires science (how different environments affect an animal's health and feelings, from the animal's point of view) and deciding how to apply those scientific findings involves ethics (how humans should treat animals). Enforcing those decisions in society involves the law (how humans *must* treat animals). There needs to be greater emphasis on ways of improving animal welfare, such as financial incentives for producers, public education, including animal welfare in the school curriculum, and research to inform government policy. Maintaining a high standard of animal welfare is essential wherever animals are managed.

Take dog breeding as an example; the demand for puppies has risen driven by COVID-19 and working from home, and the price of puppies has soared. So buy a dog and produce a litter from it and that will generate income – in theory. But the associated vet's bills are so high that there has been a surge in the establishment of canine fertility businesses with no veterinary qualified staff, which has raised significant concerns about their activities since they can operate with little in the way of regulatory oversight or accountability. Their work often involves high-value breeds like French Bulldogs, which often struggle to give birth naturally. In Scotland there are now proposals to introduce a strict licensing framework for canine fertility businesses in order to clamp down on unethical breeding practices, regulate the services offered, ensure higher standards of care, and protect animal welfare. The businesses offering canine fertility services will be licensed annually and inspected regularly by experienced veterinary surgeons to ensure compliance (Scottish Government 2024).

Where will the regulatory inspecting vets come from and how will they be trained (or even educated)? Already vets are involved in carrying out inspections of animal research facilities to ensure compliance with the Animals (Scientific Procedures) Act and inspections of slaughter houses for the Food Standards Agency. It is not easy to fill these posts while vet students are encouraged to consider specialising in one area of treatment such as oncology or orthopaedics. That brings us on to the consideration of end-of-life care for animals. The reality is that every animal (and human) is going to die, and the management of that death is critical in ensuring good welfare and minimising any suffering involved. Vets are very privileged to have euthanasia as a tool to manage this process. Animals do not sign consent forms or understand that undergoing such interventions as multiple limb amputations or unpleasant chemotherapy will enable them to live a few months longer. Death can be prolonged and tortuous; it is better to make it short and painless (Wolfensohn 2024a). But vet students are taught how to diagnose and treat; and euthanasia is perceived as failure.

21.5 THE BIGGER PICTURE – INFLUENCING POLICY AND LEGISLATION

Societal ethics and policy-making lead to legislation, balancing the values we hold for different species. Influencing policy development in such matters as animal welfare, ecological conservation, and risks to humans requires a focus on public attitudes to and understanding of science, as well as consideration of potential unforeseen consequences of the social/environmental/economic impacts of policies.

How do these considerations affect the complexity of policy development and implementation by governments, and on environmental, public, and veterinary health and welfare? Policy-makers need access to ethical and sound evidence on which to base the policies, which must be robust enough to benefit social wellbeing and societal progress. People need to be part of the decision but will not necessarily accept 'expert' opinion. Indeed, sometimes experts ask the wrong question, or don't define it clearly and thus get opposing answers, which then undermine the value of their expertise. Sometimes all the evidence and information that is needed is simply not available as it may take time to collect, but decisions by policy-makers may have to be taken urgently. Social media has a significant influence; the level of cuteness of animal stories reported has an impact, and the financial model of newspapers has changed so they are less able to investigate and subject issues to ethical review, as this will slow down the process of getting into print. Should the free press be more accountable since the media plays a significant role in confusing issues around animal welfare, with a tendency to highlight the owner's view or the animal's cuteness in order to make a good story? A single solution to promote higher animal welfare across the entire EU is unlikely due to significant regional differences and the fact that what is appropriate in each region depends on many factors (Keeling et al. 2012). Influencing policy development in such matters as animal welfare and biodiversity requires animal sciences (with a focus on public attitudes to, and understanding of, science) and also depends on the relevance of these issues to policy-making and their resonance with public perception. Influenced by the concept of cuteness, the values we hold for different species translate into policy-making, via ideas around animal welfare, ecological conservation, and risks to humans. However, there may be unforeseen consequences of the social/environmental/economic impacts of policies, and we need to be mindful of the interaction between the systems of the natural world and humans. There is a role for the veterinary surgeon in One Health: Humans, Animals, Environment. How does this fit into veterinary education? We need integrative governance of animal and sustainability concerns to develop an overarching global guidance system on all aspects of sustainable development (Wolfensohn 2024b).

There are currently five 'societal challenges' to food and farming systems: animal health and animal welfare; human health; demand and supply; social, cultural, and political challenges; and environmental and ecosystem challenges. Politics, legislation, economics, farmers, retailers, and consumer interactions all have an impact on the welfare of the animals, vets can stimulate discussion on what must be done to improve animal welfare with the increasing use of technology for animal husbandry. Breeding strategies should protect animal welfare and not pursue production outcomes and business performance at the cost of welfare. Animal welfare must be a key sustainability objective – including consideration of a good life, a humane death, and the Five Domains of animal welfare (Mellor et al. 2020), balanced with ethical, economic, and environmental considerations. We need to ensure the next generation of vets will be educated and motivated to take action and make a difference, redefining what it means to be a supervet . . .

REFERENCES

Bartram DJ, Baldwin DS. Veterinary surgeons and suicide: a structured review of possible influences on increased risk. *Vet Rec*. 2010;166(13):388–397.

Batchelor CEM, McKeegan DEF. Survey of the frequency and perceived stressfulness of ethical dilemmas encountered in UK veterinary practice. *Vet Rec*. 2012;170(1):19–22.

Fox MW. Euthanasia: doing our best for animals. *Vet Rec*. 2020;186(1):32–33.

Grimm H, Bergadano A, Musk GC, et al. Drawing the line in clinical treatment of companion animals: recommendations from an ethics working party. *Vet Rec*. 2018;182(23):664.

Hutton VE. Animal euthanasia-empathic care or empathic distress? *Vet Rec*. 2019;185(15):477–479.

Keeling LJ, Immink V, Hubbard C, et al. Designing animal welfare policies and monitoring progress. *Anim Welf*. 2012;21(S1):95–105.

Mellor DJ, Beausoleil NJ, Littlewood KE, et al. The 2020 five domains model: including human-animal interactions in assessments of animal welfare. *Animals (Basel)*. 2020;10(10):1–24.

Persson K, Selter F, Neitzke G, et al. Philosophy of a 'good death' in small animals and consequences for euthanasia in animal law and veterinary practice. *Animals (Basel)*. 2020;10(1):124.

Royal College of Veterinary Surgeons (RCVS). Code of Professional Conduct for Veterinary Surgeons. 2012. https://www.rcvs.org.uk/setting-standards/advice-and-guidance/code-of-professional-conduct-for-veterinary-surgeons.

Sandøe P, Christiansen SB. *Ethics of animal use*. 1st ed. Hoboken: John Wiley & Sons; 2013.

Sandøe P, Palmer C, Corr S. Human attachment to dogs and cats and its ethical implications. *Proceed 22nd FECAVA Eurocongress Vienna, Austria, 2016 Jun 22–25*. 2016;31:11–14.

Scottish Government. Licensing canine fertility services. *GOV.SCOT* [Internet]. 2024 Aug 16. Available from: https://www.gov.scot/news/licensing-canine-fertility-services/.

Vandeweerd J-M, Kirschvink N, Clegg P, et al. Is evidence-based medicine so evident in veterinary research and practice? History, obstacles and perspectives. *Vet J*. 2012;191(1):28–34.

Wolfensohn S. Too cute to kill? The need for objective measurements of quality of life. *Animals (Basel)*. 2020;10(6):1054.

Wolfensohn S. Euthanasia. *The Pet Profession Podcast* [Internet]. 2024a May 27. Available from: https://open.spotify.com/episode/3p18wUgXxLuPerwNf0BWkx?si=GNfiP1BWQUeV0bceYbw-EA.

Wolfensohn S. Understand and improve welfare by using the animal welfare assessment grid. *Global Synergy for Animal Welfare: From Research to Impact* [Internet]. 2024b Jul 2. Available from: https://www.youtube.com/watch?v=xOuT5f4VOtM.

Yeates JW, Main DCJ. Veterinary opinions on refusing euthanasia: justifications and philosophical frameworks. *Vet Rec*. 2011;168(10):263.

22 The Art of Veterinary Science

Kendal Shepherd

It questions the seemingly ubiquitous quest for an elusive, and certainly expensive, 'gold standard', and whether the more client- and bank-balance-friendly term 'professional competence' should be considered instead as a more practical and achievable alternative. The author uses experiences, both good and bad, and anecdotes garnered from her years working in general practice and more recently, as a legal expert witness, as well as her knowledge of the intricacies of the dog-human relationship, to illustrate and inform her view of the art and how using it to its full should enhance both professional, client and patient satisfaction.

22.1 BACKGROUND

To put this chapter and its musings in context, in 1972, I was in a year of 26 students at Bristol, only six of us female. I was told during the obligatory introductory chat with the dean of the faculty that I was unlikely to last the course as I was pretty, and there'd be a lot of distractions. I brought a first-year lecture at the Meat Research Institute to a halt by asking the flummoxed lecturer whether he really thought that bacterial contamination of the meat was the only disadvantage he could think of involved with the harpooning of whales. My first practice dictated that 'ladies wear skirts' when I turned up on the first day in trousers. Gold standards, continuing professional development, and paid maternity leave were unheard of. But I had it relatively good compared to those in the past. On sharing the harpooned whale tale with Dr Mary Stewart many years ago, she replied with her own 'women causing trouble' story. As a student, she had had the temerity to question the castration of bullocks without local anaesthetic. She was dismissed from the scene with the professorial comment, 'That's what you get by allowing women into the profession'.

Now university intake is largely female, and the profession (I refuse to call it an 'industry') has changed almost out of all recognition. But have the changes all been for the better? Despite the attributes that women have undoubtedly brought, is a predominantly female profession good for it? Has awareness and implications of the art of veterinary medicine increased as a result?

In 2002, I wrote a letter to the *Veterinary Record*, in answer to a then-current discussion about the introduction of a veterinary science degree and the competition (some argued threat), it appeared to pose to practising veterinary surgeons.

The opening paragraph read,

> It is extremely interesting to read in Professor Lance Lanyon's letter (VR November 2nd, 2002), that, in founding the Royal Veterinary College, Charles Vial de St Bel in 1790 considered the practice of veterinary medicine to be an art and that the purpose of veterinary science was to instruct and inform this art. He also placed as much emphasis upon the preservation of health as upon curing of disease. The concern of those members who seem threatened by the introduction of a veterinary science degree, would imply that they themselves are not aware of the contribution that art makes to veterinary practice. If the art of practice is taken to mean more than merely 'clinical methodology and the development of the skill of its application', then there should be no difficulty in differentiating the veterinary practitioner from the veterinary scientist and acknowledging the value of each to preserve and promote animal health and welfare.

As the said Professor Lanyon had been a young lecturer of mine during the latter stages of my less-than-illustrious veterinary student career (terminating, with some surprise successfully, in 1978), my interest was piqued, and I went on to question if both science and art were needed to fulfil one's obligations in practice, then what exactly was the art and whether it was actually being taught. I felt that my own student experience had led me to believe that future clients needed only to be impressed by my knowledge of subjects such as anatomy, biochemistry, and pharmacology, with no mention of the subtleties of art and how it could be used 'not only ensure the success of Mrs Jones's treatment of her treasured poodle, but also to lessen the impact of Mr. Jones's loss of his prized pedigree herd'.

There is reference to the application of veterinary art in 'The works of Charles Vial de Sainbel, Professor of Veterinary Medicine' (published posthumously in 1795), specifically in his essay 'General Observations on the Art of Veterinary Medicine', where he emphasised the importance of good husbandry and helping nature take its healing course rather than doing anything which might impede it. The final paragraph even recommends that the veterinary student should arm himself with a knowledge of 'stenography or short-hand writing' in order to record the minutiae of successes as well as failures. In this way, he 'would be in possession of every word that has been pronounced' and be able to 'mark with more precision his own inferences and opinions'. Setting aside the inherent assumption that all such students would be male, advice regarding accurate and detailed recording is just as, if not more, relevant today.

22.2 WHAT IS 'THE ART'?

But what did St Bel himself mean by 'the art'? He was indeed a rather good artist to which his illustration of the ideal proportions of the illustrious racehorse Eclipse testifies, but did 'the art' imply more than just making the best use of one's medical and surgical knowledge in practice? What else is required?

The Art of Veterinary Science

In the fifth century BC, Hippocrates famously wrote, 'As to disease, make a habit of two things – to help, or at least do no harm'. He went on to say, 'The art has three factors, the disease, the patient, the physician. The physician is the servant of the art. The patient must cooperate with the physician in combating the disease'.

Just one of the many quotes attributed to him, this emphasises the need for cooperation between physician and patient. Hippocrates' reflection that 'Life is short, and art is long, the crisis fleeting, experience perilous, and decision difficult' seems to mirror what an increasing number of graduates feel today. Working in general practice, particularly those owned by corporates, and experiencing daily conflict, with professional obligations as well as with employers and clients, appears to damage self-esteem and mental health, as well as bank balances. It has forced many to consider a change of career and resulted in many veterinary press articles, courses, and conference presentations on how to simply stay sane.

But Hippocrates goes on to say, 'The physician must not only be prepared to do what is right himself, but also **to make the patient, the attendants, and externals cooperate**'.

Would an understanding and appreciation of 'the art' and its use help to reconcile these current conflicts?

22.3 THE CONSULTATION

The purpose of a consultation is to diagnose and advise the scientifically correct treatment for a given patient. An understanding of the human-animal bond is vital and the effect this has upon one's ability to dispense the 'correct' treatment must be taken into account. Again, Hippocrates has relevant thoughts on the matter. 'I urge you not to be too unkind, but to consider carefully your patient's superabundance or means. Sometimes give your services for nothing, calling to mind a previous benefaction or present satisfaction. And if there be an opportunity of serving one who is a stranger in financial straits, give full assistance to all such. For where there is love of man, there is also love of art'.

Had Hippocrates been thinking of animals as patients rather than people, I have absolutely no doubt he would have considered the human an essential part of the equation. The client is, after all, the conduit by which the prescribed treatment of the animal in their care is administered and, in this regard, veterinary medicine may be more akin to paediatrics, in that babies and small children can do nothing for themselves and are entirely dependent on their caregivers.

The RCVS Guide to Professional Conduct has this to say: 'Having reached a provisional diagnosis, taking into account the animal's age, the extent of any injury and disease and the likely quality of life after treatment, veterinary surgeons should make a full and realistic assessment of the prognosis and the options for treatment or euthanasia and communicate this to the client'. Where does it say anything about taking the nature of the client themselves into account?

Liking animals is not enough in our profession: understanding and empathy with people is essential. Owners are the means through which our skill is manifest, by understanding the treatment rationale and delivering the medications accurately as prescribed, as well as by having the wherewithal to pay for our diagnostic and surgical skill (either by being well-off or having the foresight to insure their pet). How much do we need to tailor the advice we give according to their individual needs and abilities, not least the ability to pay? How much should we feel obliged to learn about a client – where they live and their lifestyle and proclivities – to be able to help them make an 'informed' choice that's right for them? Are we doing more harm than good by overloading clients with choices that are far beyond their ability to understand or pay for?

22.4 BEHAVIOUR OF THE PATIENT

As we understand more and more about how intimately humans and dogs have evolved together from the behavioural perspective, the more we realise that some behavioural insight must be required for the general practice veterinary surgeon to both diagnose and treat illness and injury properly. How a dog behaves is, after all, crucial to delivering veterinary care in the first place, and we must routinely delve a little deeper into the relationship between dog and owner to understand the unit that presents itself in the consulting room. Behavioural insight and its application must therefore be considered part of 'the art'.

Not only must the client be used as the 'go-between' in terms of delivering treatment, but behaviour counselling (my speciality being the dog) has taught me that the animal itself can be used in three-way communication and to bring appropriate pressure to bear on its owner in decision-making. 'What do you think your dog would prefer to do and why?' is a question that must always be asked and demonstrated when educating in the principles of learning and explaining what dogs do and why. Without this insight, clients cannot routinely change their dog's mind and choice of behaviour in daily life, essential to creating healthy behavioural habits. In a similar manner, encouraging clients to imagine how their pet may be feeling 'in sickness and in health' may be beneficial when discussing the pros and cons of particular avenues of treatment and their impact on the animal.

Developing personal relationships with clients over time is vital, not to become best friends, though this may happen, but to be able to predict how they may react in different situations. From the clients' point of view, it is becoming increasingly clear that the inability to see the same vet twice is a major source of irritation and complaint. From the veterinary point of view, whereas there may well be, on occasion, clients whom one feels like calling in sick to avoid seeing, the benefits of knowing one's clients well ought to far outweigh the disadvantages.

22.5 EUTHANASIA

Of all the services offered in general practice, euthanasia is possibly the most sensitive. In my experience, far more letters and cards of appreciation were received after putting an animal to sleep than any successful surgery. A down-to-earth and honest approach is essential regarding the reasons for any decision made. Particularly when discussing euthanasia, this must be without incurring any undue feelings of guilt. Even when putting an animal of one's own to sleep, some degree of guilt is always felt after this irreversible decision. Was it made too soon? Could more have been done? Above all, although cost of potential treatment inevitably has a bearing on feasibility of alternative routes, the owner should never be made to feel guilty owing to inability to pay.

However much a client wants their pet to remain alive, there should be no unnecessary prolonging of life just because we now have the facility. Some clients may grasp at the flimsiest of straws however much they cost and have great trouble contemplating euthanasia. Although a vet who also dissolves in tears is not necessarily helpful to a grieving client, neither is the exact opposite, as an experience of mine when 'seeing practice' (as EMS was then called) amply demonstrates.

An elderly couple brought in their emaciated, starey-coated cat to see one of the partners, not having consulted a vet for some time. After expressing in no uncertain terms his disgust at the condition of the cat and declaring that it needed to be euthanised immediately, he picked it up by the scruff of the neck and marched it out of the room for the deed to be done. I still recall the shock on the owners' faces as they were presented afterwards with their dead cat. At the time, the least offensive thought I could muster was that he was completely devoid of any bedside manner, and my enduring regret is that I did not have the courage to question his actions. He later rose to the dizzying heights of BSAVA president. It may well be that this episode was an anomaly, an example of how the pent-up emotions of frustration and anger can get the better of the best of us, and, in its own way, was indeed a valuable learning experience.

22.6 GUILT – A SALUTARY TALE

Guilt may of course amount to more than an internal emotion and a prosecution brought under the Animal Welfare Act illustrates both the need for honesty in report writing and implications of guilt admirably. A visit by a dog warden confirmed neighbourly suspicions that a dog had been severely neglected, and as the dog warden had no power to seize the dog and the RSPCA being unable to attend, the owner was instructed to take the dog for immediate veterinary examination. After this examination, during which the dog was described as 'emaciated', the mutual decision was reached to put the dog to sleep. The veterinary report, which was written for court, included discussion of possible differentials, including cancer and kidney failure and that blood test screening would be the next step. The fact that the client only had '£85 pounds to his name' according to the clinical notes, was omitted.

On post-mortem, however, the dog was found to have undigested food in the stomach and, according to the dog warden's report, had been more than willing and able to drink. There was no evidence of neoplasia or any other condition which could account for the emaciation.

Although the owner was quite rightly found guilty of causing suffering by failing to address the causes of weight loss, I commented in my report, 'Any suffering was indeed relieved by the attending veterinary surgeon, in that dead dogs cannot suffer. I feel it would be wrong however, should the Court be left with the impression that this dog lost his life because there was no other way that his suffering could be relieved'.

And finally, I mused, 'I do wonder what the outcome would have been had the RSPCA been available to visit, with the power to remove a suffering animal and place it under their care. It does seem to me, at best unlikely, that an irreversible decision (euthanasia) would have been made with such alacrity in a dog so evidently able and willing to eat and drink'.

22.7   THE 'ART' OF CONSULTING

In essence, the skill in consulting and decision-making involves managing clients so that what is possible from their perspective is exactly what an attending veterinary surgeon wants from their own – to find practical, welfare-oriented, and possible-to-achieve solutions to everyone's satisfaction. It is possible to deliver 'best practice' without striving for 'gold standard'. As Richard Brown says in his excellent *Vet Times* articles, 'gold standard' should be replaced with the concept and term 'professional competence' (see references). Part of professional competence should surely be to have clients who walk out of a consultation room satisfied with their 'informed choice', without feeling they have been manipulated, short-changed, condescended to, or criticised.

Would this not lessen the burden that the profession is now under?

22.8   RECORD-KEEPING

Accurate and detailed clinical notes are essential in order to ensure that vital information is not missed, not only for all members of a practice team but also for those who may need access to a client's notes outside the practice, for referral purposes or should a second opinion be sought at another practice. If Charles Vial de St Bel's advice regarding shorthand writing is anything to go by, record-keeping should also be considered part of 'the art'. When working as a GP locum, all I needed to know was what the client in front of me had been told and what they understood about the treatment their pet was undergoing. I could then hit the ground running in a consultation. Yet, then as now when reviewing veterinary histories for recent legal cases, all too often the histories are heavy on vaccine reminders, flea preparations, wormer dispensing, and payment details, but remarkably light on giving me the content and flavour of a consultation.

It used to be obligatory for veterinary history to follow an animal should clients wish to change practice. Apparent, to my mind ill-advised, relaxation of the rules of supersession has enabled clients to flit from practice to practice, often dictated by relative costs and convenience, with no obligation, even for the sake of one's own safety, to be appraised of previous veterinary history. I recall, when insisting on obtaining veterinary records regarding a behaviour case and seen while working for Roger Mugford, finding out that written in bold across the record card was the vital information 'IF MR X PHONES, DO NOT PTS!' What did *that* tell me about relationships at home and the bearing it may have on the dog's treatment?

A recent RSPCA prosecution illustrates how lack of awareness of social background, inadequate and misleading detail in consultation notes, and subsequent poor communication between colleagues impacted, to my mind at least, very unfairly on the accused.

Two 15-year-old dogs were seized on welfare grounds as suffering from a chronic and inadequately investigated skin condition, which proved to be owing to a flea infestation. One dog was simply irritated by fleas, and the second, a litter mate, showed a true allergic reaction. Within two weeks in RSPCA care, having been removed from the flea-infested house and appropriately treated, both dogs' skins were restored to health. In contrast to the expected finding in such cases, where there is often a paucity or complete lack of veterinary history, these dogs had over the years been taken multiple times for veterinary examination. The owner was hardly ever seen by the same vet twice. Their records revealed far more financial detail than consultation notes, and what little there were had hardly any reference to fleas, concentrating instead upon one dog's anal furunculosis and the other's possible differentials for the 'skin condition'.

The owner, now 30, had been diagnosed with autism at the age of 15 and more recently with ADHD, the conflicting symptoms of which included an obsessive need to attend to instructions and lack of being able to organise thoughts or actions, as was evident throughout the sad history.

My report read, 'I do wonder what the purpose of prosecution is in this particular case. There is no question that the dogs, as well as the environment they lived in, needed proper thorough treatment for fleas. There is also no doubt that removing them to be examined and successfully treated was the most expedient thing to do as both medication of the dogs and removing them from the source of fleas, in the absence of thoroughly fumigating the house, was achieved in a very short space of time. In effect, this also enabled a second opinion on XXXX's condition to be sought, in the light of the vets appearing unable to make up their collective minds. It may even have been that, if the owner's full set of circumstances and personal difficulties had been appreciated and approached empathetically, she may have been persuaded to sign the dogs over permanently for their own good'.

22.9 STUDENT SELECTION

One has to question whether the right students are being accepted to universities in the first place. Whatever their gender, disillusionment, dissatisfaction, and the inability to cope with the realities of general practice currently abounds, evidenced by the rate at which young vets are leaving the profession. Might this indicate not that conditions have worsened (when in fact, in practical terms, they have never been better) but that the selection process is too dependent on academic success rather than considering the all-round attributes needed to produce veterinary surgeons who can successfully stay the course. If the attainment of 'gold standard' is a graduate's sole ambition, they are possibly not suited to the realities of general practice.

Continuing professional development existing as an immediate burden after graduation does not help and, in my opinion, is unnecessary as a professional obligation for at least the first five years in practice. What have students been learning at college if, despite increasing complexity and breadth of knowledge, it is still considered insufficient to fit them for general practice? Could it be that giving the impression the newly qualified vet still has so much to learn, and is somehow rendered inadequate thereby, contributes to lack of confidence and feelings of incompetence?

22.10 ACCEPTING HELP WITHOUT LOSING FACE

In my last full-time general practice, I saw mainly small-animal clients, but out-of-hours on the one in four rota, I had the occasional large-animal call-out. Upon arrival, I was greeted by an extremely gruff farmer who was quite obviously having extreme difficulty hiding his disappointment at seeing all 5'1½" of me appear to attend to his cow in thus far unproductive labour. I quickly diagnosed a uterine torsion, all the while fighting to recall how to cast a cow. How grateful I was for almost telepathic communication with an able cowman who asked if I wanted to use Reuff's method before I had to admit any lapse in memory. Moreover, he seemed to have the most welcome knack of making all his moves seem like my idea. He waited without a hint of impatience while I worked out the correct direction to roll a cow to untwist the uterus, and after two attempts, the calf could be delivered. The most difficult part was hiding my astonishment at the success and instead giving the impression that I did it every day.

Sadly, the calf was dead: a live animal would have iced the cake. All the same glowing inside, I washed up and took my leave, wanting to hug the cowman and receiving a slightly less grumpy farewell from the farmer. A few days later, my boss forwarded on to me how the farmer had rather grudgingly admitted to him how impressed he'd been.

22.11 'HAVING A GO'

My experience of general practice seems now to have been relatively unencumbered by the woes that beset current members. With no obligation to follow set protocols or corporate dictator breathing down my neck, I may well have been in a better position to experiment (in other words, turn theory into practice) than current new graduates seem to be. There were very few referral centres even if I'd felt unsure about what to do and how to do it. Neither was there any pressure to meet a 'gold standard', even less to bamboozle clients with all the available options and attendant costs. Being prepared to have a go with a decent textbook and ever-reliable nurse on hand was the norm.

The Art of Veterinary Science

In my early days, I vividly recall breaking the speed limit to my parent's house to collect one of their Great Danes to be used as an emergency blood donor. One Sunday, a practice nurse had presented her own elderly dog, quite casually under the circumstances, having correctly diagnosed that Kipper had a ruptured splenic tumour. After diving straight in to successfully remove the spleen (on the way being told to ignore the rattling stones in the stomach as she 'always vomits them up'), it became worryingly obvious that she was still bleeding post-op, hence the urgent need for blood.

Leaving a note for my parents as to the dog's whereabouts, I shouldered the oversized dog into my undersized Mini Clubman and made a return dash to the surgery. With no blood collection bags or anticoagulant to hand, I had a relay of nurses taking blood from him to be immediately delivered by syringe to the patient, while I rectified my previously inadequate ligatures via a second exploratory laparotomy. I had been assured that, as long as the blood was collected and delivered smoothly, there should be no problem with clotting. As the donor continued to be his goofily placid self and the patient comatose, the procedure went without a hitch.

By some miracle, the dog survived to duly regurgitate her habitually swallowed stones. The long-suffering Great Dane was used on one other occasion, though this time under less strenuous circumstances.

There is nothing better than experiencing what can be done with the bare minimum of equipment to inform 'the art'. Working in Crete in the 1980s taught me how much one can do on a moped, with a stethoscope, thermometer, and bottle of Euthatal on board. Vaccinations, antibiotics, and other medications could be readily obtained from a pharmacy, as could giving sets and drip bags, and the local hospital persuaded to x-ray, if absolutely necessary. Before my arrival in Agios Nikolaos, the closest thing to a vet was the local meat inspector who used to administer vaccines and the nearest private vet nearly 70 kilometres away in Heraklion. With no competition, anything I could manage was a bonus.

Now I wonder whether there is a need for third-world vetting to become a speciality, the veterinary equivalent of a war doctor, to help combat the seemingly inexorable advance of unaffordable complexity and to combat the current need to hide behind evidence-based medicine, as well as to inform the basic art and skill of veterinary science. But the current issue of BSAVA's *Companion* magazine arrives, not to extol the virtues of thinking outside the box and taking the odd risk, which such a course would inevitably entail, but how 'assisted decision-making' is required when prescribing antibiotics and the publication of the 'Protect Me' guidance. Oh, and an article arguing for sentience in bees.

How times have changed.

REFERENCES

Brown R. Vet profession's wrong turns. *Vet Times* [Internet]. 2023a Aug 29. Available from: https://www.vettimes.co.uk/article/vet-professions-wrong-turns/.

Brown R. Vet profession's wrong turns, part 2: possible solutions. *Vet Times* [Internet]. 2023b Sept 5. Available from: https://www.vettimes.co.uk/article/vet-professions-wrong-turns-part-2-possible-solutions/.

Vial de Sainbel C. The works of Charles Vial de Sainbel, Professor of Veterinary Medicine: to which is prefixed a short account of his life. Including also the origin of the Veterinary College of London. *Wellcome Collection* [Internet]. 1795. Available from: https://wellcomecollection.org/works/xku9ppne/items?canvas=9.

FURTHER READING

Gardiner A. The 'dangerous' women of animal welfare: how British veterinary medicine went to the dogs. *Soc Hist Med*. 2014;27(3):466–487.

Koronakis-Rohlf and Batzini. *Greek wisdom – the foundations of medicine: an anthology of quotations*. Athens: Topos Books; 2020.

Shepherd K. *Demystifying dog behaviour for the veterinarians*. 1st ed. Boca Raton: CRC Press Taylor & Francis Group; 2021.

Stewart ME. *Companion animal death*. 1st ed. Oxford: Butterworth-Heinemann; 1999.

23 Veterinary Academia, Clinical Specialisation, and Animal Welfare

R. Eddie Clutton

23.1 INTRODUCTION

The extent to which members of the Royal College of Veterinary Surgeons (RCVS) can adhere to their declaration to ensure the health and welfare of animals committed to their care depends on the member's circumstances and their role within the profession. Conscientious small-animal and equine practitioners can achieve these goals on an individual animal basis and with every consultation. Farm animal vets might achieve relatively minor benefits for individual animals, but these may become immense when translated to herd or flock level. In caring for animals used in experiments, laboratory animal veterinarians ensure the quality of scientific data and the safety of subsequent medical innovations. However, the potential to do good things for animals is arguably greatest amongst veterinary academics – as researchers and educators. Meaningful advances in animal welfare science, pain recognition and management, animal behaviour and consciousness, quality of life (QOL) assessment, and animal and veterinary ethics are most likely to result from the efforts of committed researchers. Thereafter, the effective dissemination of new findings improving animal welfare is required for achieving real-world results, and whilst presentations at scientific congresses and the publication of scientific reports are important for influencing events at higher levels (and advancing academic careers), motivating veterinary undergraduates to practise ethically, by repeatedly emphasising what their constant endeavour must be, is probably more likely to get health and welfare to the animals that need it.

Unfortunately, when veterinary academics are unconsciously indifferent to animal welfare or deliberately allow their constant endeavour to pursue less honourable objectives than an animal's wellbeing, then things can go wrong on a grand scale. This chapter examines the possibility that some elements of veterinary academia and its bed-mate clinical specialisation may have had (and continue to have) adverse effects on animal welfare.

23.2 VETERINARY SCHOOL CURRICULA

Veterinary schools are expensive operations and over the last few decades have come to rely increasingly on revenue from full fee-paying non-domestic students attracted from North America and elsewhere. One of the numerous ways to attract such students is to offer courses that the naïve undergraduate may believe facilitates their intended career path. Not infrequently, this involves niche interests based on misleading impressions of the profession given by television (Lamb 2018) and other media. Thus, some undergraduates see themselves in the companion animal sector performing leading-edge (though unproven) surgery, while others imagine working in marine mammal conservation or propagating bearded dragons. Consequently, important though less appealing subjects, e.g. epidemiology, public health, pig, poultry and fish medicine, ethics, and anaesthesia, become deprioritised in the curriculum, and veterinary education is nudged towards the favoured paths of non-domestic students rather than what the nation, planet, or most animals require. Consequently, farming communities in the Highlands and Islands of Scotland find themselves without vets – while the pet rabbit owners of Edinburgh find themselves spoilt for choice.

Veterinary schools recruit specialist clinicians to promote popular courses of limited global value. By doing unique things to animals, clinical specialists elevate the school's profile, so they are rewarded financially and receive academic accolade. The latter seldom reflects the meaningful contribution to scholarship expected of non-clinical faculty members, so it is divisive and devalues the achievements of true academics. This is aggravated when clinical academic specialists are designated affiliates because they then receive academic award whilst avoiding academic responsibilities, e.g. doing meaningful research, publishing material of value, attending more meetings, and marking undergraduate exam scripts. The effects of specialist clinicians on undergraduate education are profound and not always conducive to ensuring the health and welfare of animals (see the following discussion).

In an ideal world, veterinary school education would be redirected towards global needs, e.g. meeting one-health initiatives, promoting food animal welfare and production, or refining animal experiments, rather than populating referral companion animal practices in affluent countries with clinical specialists. That said, global versus local objectives could be integrated: students with small-animal leanings could cut their teeth on 'capture, vaccinate, neuter, and release' projects in developing countries. Those destined for work in the racing industry could spend time ensuring the health and welfare of equids (and bovids) wherever the working capacity of these species is critical in supporting human standards of living. Ultimately, career choices lie entirely with graduates, but vet schools could go some way to directing them down avenues where they can achieve greater things for animals and society in general, and more fulfilling careers for themselves.

The current competition to attract foreign students sets vet schools against each other and encourages the development of 'attractive' rather than useful study programmes. This might be solved by establishing a uniform veterinary curriculum across all United Kingdom (UK) vet schools. The world needs humanely produced animal protein somewhat more than pets which struggle to breathe. Some veterinary school leaders need to recognise this and graduate classes which can meet the broader challenges. A greater involvement of animal welfare scientists, ethicists, and ecologists in the veterinary curriculum may prove helpful in this.

23.3 CLINICAL SPECIALISATION

The first professional organisation devoted to a veterinary speciality was probably the Association of Veterinary Anaesthetists of Great Britain and Ireland in 1964. The British Veterinary Radiology Association established itself a year later. In response to this, the RCVS established certified training programmes with qualifications for recognised specialities; this encouraged specialists to become educators within an expanding veterinary curriculum. During the 1990s, the responsibility for veterinary specialisation passed to the European Board of Veterinary Specialities (EBVS), an event which probably saw the purpose of veterinary specialisation changing from improving animal health and welfare through specialisation, to developing specialisation and promoting veterinary specialists for its and their own sake, respectively.

The reasons for this are reasonably clear: when the health and welfare imperatives of the RCVS declaration are lost (many EU veterinary graduates are not required to declare a commitment to animal welfare), then other 'drivers' prevail. The form these alternatives take depends on the discipline itself: in bovine reproduction or equine orthopaedics, the goals remain to improve cattle breeding and the horses' capacity to compete, respectively. Where animal purposes are less obvious, e.g. companion animal ownership, goals become opaque and open to interpretation. The conscientious specialist will continue to use his or her skills to improve their patients' QOL although others may prefer to prioritise longevity. To some, specialisation may mean developing different ways to solve common problems in congenitally deformed and dysfunctional animals, rather than prevent them from being bred in the first place. Others may believe that specialisation confers a right to test ideas on client animals in the pursuit of clinical novelty and personal accolade irrespective of the boundaries of recognised (or routine) veterinary practice. Unimaginative veterinary specialists seem to follow paths previously created by medical pioneers, unaware that the needs of human and animal patients are quite different. When companion animal specialisation is unconfined by animal health and welfare commitments, there is a natural and inexorable gravitation towards overtreatment with its associated potential to harm animals and their owners. This is all the greater when it occurs in an educational environment (see the following) because the harms are exponentiated and other people may suffer.

The harms of overtreatment are speciality-dependent, being arguably greater in surgery (Quain et al. 2021), oncology (Ware et al. 2019), intensive care (Fordyce 2017), and anaesthesia. A detailed justification for this statement is beyond this chapter's scope but will be limited to a few key facts. First, advanced complex and invasive surgery raises concerns because there is little or no information on post-surgical chronic pain syndromes in domestic animals. These are devastating in human patients undergoing amputations, thoracotomies, mastectomies, herniorrhaphies, and sternotomies, amongst others (Searle & Hopkins 2009), and there are no compelling biological reasons to believe they do not afflict animals. Human survivors of intensive care not infrequently suffer incapacitating post-traumatic stress disorders, the causes and risk factors for which are poorly understood (Burki 2019). Consequently, one wonders with what confidence veterinary intensive care specialists can assure owners that their animals are not experiencing similar psychological adversities. Moving to oncology: given the likelihood that animals probably don't understand the significance of a cancer diagnosis (particularly when there are no clinical signs), then most veterinary oncological procedures are in breach of the *primum non nocere* principle. Finally, veterinary anaesthetists may be complicit in overtreatment when they make questionable procedures possible in higher-risk, e.g. older, animals, although motives will vary. Those indifferent to welfare considerations will obey managerial orders to complete operating lists without question, concern, or conscience. In contrast, more typical anaesthetists may fear the consequences of refusing to participate in what they perceive to be cruel and unethical interventions (see later) but participate nevertheless. Others may genuinely feel they are contributing to a *bona fide* attempt to improve an animal's QOL. Anaesthetists attracted by new and exciting technical and/or intellectual challenges should first ask whether the intervention is in the animal's best interests and, if any doubt exists, examine their own consciences and their choice of post-graduate speciality.

Adverse welfare consequences of specialisation can be managed in at least four ways. First, all specialist colleges should assert that the pursuit of animal health and welfare is their principal objective. As part of this, colleges should accept euthanasia as a suitable therapy for 'unlikely to survive' cases and accept exam-credentialing submissions describing humane terminations rather than reports of heroic yet futile cruelty (see Chapter 28 on the death of veterinary euthanasia). Third, colleges should include modules on animal and veterinary ethics, and animal welfare science, as part of their curricula. Fourth, the specialties should be encouraged to adopt a more holistic form of specialisation – in reality, an active de-specialisation which is gaining popularity in contemporary medical practice (Swire & Brown 2023).

23.4 CLINICAL SPECIALISATION AND UNDERGRADUATE EDUCATION

Clinical experts teaching popular subjects in veterinary schools often become clinical role models for the fee-paying students they attract but, when indifferent to animal welfare, possess the potential to set bad examples beyond the 'normalisation' of overtreatment. For example, they may encourage innovation in areas of clinical novelty rather than animal health and welfare. This attracts students because the former is superficially more exciting, dynamic, and heroic than the latter, which often involves either doing nothing at all, e.g. box- or cage-rest, euthanasia, or something complicated, e.g. epidemiology. Other poor clinical examples, e.g. performing BOAS surgeries rather than outbreeding brachycephaly, have already been mentioned, along with pursuing the quantity rather than quality of an animal's life, conducting unethical and unapproved clinical trials or experimental surgical procedures on client-owned animals, and following anthropocentric avenues with little or no hope of animal benefit.

As role models for veterinary undergraduates, academic clinical specialists who do not openly promote animal health and welfare run the risk of establishing bad habits as a norm to be accepted and propagated by generations of graduating veterinarians (McGurgan et al. 2024). Such problems might be prevented by regular attendance at CPD courses titled, for example, 'Animal health and welfare – the basics for veterinary specialists'.

23.5 GOLD STANDARD CARE

An example of welfare-indifferent specialisation is gold standard care (GSC). A powerful catalyst for both overdiagnosis and overtreatment, it is difficult to know when GSC first arose or what precisely it is. The GSC zygote probably formed when undergraduates were first taught that their professional advice should be based on a recitation of all available treatment options rather than what they themselves would do were the animal their own. This non-paternalistic approach to veterinary consultation has numerous drawbacks. First, it is not what clients expect: many pay for sincere advice in the form of an honest answer to the question 'What would you do if this were your animal?' Providing a range of options may embarrass clients who struggle to understand what they are told; this means their eventual consent may not be informed. Second, referring to the most advanced, innovative, complex, and expensive option as gold standard – which is what the term usually seems to mean – leaves the client in no doubt that all other options are sub-optimal. Whether intentional or not, this is likely to add guilt to the client's embarrassment, particularly if they are poor and their animal is uninsured. It is not surprising to realise that promoting gold standard options expedite many specialist goals. For example, it provides leverage for aspiring academics to recruit material for case reports (a credential for board examinations) or for established academics to conduct clinical research on a client's animal. It also provides opportunities for some to perform untested treatments with or without untested materials or devices.[1] Unsurprisingly, GSC is also likely to demand greater professional fees, with a large overdiagnosis element caused by the running of tests with little clinical value. Despite these 'advantages' to the specialist, there appears to be an encouraging increase in a general unease with GSC amongst UK veterinarians (Skipper et al. 2021). Another potential advantage of the imminent CMA enquiry (British Veterinary Association 2024) might be the restoration of veterinary professional pragmatism over GSC, whereby animals receive care according to their needs, their condition and its prognosis, and with a full and sensitive consideration of their owners' wishes and circumstances.

23.6 STUDIES USING CLIENT-OWNED ANIMALS

Clinical specialisation depends on innovation and the continuous refinement of methods, i.e. research. Some argue this is most useful when conducted on client-owned animals because being 'the real thing' their ailments are natural and not inflicted experimentally. However, there are problems with this, especially when the researcher has limited scientific training and is indifferent to animal welfare and ethical considerations. In the worst-case scenario, the animals of poorly informed yet consenting clients may become involved in poorly designed projects of low clinical relevance without any guarantee that the treatment received is not worse than standard therapy. There is, therefore, a greater need for independent and robust ethical review when pets are involved in clinical trials, not least because such trials are likely to involve the potentially competing interests of the specialist clinical researcher, the owner, their animals, and possibly commercial sponsors. Independent and robust review is the responsibility of institutional veterinary ethical review committees (VERCs). These are likely to benefit from adopting some elements of the animal welfare and ethical review boards (AWERBs) which are a legal necessity tasked to ensure the ethical use of animals in biomedical research.

Companion animal projects that pose any risk of harm to any animal must first undergo harm-benefit analysis, allowing the harm-benefit ratio (HBR) to be estimated. This involves weighing the potential harms facing participating animals against the anticipated scientific benefits of the research and the likelihood of a successful study outcome. Research which harms animals and is of limited benefit and/or little clinical significance must not be allowed. For approved projects, ongoing independent oversight is necessary to ensure that harms are minimised and benefits maximised and ends with a retrospective assessment of the actual harms and benefits encountered. Such processes have established safeguards for laboratory animals and are equally important in veterinary clinical trials because animals cannot give their informed consent to participate.

Clients consent to their animal's involvement in clinical trials after being fully informed of all relevant details, including the potential for their animal to suffer more than they would have done had they undergone standard treatment. While it is hoped that untested therapies will be better than existing treatments, clients must be warned that they may be worse, have unexpected side effects, or be hazardous. The appropriate (scientific) use of placebo in trials also raises ethical concerns because placebo allocation will, at best, delay and, at worst, deny an animal's access to effective therapy. Providing such information without bias may be difficult for some specialist investigators, in which case the VERC may suggest alternative methods. Additionally, the VERC must approve the wording of the study-specific consent document.

Humane endpoints (HEPs) are established before potentially noxious studies begin, in order to minimise any harms the animals later experience. HEPs are sets of clear, predictable, and unambiguous clinical signs that indicate a level of animal suffering that is not scientifically justified, authorised nor equivocal. Reaching HEPs during a study triggers the immediate end of the animal's suffering by either (i) withdrawing the animal from study and providing relief, e.g. analgesics, or (ii) killing it humanely. Euthanasia offers crucial protection for animals used in research, but when research subjects are pets rather than laboratory animals, setting and adhering to immutable endpoints becomes difficult. A pet animal's fate will not depend on objective assessments made by experienced animal care technicians with a legal mandate to minimise suffering, but by the owner and the clinical specialist managing the project. Under these circumstances, animals may experience extended suffering while their owners wait, potentially in vain, for an unproven treatment to work. The potential for conflicts of interest is clear.

Preventing the misuse of client-owned animals during clinical trials by over-enthusiastic clinical specialists is best achieved by a robust VERC operating with the full support of senior management and reported to by both the clinical investigators and institutional research assistants. The latter, aware of the conditions of the project's approval, must report infringements to the committee. Problems arise when clinical trial supervisors exploit their positions as members of senior management, or worse, the VERC itself. Under these conditions, staff may feel threatened and disinclined to raise concerns although as veterinary surgeons or nurses, they may be professionally bound to do so. Consulting the RCVS's Ethical Review Panel may be one option to consider when these difficulties arise; registering an official 'concern' with the RCVS Concerns – Professionals (rcvs.org.uk) remains another.

23.7 CLINICAL ETHICAL REVIEW COMMITTEES

Most clinical specialists (and indeed, most non-specialist veterinarians) understandably want to extend specialty boundaries, to innovate, refine, develop new ideas, and/or acquire new skills. Occasionally, pursuing these natural tendencies may cross thresholds that result in animal suffering. This may be accidental when the specialist's judgement is affected by sheer enthusiasm, or it may be callously deliberate. 'Going too far' readily results in 'overtreatment' and repeatedly raises the question 'Just because we can, should we?' Conscientious vets, aware of the welfare costs of over-overtreatment and working with similarly minded-colleagues, are likely to be self-regulating. A workplace devoid of egos and competitiveness, which supports civil communication and expects mutual respect for all team-members, will facilitate self-regulation. Such conditions may not be found in some clinical companion animal practices or academic environments where the risk of overtreatment is high and the need for ethical oversight is urgent (Fordyce 2022).

Veterinary teaching hospitals are staffed by people with different goals and moral sensitivities. Senior, usually specialist clinicians promote, develop, and teach their speciality while residents are there to learn it. Anaesthetists, imagers, and nurses attempt to support the senior clinicians in their mission. Case management is almost always directed by the senior clinician because it will be for his or her skills that the case was referred. This primary clinician will also hold the principal consultations with the client and the referring vet and, in this role, they will convey the information required for the client's informed consent. A conflict of interest arises here if the primary clinician encourages treatment for reasons other than improving the animal's outcome and major problems can arise when professional opinions over what is in the animal's interests differ. Primary clinicians may believe that theirs alone is the right to plot a case's clinical course, but their clinical and moral decision-making processes may not be flawless. Clinical decisions are only properly challenged by others in the same speciality with similar experience levels. However, disputing a specialist's ethical judgement is more difficult because empathy and sympathy with an animal's suffering are not examinable, i.e. board certifiable, and individuals, including nurses and students, may have strong and defensible reasons for why they think some aspects of clinical case management may be unwarranted, unfair, cruel, and wrong. In these situations, it is not acceptable for the primary clinician's morality to automatically prevail (although supported by senior management, it often does). Being a senior clinical specialist in, for example, veterinary oncology does not confer automatic authority in ethical decision-making when it comes to the treatment of animals with malignancies, particularly when the motivation for doing so arises for reasons other than the promotion of animal health and welfare. This leaves conscientious objectors – often anaesthetists and nurses – with two options: either they feel compelled to stay silent yet participate in procedures they believe to be wrong – and to subsequently suffer moral stress (Batchelor & McKeegan 2012) – or they refuse to participate and accept the consequences to their careers and salaries. The latter seems even more hazardous and likely when individuals in senior management are themselves specialists in areas of ethical concern, e.g. veterinary oncology, experimental orthopaedics, and intensive care.

Problems arising from different moral sensitivities within the veterinary team may be resolved by clinical ethical review committees (CERCs). These differ from the VERC insofar that they judge individual cases suffering possible overtreatment rather than the HBRs of clinical research proposals. The *modus operandi* of institutional CERCs must vary to meet the needs of different institutions, but one possible process could run as follows. Anyone, including students, concerned with the wellbeing of an animal undergoing treatment at the facility could anonymously (or otherwise) report their concerns – while identifying the associated clinical specialist – to a designated CERC representative for students, nurses, or junior academic staff. These would rapidly judge the validity of the concern and if considered appropriate, pass it on to the CERC. The CERC, ideally consisting of a senior clinical chairperson, an ethicist, an animal welfare scientist, an anaesthetist, and nursing, student, and junior academic representatives, as well as a few animal-owning lay members, would then co-opt a member of the speciality under consideration (but not the individual cited in the complaint) to deliberate the case. The cited specialist would then be invited to discuss these deliberations after which a decision would be made with respect to the animal's future.

As with VERCS, CERCS need to be independent, autonomous, and protected from vindictive senior managers whose own practices may become causes for concern and the subject of ethical, i.e. CERC examination.

In situations in which a CERC-based process is infeasible, e.g. when a prompt decision is required and/or when important committee members cannot be convened in time, the use of the veterinary ethics tool (VET) (Grimm et al. 2018) is strongly recommended.

23.8 THE MORAL DISASSEMBLY OF VETERINARY GRADUATES

Whilst contemplating a potentially lifelong career in veterinary medicine, many veterinary undergraduates develop rational ethical foundations and beliefs with respect to animals and their future profession. These foundations may undergo some modification during five years of veterinary education, but many will remain unchanged or become consolidated by the end of this period. Unfortunately, many graduates then enter a workplace where these ethical principles are progressively dismantled and, concluding that they have made a mistake, leave the profession to do something unrelated to veterinary medicine – or worse (Dolby 2022). Disillusionment is not the only reason for the attrition rate amongst fresh veterinary graduates in the UK (RCVS 2022) but is one worth exploring.

Logically, recent graduates would not face ethical deconstruction if the veterinary profession shared a common moral compass calibrated with a single, unambiguous magnetic north. Arguably, it does, in the declaration 'ABOVE ALL, my constant endeavour will be to ensure the health and welfare of animals committed to my care', and any confusion as to what that might mean can be dispelled by reading Sean Wensley's chapter (number 37) on vets speaking for animal welfare. Achieving stronger moral alignment between graduating vets and those at the coalface is most likely to succeed by revising veterinary education rather than restructuring attitudes in the real world, although both can occur simultaneously. Two revisions worth examining are (i) to incorporate more ethics into the core curriculum and (ii) to increase the duration of required extra-mural studies. Unfortunately, both demand time, of which there is usually little to spare. A more efficient strategy would be for clinical specialists – as professional role models – to unambiguously prioritise and promote animal welfare in the practise, teaching, promotion, and demonstration of their particular speciality. Those who protest that they already do so will presumably have little problem in encouraging their head of school to establish an institutional CERC who might then determine whether their protestations are justified or evidence of delusion.

23.9 CONCLUSION

Veterinary academics and clinical specialists are in an ideal position to ensure veterinary graduates are committed to animal health and welfare and possess the skills and knowledge to realise these commitments. Unfortunately, specialisation *per se* can create distractions which may paradoxically exert a subverting effect. As subjects taught within the veterinary curriculum, animal and veterinary ethics remain relatively undeveloped compared with traditional and popular subjects like surgery and medicine (De Briyne et al. 2020). However, progressive incorporation of ethics and welfare within the undergraduate course and integration with related subjects might bring an end to veterinary overtreatment, overdiagnosis, and other excesses.

NOTE

1 These run counter to the RCVS's Guide to Professional Conduct because 'untested' means 'efficacy unestablished', which in turn means the RCVS-required assurances that the untested procedure will improve an animal's health and welfare cannot be made with confidence.

REFERENCES

Batchelor CE, McKeegan DE. Survey of the frequency and perceived stressfulness of ethical dilemmas encountered in UK veterinary practice. *Vet Rec.* 2012;170(1):19.

British Veterinary Association. Joint response to the Competition and Markets Authority consultation on veterinary services for household pets in the UK. *British Veterinary Association Media* [Internet]. 2024 Oct. Available from: https://www.bva.co.uk/media/5686/submission-to-cma-oct-2023.pdf.

Burki TK. Post-traumatic stress in the intensive care unit. *Lancet Resp Med.* 2019;7(10):843–844.

De Briyne N, Vidović J, Morton DB, et al. Evolution of the teaching of animal welfare science, ethics and law in European veterinary schools (2012–2019). *Animals (Basel).* 2020;10(7):1238.

Dolby N. *Learning animals curriculum, pedagogy and becoming a Veterinarian.* 1st ed. Boca Raton: CRC Press; 2022.

Fordyce PS. Welfare, law and ethics in the veterinary intensive care unit: (a discussion of the different types of suffering that patients may endure in the veterinary intensive care unit, the legal limits to that suffering, and the ethics underpinning at what point that suffering becomes 'unnecessary'). *Vet Anaesth Analg.* 2017;44(2):203–211.

Fordyce PS. We need ethical review processes for extreme clinical companion animal practices. *Vet Rec.* 2022;190(8):330.

Grimm H, Bergadano A, Musk GC, et al. Drawing the line in clinical treatment of companion animals: recommendations from an ethics working party. *Vet Rec.* 2018;182(23):664.

Lamb H. Are TV vets good or bad for the profession? *Vet Rec.* 2018;183(2):73.

McGurgan P, Calvert K, Celenza A, et al. The Schweitzer effect: the fundamental relationship between experience and medical students' opinions on professional behaviours. *Med Teach.* 2024;46(6):782–791.

Quain A, Ward MP, Mullan S. Ethical challenges posed by advanced veterinary care in companion animal veterinary practice. *Animals (Basel).* 2021;11(11):3010.

RCVS. RCVS workforce summit 2021. *RCVS News & Views* [Internet]. 2022 Mar 14. Available from: https://www.rcvs.org.uk/news-and-views/events/workforce-summit-2021/.

Searle R, Hopkins PM. Pharmacogenomic variability and anaesthesia. *Br J Anaesth.* 2009;103(1):14–25.

Skipper A, Gray C, Serlin R, et al. 'Gold standard care' is an unhelpful term. *Vet Rec.* 2021;189(8):331.

Swire C, Brown H. Balancing generalism and specialism: what can the vet profession learn from human medicine? *Vet Rec.* 2023;193(9):375.

Ware J, Clutton E, Murphy K, et al. Should we be euthanising cancer patients? *Vet Rec.* 2019;185(18):574.

24 What are General Practitioners Good for?

Brennen McKenzie

Primary care vets must be trained to practice evidence-based medicine and to offer an appropriate spectrum of care options within the highly variable, often resource-constrained general practice environment. Maximising the potential of GPs does not mean disdaining specialists or not referring cases when appropriate. It means delineating the domains of primary and specialty practice rationally and supporting general practitioners in developing their knowledge and skills and providing high-quality care while still utilising specialty services when these are truly necessary for the patient.

> *We must provide an outlet for the creative faculties . . . And it is this challenge which is recognized by every graduate who turns away from practice, disillusioned by his or her inability to find satisfaction in a situation where . . . the expectations of training are dashed by the reality of practice. Somehow, we must change the system lest the process of education leads to an increasing number of square pegs looking for a home in a world of round holes . . .*
>
> *We must seek to elevate the status of the practitioner, not only that his position is elevated in the eyes of the academic but, more importantly, in the minds of practitioners themselves. Too often we hear that a practitioner cannot be expected to teach or to research. This is the philosophy of despair.*
>
> Peter Rossdale (**Rossdale 1978, 327**)

If I'm being honest, the first couple of years of vet school were a bit tedious. I was a career-change student, about 10 years older than most of my classmates. I had behind me years of struggling to find a career that was meaningful and challenging yet also economically viable. In that context, being back in school wasn't such a bad thing. And unlike a lot of my classmates, I hadn't always dreamed of being a vet, so I didn't experience the shock of achieving a lifelong dream only to find it was imperfect. But hours and hours spent memorising facts, many of which I suspected I would never need again (and I was right!), wasn't exactly thrilling. I did OK, but I didn't stand out. Until I got to clinics.

When I started my clinic rotations, everything came to life for me. The process of clinical reasoning, of collecting and sifting through the information available to find the salient patterns and then matching those to the tools I had available was fascinating and satisfying. Doing medicine was enormously better than learning about medicine! I may not have been the smartest or most talented in my class, but I turned out to be pretty good at the clinical aspects of veterinary medicine, and my teachers noticed.

One day, an internal medicine resident came up to me while I was studying in a hospital hallway. She wanted to tell me that she and some of the other residents and faculty members running the rotation had been talking about me. They had concluded that I absolutely had to do a residency because, in her words, 'You're too smart for general practice'.

Of course, my first reaction was an ego-driven flood of dopamine and self-satisfaction. I appreciated the complement, and it reinforced my suspicion that I was actually pretty good at this stuff. But when I had some time to think a bit more about the remark, I started to take a darker view of it.

Roughly 12% of US veterinarians are board-certified specialists (AVMA 2021a, Jul, 2021b, Dec). That number was surely lower when I graduated 25 years ago! With this context, one view of the resident's complement could be that specialty practice is for the best and brightest, and the rest of us have to settle for the less intellectually challenging life of primary care medicine. Being a GP, in this frame, is a consolation prize or a fallback position for the majority of us who don't make the cut.

By temperament I'm certainly a nerd, and I likely would have pursued a specialty certification (probably in emergency and critical care) and maybe an academic career if that had been possible. But at the time I graduated, I was 35 years old, I had a six-month-old daughter and a spouse who had indulged my search for a career long enough. I also had $160,000 in loan debt (a pittance by today's standards, of course, but easily in the top 3% of vet school debt back then). Internship and residency weren't realistic, and it was time to get a job.

So did I settle for a lifetime of routine and drudgery? Nothing but vaccines, spays and neuters, and anal glands until I retired? Or maybe, at best, the challenge of entrepreneurship and running a small business? Am I the old guy who hasn't added a new procedure, drug, or piece of equipment to his toolbox since most new grads were born and doesn't see why the way we did things in the 'good old days' needs to change? Well, not exactly.

I have found many ways to sustain my engagement and enthusiasm with medicine, to challenge myself and grow, both professionally and personally, in my work. Most importantly, I have maintained a commitment to high-quality, evidence-based medicine (EBM), and I have been able to help my patients and clients and even contribute to the growth of the veterinary profession. All as a lowly GP. So how did I do that?

To start with, when my first practice didn't meet my expectations for quality of care or opportunities to learn, I started doing relief work at local emergency hospitals to take on more challenging cases. In the absence of a mentor willing and able to teach me, I looked for every opportunity to learn the hard way. It was pretty scary being on alone at night right out of vet school. It wasn't how I would have chosen to learn, but such a sink-or-swim approach seemed all that was available to vets not destined for internships and residencies in those days.

What are General Practitioners Good for?

Once I had a few years in practice, I managed to talk my way into an exceptional hospital, which I have long considered a model of what is possible in general practice. We have been an independent 24/7 practice with up to 30 veterinarians, almost all GPs, and many extremely talented technicians, including some with VTS specialty certification. Individual veterinarians were encouraged and supported in pursuing their interests, which allowed me to offer abdominal ultrasound and echocardiography, endoscopy, chemotherapy, and a high-level of surgical and medical care to my patients.

While working in this rich environment, I have constantly striven to 'up my game'. I got involved in the Evidence-Based Veterinary Medicine Association (EBVMA), helping to lead this organisation made up largely of academic veterinarians. I have published and spoken on evidence-based medicine and promoted it to primary practice clinicians around the world.

I have also been lucky enough to have the opportunity to teach veterinary students in practice. Many come to clinics with a wealth of facts crammed into their heads and little idea how to organise and use them effectively to help patients. As much detailed content knowledge as they get from each specialist they train with, many students get very little process knowledge.

Clinical reasoning skills, the ability to take all the knowledge they have ingested over the years and both organise and use it effectively to make decisions in real time across a broad set of medical domains and patient populations, is something few veterinary students I see have had the chance to think deeply about or practice. This is one area in which the general practitioner is pre-eminent; the pragmatic evaluation of available information and application of available resources to solve clinical problems within the inevitable constraints of time and money. The broader the range of problems you have to solve and the more limited your tools for solving them, the more efficiently and creatively you have to think!

I have also continued my formal education, completing a master's degree in epidemiology. Even at this stage (don't you dare say 'venerable'!) of my life and career, I am seizing opportunities to learn and grow. I have shifted to part-time clinical practice so I can take on a role in canine ageing biology research. I still do spays, neuters, vaccines, and anal glands, but that is hardly a fair summary of my career as a GP.

Of course, my path isn't the right or the only way to make life in primary care practice meaningful and challenging. It is just one example of many possible paths. But I think it belies the notion that academic veterinarians all too often inculcate in their students that being a GP is a dead end, a second class of veterinary career.

I still run into this view from time to time. When doing an advanced echocardiography training course, I was chastised for even thinking I should be able to offer this service by the other students (all internists). A few specialists have been offended when I questioned their recommendations, even when I could present clear research evidence to support my concerns and their position relied entirely on their clinical experience and authority as diplomates. And the medicine resident who encouraged me to pursue specialisation so many years ago was not the last to suggest, with the best intentions, that my knowledge and abilities were somehow inconsistent with my role as a GP. I doubt that I am the only primary care veterinarian to have such experiences.

So how should we think about the role of GP? How should we see ourselves fitting into the profession, and how should students and academics learn to understand our role? What strengths and limitations characterise the general practice role, and how do these complement the academic and other veterinary roles? All of these are deep and hard questions with no simple answers, but I will offer a few thoughts.

Because primary care practice is where the vast majority of patient care happens, our profession has an ethical responsibility to prepare GPs for providing high-quality, evidence-based care. Many of the students I teach and the new graduates I mentor seem to come out of the veterinary educational system with the idea that they should handle only minor problems and refer anything challenging. The definition of what is appropriate for GPs to manage seems to shrink yearly. It's not just the shock I still sometimes see when I talk about performing an echo or an endoscopy in primary practice. I have had new graduates who felt it was inappropriate to interpret a radiograph or diagnose a mast cell tumour on cytology without specialist input. The message they often seem to get from their teachers (nearly always academic specialists) is that if a specialist can do something then a GP shouldn't do it.

Of course, this extreme view is not consistent with practical and economic reality. The obvious problem of insufficient specialty capacity and the inability of many pet owners to afford the cost of specialty care is an obvious flaw in this model. However, I believe there are other flaws to this view that are even graver.

One is that such 'dumbing down' of general practice to routine wellness care and management of only minor health problems diminishes the quality of care patients receive. It creates a self-fulfilling prophecy. If we teach veterinary students that talent, intelligence, and ambition can only be satisfied in specialty practice, then people with those attributes will eschew general practice. If we don't teach GPs that they should be practising high-quality EBVM because only specialists can do that, then it will become true.

Another problem with primary practitioners gradually ceding diagnosis and treatment of serious problems to specialists should be abundantly clear from even a casual glance at the human healthcare system. The hyperspecialisation of human medicine has led to absurdities.

I once started explaining the nature and management of a cranial cruciate ligament rupture to a client when he stopped me with a chuckle. He was an orthopaedic surgeon. After four years of undergraduate education, four years of medical school, an internship, and more than one residency, his entire career consisted of six procedures on the human knee. A brilliant and arguably overeducated man had been reduced to a highly paid, very specialised carpenter.

My own mother has a laundry list of medical problems common in the elderly. Her primary care provider (PCP) handles virtually none of them, simply referring her to a different specialist for every issue. As her advocate, I have to coordinate care among the PCP, the endocrinologist, the diabetes care manager, the dermatologist, the stroke rehab physician, the orthopaedic surgeon, the occupational and physical therapists, and an occasional ER physician. Apart from the caregiver burden this imposes, the number of errors I have to catch in handoffs between doctors and the gaps in care when a problem fails to land in anyone's designated territory significantly reduce the overall quality of healthcare she receives.

Is this the model we wish veterinary medicine to follow? Laying aside the economic realities that would impede full adoption of the hyperspecialisation, is this even a model we should aspire to? I would argue it is not, yet that is the direction we would head in if the lessons many of my students and new graduates take away from their training were implemented.

The strengths of the primary care practitioner are many. We have a holistic view of the patient throughout the life cycle that is usually unavailable to the specialist. While our knowledge base is inevitably shallower than those in specialty practice, it is broader, allowing us to integrate multiple medical conditions, husbandry and other owner variables, individual temperament, life stage, and many other factors into the management of specific healthcare problems. I would argue that this approach typically allows for better overall patient care, especially when cases are complex with multiple concurrent morbidities.

GPs are also consummate problem solvers, accustomed to making do with limited information and resources. If this ability is not only honed by experience but strengthened by the application of evidence-based medicine techniques and training in clinical reasoning, it becomes a powerful tool. Specialists are undoubtedly knowledgeable, talented, and creative thinkers, but depth of expertise comes at a price; the loss of a broad perspective and a tendency to follow familiar patterns within a domain even if elements of the context outside of that domain might suggest a different approach.

Finally, there is the obvious issue of accessibility and affordability I have already mentioned. Too many companion animals already go without care because their owners cannot afford it. The recent enthusiasm for the concept of a spectrum-of-care approach is a tangible recognition that the perfect should not be the enemy of the good, and that the most intensive and technologically advanced care is not always accessible, and it is not always the only way to achieve the desired outcome for patients and their owners. GPs are ideally qualified by role and experience to find the optimal balance of patient needs and owner resources. Increasing the reliance on specialists without a fundamental shift in the economic model of veterinary medicine will simply make care less available to more patients.

Apart from the benefits to patients and clients in supporting high-quality care in general practice, encouraging GPs to value themselves and their work and to stretch themselves professionally is important to maintaining a talented and satisfied veterinary workforce. We all know that our profession is struggling right now, with vets bearing the stacked burdens of high workloads, huge debt, and the many physical and emotional challenges of the job. Constraining people to smaller, and smaller boxes, as GPs or as specialists, is just creating more round holes for Dr Rossdale's square pegs. Channelling the most ambitious and talented students into specialty practice or academia and denying those who do go into general practice the opportunity to fully engage their intellect and creativity in their work can only exacerbate the problems our profession is facing with burnout and job dissatisfaction.

How, then, can we encourage all of our students and new veterinarians to maximise their potential, provide the best possible care for our patients, and avoid the pitfalls of hyperspecialisation that bedevil our colleagues in human medicine? As I have already implied, I think evidence-based medicine is a key part of the answer!

Teaching all veterinarians, regardless of their eventual area of practice, to practice EBM would be a good start. While some effort to do this is already part of the curriculum, I cannot say that most of the students or new graduates I see have really absorbed the core concepts of critical thinking and reasoning that underlie EBM. We are still emphasising memorisation and regurgitation of facts over rational, effective reasoning strategies.

My students are better able to search the literature and use electronic information tools than my generation, but they don't often seem to understand what these tools are for. They still seem to rely primarily on authority and the dicta of their mentors for guidance rather than using the information they have learned to support critical reasoning. When I question the rationale for a particular treatment choice, all too often the response is still 'That's what Dr X said to do'.

Teaching vets to think critically and independently and to rely on critical appraisal of controlled evidence as far as possible can only improve the quality of clinical reasoning and patient care. It also has the advantages of strengthening one's confidence in one's recommendations and practices, and reducing the tendency to defer to academics or specialists, which drives a lot of the relinquishing of cases and problems that could appropriately be retained in the general practice setting.

EBM also helps to delineate the role of generalist and specialist. In areas where there is strong evidence to guide diagnosis, prognosis, and management, there is less need for the deep and narrow experience of the specialist. Conversely, when a problem is uncommon or not well understood and there is little reliable evidence concerning it, a specialist's strengths become critical.

As an example, the vast majority of the heart disease cases I see in practice are myxomatous mitral valve disease (MMVD). This is a relatively well-understood condition with clear diagnostic and staging criteria and strong consensus guidelines available to inform treatment. I use echocardiography to support my management of MMVD cases. In my career, I have done over one thousand echocardiograms, and about 85% of these have been MMVD cases. There is no reason that the greater expertise and experience of a cardiologist should be necessary to diagnose, stage, and manage this condition in most patients with typical presentations.

My use of this tool fits well into the role and competency of the general practitioner. And the skills I have developed evaluating MMVD patients have helped me utilise the tool in other ways that improve patient care. I don't need to call in a cardiologist to identify a right atrial mass prior to subjecting a patient with haemangiosarcoma to a splenectomy. I can identify and manage pericardial effusion without the delay of waiting for a specialist or transferring the case. All of these are reasonable and natural elements to primary care.

On the other hand, there are absolutely cardiac cases that fall outside my competency and which I should, and do, refer. I don't ultrasound young animals with murmurs because many will have uncommon congenital anomalies I am not qualified to identify or manage. And whenever there is a case that does not fit well into a clear and evidence-based diagnostic pattern, or when I find something I have not seen before, I don't charge the client for my scan and I call in a specialist who is better equipped to evaluate and handle the case.

Maximising the potential of GPs does not mean disdaining specialists or not referring cases when appropriate. It means delineating the domains of the two rationally rather than by tradition or by organ system. EBM is a useful way to support primary care practitioners in developing their knowledge and skills, maintaining their job satisfaction, and providing high-quality care while also utilising specialty and academic services when these are necessary and will benefit the patient.

Of course, even I recognise that EBM can't solve all of our problems. The lessons my students and new graduates are absorbing about their place in the profession are predominantly cultural lessons, expectations of the whole community as envisioned by a small subset of the profession. Academics don't complain to their students about the failings and misjudgements of GPs because they are mean people. They do so because they see a skewed sample of cases that end up at the university. The most unusual, most difficult problems and those that have not been solved by primary care practitioners are most of the cases that make it to the teaching hospitals. All the cases we manage successfully, often within strict constraints of money and other resources, are invisible to those who teach students how to view the general practice role.

As a profession, we have to think deeply about how we understand the categories of general practitioner, specialist, and academic. If we want to avoid the excessive costs and harm to patient care that have come from hyperspecialisation in human medicine, and if we want to provide satisfying and challenging careers for all new veterinarians, we need to avoid the trap of seeing academia and specialty practice as the brass ring and primary care as a consolation prize.

REFERENCES

American Veterinary Medical Association (AVMA). Veterinary specialists 2021. *AVMA Reports* [Internet]. 2021a Jul. Available from: https://www.avma.org/resources-tools/reports-statistics/veterinary-specialists-2021.

American Veterinary Medical Association (AVMA). U.S. veterinarians 2021. *AVMA Reports* [Internet]. 2021b Dec 31. Available from: https://www.avma.org/resources-tools/reports-statistics/market-research-statistics-us-veterinarians-21.

Rossdale PD. Combining research with veterinary practice. *Can Vet J*. 1978;19(12):327–330.

25 Do Vets Need to Love Animals?

Kathy L. Murphy

25.1 INTRODUCTION

My mother says that from the first time I was asked that pivotal childhood question 'What do you want to be when you grow up?' I said I wanted to be a vet and never changed my mind. Many commented, along my career journey, that I was lucky to have such clarity and focus from a young age. It certainly made choosing subject options at school easy and provided motivation for study and resits. I have never regretted my career choice and have been fortunate to work with a range of species across clinical practice and academia in different countries – in first opinion, referral, and laboratory animal practice. In light of a late diagnosis of autism and attention deficit disorder in my fifties, I will say, though, that I came to view my 'focus from a young age' as slightly more complex than luck. Another comment I frequently receive when sharing what I do for a living is 'You must love animals'. Sometimes, it is posed as a question but often stated as an obvious prerequisite for being a vet, which I find odd given that people's first response to doctors is not usually 'You must love people'.

Whether veterinarians need to (or *must*) love animals seems simple at first glance, perhaps. Indeed, the career advice that I, and many others, received throughout schooling was that being a vet was at the top of the list if you were academically bright and an animal lover. Gallagher et al. make a compelling argument supporting non-romantic love as a core value in veterinary medical practice (2018). Of course, love can mean different things to different people. However, the Oxford English Dictionary definition of love 'A feeling or disposition of deep affection or fondness . . . manifesting itself in concern for [another's] welfare' seems highly applicable to the veterinary profession – after all, how could one provide optimal care without a deep concern for the welfare of the animals? Animal welfare is at the heart of everything we do in veterinary medicine, or at least it should be.

Renowned Emeritus Professor of Animal Welfare Donald M. Broom has argued throughout his career that veterinarians have a crucial role in assessing and ensuring the welfare of animals. His work emphasises the importance of identifying factors necessary (must be present for good welfare) and sufficient (alone can guarantee good welfare) when evaluating and ensuring the wellbeing of animals. If love manifests itself in concern for another's welfare (per the Oxford English

Dictionary definition), it seems entirely appropriate to ask whether love is necessary and/or sufficient for good animal welfare.

25.2 IS LOVE NECESSARY FOR GOOD ANIMAL WELFARE?

Plenty of people do not identify as animal lovers; my parents are an example. However, that does not mean they lack compassion or empathy for animals. I saw my parents (however reluctantly) provide my pets with excellent care when called upon. They were driven to understand and fulfil the pets' needs and go above and beyond to improve their welfare. My mother built a vast three-dimensional maze for my pet rats (Wooster and Dini [Houdini]). The maze took up a decent chunk of my university bedroom and outlasted the rats, and all of this despite her confessing that she hated rats and that their tails gave her the creeps. Similarly, vets may not have an emotional attachment which could be described as love to every animal or species they treat. However, in such situations, I have witnessed the provision of excellent care and commitment to improving animal welfare and wellbeing first-hand.

In many circumstances, loving animals may benefit a vet and their patients, facilitating connections, trust, passion, and commitment to the work, but ultimately, what matters is the *actions* taken to improve animal welfare. Effective actions come from knowledge, compassion, empathy, and a commitment to welfare and do not necessarily depend on deep affection or fondness. The pragmatism that can come from a less emotional approach to clinical decision-making may be a benefit, particularly when faced with ethical dilemmas. In addition, other veterinary team members often provide loving patient care, reducing or eliminating dependence on an individual veterinarian identifying as an animal lover or meeting pre-existing expectations for the most appropriate expression of love. Moreover, whilst having a caring and empathic workforce is generally positive, high levels of empathy can sometimes result in emotional contagion, where one team member's emotional strain can spread to others, amplifying overall workplace stress. These examples are just a few of the many factors that highlight the importance of diversity within a clinical workplace.

25.3 IS LOVE SUFFICIENT FOR GOOD ANIMAL WELFARE?

Having a deep affection and fondness for another does not necessarily prevent harm. Humans often make irrational decisions in the name of love, which can extend to their treatment of animals. I have encountered many situations where harmful action or inaction has caused suffering despite love for the animal being present. I was once asked to join a colleague attending a pony that had suffered a catastrophic and unrepairable fracture of the forelimb. My colleague had advised euthanasia, but the client refused, saying that they loved the pony too much to do that. My colleague had made the pony as comfortable as possible, hoping that the client just needed a bit of time to process what was happening. Despite both of us explaining how much the pony was suffering, and the referral hospital agreeing on the phone that euthanasia was the only kind option, the client continued to refuse, saying she loved the pony too much. The client's emotional connection with, and love for, the pony was as undeniable as it was painful to watch. Eventually, with the support of family members and local police officers, the pony was euthanised, but it took longer than it needed to. There were no winners that day.

There are many examples of love not being sufficient for good animal welfare. The obese family pet 'killed with kindness'. Pet guardians who clearly love their pets, or vets who clearly love animals, withholding analgesia, unable to accept that the animal is in pain or to appreciate the suffering involved with painful conditions such as arthritis. Animal hoarding and some rescue situations involving animals not having their basic needs met due to mental ill-health or insufficient knowledge, facilities, or funding. The breeding and promotion of dogs with exaggerated features which are known, or can reasonably be assumed, to cause suffering. Veterinarians' involvement in all of these challenging dynamics raises yet further questions about the intersection of love for animals and professional obligations.

Having taken a break from companion animal practice for some years before returning to do a residency in veterinary anaesthesia and analgesia, I was shocked to see how much patient suffering had become normalised in the name of innovation and advancement. Patients with multiple debilitating conditions, experiencing the stress of diagnostic tests that made little or no difference to their condition or quality of life; invasive, unproven, or even experimental procedures, often requiring a stressful and painful stay in intensive care, sometimes with an unknown prognosis, or worse still, a known poor prognosis or high likelihood of post-operative complications or chronic pain. The vast majority of vets I met in those environments very clearly loved animals, and when asking about the justification for a planned intervention, I would usually receive one of three responses: (i) 'It's what the owner wants', (ii) 'The animal is going to die if we don't do anything', or (iii) 'We can't advance if we don't practise'. Such pressures, or conflicts of interest, are also found in human medicine. In a survey of over two thousand American physicians, more than 95% were of the opinion that overtreatment occurred in the medical profession, with 59% citing patient pressure, 84% citing fear of litigation, and with skills acquisition identified as a potential conflict of interest, along with notoriety, publications, and financial gain (Lyu et al. 2017). In their 2018 report 'Talking about dying: How to begin honest conversations about what lies ahead', the Royal College of Physicians highlight the importance of having honest conversations with patients (in human medicine) about death, treatment options, and resuscitation status, making the point that a better death is more dignified for the patient and gives bereaved families a better experience of death (Bailey & Cogle 2019). I sometimes found that similar conversations were lacking for the veterinary cases I was involved with during my residency. Where they *did* occur, they often leaned towards the view that euthanasia or palliative care represented failure.

25.4 THE DUAL ROLE OF THE VETERINARIAN

Veterinarians often have to balance what is best for the animal with what is best for the human – considering factors like financial hardship and caregiver burden on the one hand and complex issues, such as the effect of their own conflicts of interest, biases, and the potential for therapeutic misconception on the other. Therapeutic misconception (the mistaken belief that decisions about animal care are being made *solely* for the animal's benefit, i.e. without bias or conflict of interest) may result in misinformed consent or lead pet guardians to seek out inappropriate, novel, or experimental treatments with a higher likelihood of harm than benefit. Consideration of the human element in this dual role when balancing best interests in this way, rather than focusing solely on the animal's needs, is fundamental to creating sustainable solutions and, ultimately, for the avoidance of harm. In my experience, such consideration utilises the very best of one's knowledge, critical analysis, compassion, empathy, resilience, self-awareness, and communication skills. Add to that the time pressure of a 15-minute appointment slot – as is customary in general practice in the United Kingdom (UK) – plus the need to resolve any conflict and process one's own emotions while wiping down the examination table, and it is starting to look like the school career advisors glossed over too much when they distilled the requirements for the job down to 'academically bright and an animal lover'. In that context, it is less surprising that the Royal College of Veterinary Surgeons (RCVS) Workforce Summit 2021 found job dissatisfaction to be the critical driver for vets leaving the profession, with 45% of leavers having been in the profession for four years or less (RCVS 2022).

25.5 THE CHANGING LANDSCAPE OF THE VETERINARY PROFESSION

The reality of clinical practice has been further complicated by a shift towards corporatisation over the past 25 years. Potential benefits and risks are associated with this continuing trend, and the issues are complex. As society increasingly values animals as members of the family, the emotional vulnerability of clients creates fertile ground for high cost veterinary care (Brockman et al. 2008). My blood runs cold when I see global financial organisations predicting that the veterinary sector financial market will more than double by 2030 (Morgan Stanley 2024) and encouraging aggregation and *'acquisition zoomies'* (KPMG 2023). Shareholders benefit from financial growth, but at what cost, and what happens to the industry once the bubble bursts and investors move on? Is there even a place for profit generation in caring professions, when we consider that clients are paying for the cost of their services plus whatever is needed to maximise growth of the company? The primary focus of the veterinary profession should be on the wellbeing of patients and clients in the communities they serve, not on the feeding of shareholders. One of the risks of the commercialisation of care is that it can erode trust between professionals and the public, as the public perceives that financial gain is prioritised over their wellbeing. In their 2024 review of over fifty-six thousand responses from the public and the veterinary industry, the UK Competition and Markets Authority (CMA) outlined significant public concerns related to the cost of veterinary care and some of the impacts of the corporate model, prompting a formal Market Investigation (CMA 2024). These issues, whilst important, may seem irrelevant to the topic of love in veterinary medicine, but bear with me.

Regardless of whether vets (and other veterinary professionals) *need* to love animals, in my experience, most identify as animal lovers. In an ideal world, this love would increase job satisfaction and benefit the individual. So what is the cause of this apparent disconnect with the high levels of dissatisfaction within the profession? One argument against love as a core value in caring professions is the risk of compassion fatigue and burnout for workers, both recognised as serious issues across the veterinary profession (Foote 2023). Could animal-loving vets be more vulnerable to burnout? Perhaps. Unpacking the factors contributing to healthcare worker burnout is outside of this chapter's scope, but many are workplace-related (Dyrbye et al. 2017). Workplace culture, therefore, becomes essential for job satisfaction and, ultimately, standards of care. Is expressing love, compassion, and empathy possible if you do not feel cared for and valued yourself? Moreover, if so, what is the personal cost? Despite the healthy financial growth of the industry, the shift towards corporatisation does not appear to be associated with improvement in workplace culture, at least in the UK.

In a survey of veterinary nursing staff, 96% of respondents agreed or strongly agreed that workplace bullying was a serious problem. Individuals with a mental health condition, multiple disabilities, or chronic conditions or those who identified as neurodivergent were particularly likely to experience discrimination, bullying, and harassment (Plowden Roberts et al. 2024). Workers deal with the stress of increasingly frequent redundancies in the face of unprecedented workforce shortages, excessive workload, and financially driven key performance indicators. Many report routinely carrying out unpaid overtime, which they feel driven to do because they care so deeply for their patients and the standard of care they receive. The increasing use of non-disclosure agreements (NDAs) when dealing with worker complaints, terminations, and resignations undoubtedly stifles awareness and open debate of these issues. Being an animal lover brought so much meaning, passion, and fulfilment to my career, but during the very brief periods I experienced toxic workplace environments, that same love for animals was the greatest stressor. For me, compassion fatigue became a protective mechanism, protecting me from the pain of failing my patients and feeling inadequate at making a difference (however untrue that may have been).

During the summer of 2024, industrial action by veterinary support staff of a UK private-equity-backed veterinary group highlighted salaries below the UK national living wage. Eighty percent of staff reported regularly borrowing money to meet basic living costs, and five percent reported using food banks (Wall 2024). Whilst the wages of veterinarians are considerably better than those of other veterinary professionals, they have not consistently kept pace with inflation, and vets earn significantly less than is usually estimated by the general public. The level of pay incentive received is, of course, crucial for the freedom of an individual to reduce or control working hours or work intensification, make work-life balance accommodations, visit friends and family, fund childcare, hobbies, their own pet guardianship, take career breaks, and make other choices to support wellbeing and protect against burnout and compassion fatigue. One risk of a few large employers dominating the labour market is the exertion of monopsony power, meaning they have the power to set wages below competitive levels due to worker dependency because they own many neighbouring practices. Bringing us back to the question at hand, it is critical that ethical debate on love for animals as a core value for the veterinary profession includes consideration of the fundamental factors contributing to workplace culture in modern-day veterinary practice. Without this, debate is highly problematic and, at its worst, could be considered a form of toxic positivity.

25.6 THE COMPLEXITY OF HUMAN-ANIMAL RELATIONSHIPS

One of the more radical transitions I experienced in veterinary medicine was moving from general practice to laboratory animal practice. I did so for several reasons, not least because I would be making a difference for society's most vulnerable population of animals. What fascinated me was the change in people's perception of my value as an animal lover. I was used to people saying, 'I couldn't do your job because I love animals too much to put them to sleep'. A comment I found tricky to respond to, the implication being that I must not love animals as much as they do. 'I suppose you become hardened to it' was a frequent follow-up. In my case, this was an oversimplification because the reverse was also true. As I became more competent and confident at providing a predictably *good* death, I could be more present to the layers of emotion involved in this unique moment and often cried alongside the client, empathising with their loss. The same was sometimes true in laboratory animal practice, and I frequently witnessed researchers and animal care staff whose affection and love for the animals they cared for would be most tangible at this time. That was what fascinated me; I was the same person with compassion, empathy, and a passion for making a difference, but with the change of professional context, I had gone from experiencing an assumption of love for animals to an assumption of indifference, as if my choice of specialty indicated deficiency or failure of some kind. Some of the most misinformed and hurtful assumptions came from within the veterinary profession.

25.7 GOVERNANCE, PRAGMATISM, AND THE LIMITS OF LOVE

We are all vulnerable to misinterpretation of others' intentions or character. A healthcare provider's warmth, empathy, and good communication can lead patients to trust them more and assume good intentions and medical competence (Kraft-Todd et al. 2017). This type of cognitive bias, sometimes called the halo effect, underpins the importance of a provider's bedside manner and has been associated with positive effects on patient compliance and clinical outcomes (Di Blasi et al. 2001). For a veterinarian, a good bedside manner is usually taken as a love for animals and reassurance of acting in the client's best interest. Of course, this may be true, and it often is. However, this cognitive bias creates vulnerability in situations with competing motivations and undeclared (or unrecognised) conflicts of interest. Some terrifying examples exist from human healthcare.

In his biography titled *The Good Doctor*, author Wensley Clarkson describes the general practitioner Harold Shipman as 'a doctor whose superb bedside manner helped him gain the confidence of hundreds of patients before he cruelly cut them down'. Dr Shipman utilised his 'Godlike reverence and respect' to murder an estimated 250 patients before his arrest in 1998 (Smith 2002). More recently, in 2023, Paolo Macchiarini, a celebrity surgeon and regenerative medicine researcher nicknamed Super Surgeon, who pioneered the world's first artificial trachea, was sentenced to 2.5 years in prison for aggravated assault. This followed the death of three patients from surgical complications years after their procedures, a court having ruled that he knew the surgeries were unlikely to succeed and had disregarded the risks to the patients. The case has multiple ethical ramifications, highlighting inadequate controls around novel and innovative procedures and risks associated with celebrity status and the halo effect in healthcare (Teixeira da Silva 2017). It is sombre to reflect back on the responses I received during my residency when questioning the justification for controversial or innovative veterinary interventions – (i) 'It's what the owner wants', (ii) 'The animal is going to die if we don't do anything', or (iii) 'We can't advance if we don't practise' – and wonder to what extent similar thought processes contributed to the decision-making process for these human healthcare procedures.

In clinical practice, every procedure comes with a risk of stress and poor welfare outcomes despite the best intentions. Clinicians must ensure that neither love nor 'superhero syndrome' blinds them, or their clients, to the realities of their work. A pragmatic assessment of the risks and potential benefits of the procedure must govern their actions. Ultimately, when we decide on a particular course of action, we *predict* that the outcome will not only outweigh the stress and suffering induced as part of the process but also improve the animal's long-term quality of life. This pragmatic approach is critical to ensuring that care promotes positive welfare outcomes. When this is not the case, reflecting on the resulting *prediction error* is essential. In laboratory animal practice, outcomes are monitored throughout the animal's life, with data being available for retrospective analysis years after death. Lifelong clinical governance of this type is a challenge in companion animal practice, where novel or innovative procedures are commonly carried out in secondary centres with limited ability to follow up once the patient is discharged. Overcoming this challenge would enable clinicians to improve the predictive power of their clinical decisions, facilitate fully informed consent, and protect animals against the unintended consequences of innovation and advancement.

25.8 CONCLUSION: LOVE AS A POTENTIAL ADVANTAGE BUT NOT A NECESSITY

In conclusion, while love for animals can be an advantage in veterinary practice, it is neither necessary nor sufficient for high standards of welfare. Love for animals must be complemented by understanding the broader context in which veterinary care is provided – including the welfare of both animals and the humans who care for them. Veterinarians must navigate the complex intersection of animal welfare, human emotions, and practical realities of the profession with an overarching pragmatic perspective. Within that perspective – and given the wide range of sectors, specialities, and types of work within the veterinary industry – diversity in approaches is not only beneficial but also essential for excellence in animal and client care.

REFERENCES

Bailey S-J, Cogle K. Talking about dying: how to begin honest conversations about what lies ahead. *Royal College of Physicians Media* [Internet]. 2019 Oct 18. Available from: https://www.rcp.ac.uk/media/ubgpwfoj/ofh-talking-about-dying.pdf.

Brockman B, Taylor V, Brockman C. The price of unconditional love: consumer decision making for high-dollar veterinary care. *J Bus Res*. 2008;61(5):397–405.

Competitions and Markets Authority. CMA identifies multiple concerns in vets market. *GOV.UK* [Internet]. 2024 Mar 12. Available from: https://www.gov.uk/government/news/cma-identifies-multiple-concerns-in-vets-market.

Di Blasi Z, Harkness E, Ernst E, et al. Influence of context effects on health outcomes: a systematic review. *Lancet*. 2001. 357(9258):757–762.

Dyrbye LN, Shanafelt TD, Sinsky CA, et al. Burnout among health care professionals: a call to explore and address underrecognized threat to safe, high-quality care. *National Academy of Medicine Perspectives* [Internet]. 2017 Jul 5. Available from: https://nam.edu/burnout-among-health-care-professionals-a-call-to-explore-and-address-this-underrecognized-threat-to-safe-high-quality-care/.

Foote A. Burnout, compassion fatigue and moral distress in veterinary professionals. *Vet Nurse*. 2023;14(2):90–99.

Gallagher A, Watson F, Fitzpatrick N. Love as a core value in veterinary and medical practice: towards a humanimal clinical ethics? *Clin Ethics*. 2018;13(1):1–8.

KPMG. Veterinary M&A industry trends. *KPMG Mergers and Acquisitions* [Internet]. 2023 [cited 2024 Sept 4]. Available from: https://kpmg.com/us/en/articles/2023/veterinary-industry-trends.html.

Kraft-Todd G, Reinero D, Kelley J, et al. Empathic nonverbal behavior increases ratings of both warmth *and* competence in a medical context. *PLoS One*. 2017;12(5):1–16.

Lyu H, Xu T, Brotman D, et al. Overtreatment in the United States. *PLoS One*. 2017;12(9):1–11.

Morgan Stanley. The pet industry has plenty of lives left. *Morgan Stanley Research* [Internet]. 2024 Jul 12. Available from: https://www.morganstanley.com/ideas/pet-care-industry-outlook-2030.

Plowden Roberts C, Robinson D, Rosolin B. Disability and chronic illness in veterinary work and education: a survey exploring experiences of disability, chronic illness, mental health and neurodiversity in the veterinary sector. *Institute for Employment*

Studies [Internet]. 2024 Jul. Available from: https://www.employment-studies.co.uk/sites/default/files/resources/summarypdfs/Disability%20and%20Chronic%20Illness%20summary%20report%20final.pdf.

RCVS. Recruitment, retention and return in the veterinary profession. *RCVS Workforce Summit 2021* [Internet]. 2022 May 2. Available from: https://www.rcvs.org.uk/news-and-views/publications/recruitment-retention-and-return-in-the-veterinary-profession/retention-recruitment-and-return-in-the-veterinary-profession-preliminary-study-updated-2022.pdf.

Smith D. Not by error, but by design-Harold Shipman and the regulatory crisis for healthcare. *Public Policy and Administration*. 2002;17(4):55–74.

Teixeira da Silva JA. Ethical perspectives and ramifications of the Paolo Macchiarini case. *Indian J Med Ethics*. 2017;2(4):270–275.

Wall T. Vets extend strike in first industrial action to hit Britain's pet-care sector. *The Guardian* [Internet]. 2024 Aug 18. Available from: https://www.theguardian.com/lifeandstyle/article/2024/aug/18/vets-extend-strike-in-first-industrial-action-to-hit-britains-pet-care-sector?CMP=share_btn_url.

26 It is Time to Ditch the Gold Standard

Tanya Stephens

The term 'gold standard' is not one that lends itself to veterinary medicine, which accepts the reality of limitations of knowledge and seeks to add to knowledge and improve the way veterinarians practise.

Rather the term 'gold standard' is a historical term borrowed from economists and signifies a monetary standard. Subject to endless debate it was dumped a long time ago for a better system. For some unknown reason the term emerged in medicine in the 1960s and has taken hold with thousands of published papers mentioning the 'gold standard' which seems to have been misinterpreted as a set standard of excellence. The actual definition remains illusionary.

The concepts of 'spectrum of care', 'contextualised care' and 'pragmatic care' (that is being a veterinarian) have most likely arisen from the realisation that the mythical 'gold standard' is unattainable. This is especially so when the so-called gold standard is equated to meaning 'unaffordable' at a time of concerns around costs of veterinary services. Interestingly the definition of spectrum of care is virtually identical to that of evidence-based veterinary medicine.

Aiming for the so-called gold standard can have unintended consequences as unrealistic standards and expectations can lead to angst and poor mental health especially in new graduates because of a conflict between taught gold standards and the reality of practice where there is no such thing.

26.1 BACKGROUND

It was 2:00 a.m. and I couldn't sleep. It wasn't anything I had eaten or too much tea or the husband and dog snoring as, yes, along with 43% of pet owners surveyed in Australia (Animal Medicines Australia report 2022), our dog Ralph sleeps in our bedroom. It was the annoyance I couldn't dispel over reading yet another mention, this time in the latest Vet Record (Collins 2020) about the gold standard. I sat up in bed and wrote a response ('it is time to ditch the gold standard'), sent it to the Vet Record, and went to sleep. I was pleased to see my letter published (Stephens 2020).

My letter states that I also have concerns about overdiagnosis and overservicing in the profession as mentioned by Collins and I agree with Collins that veterinarians are becoming unaffordable. The term 'gold standard' mentioned in Collins's letter led to my middle-of-the-night letter writing rant. As a practitioner, I cringe at the mention of the words 'gold standard'.

Medicine is an inexact science and we should not be talking about a mythical and undefined gold standard. We know from surveys that unrealistic standards and expectations lead to angst and poor mental health in the veterinary profession, especially in new graduates. There is a conflict between stated gold standards and the reality of practice where there is no such thing. This shifts the blame when things go wrong, which they invariably do, onto the individual, instead of the profession.

Instead, I wrote that we must focus on using evidence-based veterinary medicine (EBVM) and good professional ethics that accept the reality of limitations of knowledge, and aim to add to knowledge and improve the way we practise. We know that the use of EBVM has better outcomes for animals and their owners and veterinarians.

I agree with Collins that there is indeed plenty of evidence that the costs of veterinary services are an issue and lead to reduced veterinary practice visits and the abuse of veterinarians which is clearly an animal welfare and veterinary welfare concern.

I go on to state that veterinary procedures should be based on good evidence, be justifiable and performed in the best interests of animals and their owners. Overdiagnosis and overservicing should be avoided at all costs to ensure that the profession maintains its standing and its social licence to operate, whilst also leading to better welfare all round.

26.2 THE MYTHICAL GOLD STANDARD

The term 'gold standard' irritates me as it is not a term that lends itself to veterinary or human medicine. Engineering, perhaps, as you can't have bridges falling down. The term is contrary to what we know about veterinary medicine and veterinary professional ethics, which acknowledges the limitations of knowledge whilst seeking to increase it. It also signifies, to me, something that is perfect and practice isn't like that and the last thing I need is for someone to tell me I'm not practising to a gold standard, especially as it has never been defined.

The gold standard may originally have been meant to signify best practice but it has surely been misinterpreted to be a set standard of excellence. To my mind it has nothing to do with veterinary practice. If practitioners are aiming for a mythical gold standard, they will be most likely disappointed as practice isn't like that. It's messy and things go wrong, and mistakes are made and pet owners can be difficult, and cats scratch.

The concept of a gold standard implies a level of perception that can never be attained by any biological test or clinical diagnosis and has unfortunate consequences, especially for newly minted veterinarians.

Clarke and Knights in 2018 discuss how unrealistic standards and expectations lead to angst and poor mental health in new graduates. There is a conflict between taught standards and the reality of practice where there is no such thing.

They used the Largescale 2015 survey of veterinary students and graduates by the BVA and the RCVS to show that many suffer from anxiety, depression, doubt, and sadly even contemplate suicide. According to the survey just 34% of graduates from five or more years ago considered their degree had prepared them very well, and only 46% say they would choose vetting as a career again. The survey also shows that veterinarians and clients had an unrealistic view of medicine as a panacea for all ills. The teaching of a clear separation between right and wrong answers, and faith in scientific and objective knowledge supports this ideal.

Clarke and Knights go on to say that the 'limitations of science – particularly in relation to certainty and predictability – tend to be unacknowledged in veterinary practice. This leaves many veterinarians pained by the occurrence of what they see as failures. Rather than acknowledging the limitations of medicine that can never fully deliver on its promise, veterinarians will tend to blame themselves . . . it is not enough simply to teach young veterinary surgeons about resilience and coping. This merely disguises these public matters by transferring the responsibility for failure from the profession back onto the individual. And this will only intensify the doubts and anxieties that vets seem already to have in abundance'.

Veterinarians and veterinary students should recognise the limitations of knowledge, the reality that there is no gold standard, and be directed towards the increasing numbers of EBVM resources such as systematic reviews and to take a good look at the EBVM Manifesto launched in 2020. As the Vet Record's senior clinical research editor at the time, Tom McNeilly, stated, 'In order to achieve the optimum health and welfare of animals, it is critical that we use current best evidence to make decisions about the management of animals in our care. This requires the generation of robust scientific evidence, being proactive about making this evidence available to end users in an understandable format and being able to quickly adapt best practice guidelines if and when the evidence changes'. Importantly, veterinarians need to acknowledge that the mythical gold standard is definitely not the same as using best evidence.

26.3 WHAT IS THE GOLD STANDARD ANYWAY?

A Google search for a definition of the 'gold standard' and where the saying originated seemed a good place to start. It appears that I'm not the first to complain about the term. There was a letter in the *British Medical Journal* complaining about it back in 2005. Claassen (2005) states that 'medical scientists have become confused about the true meaning of the term "gold standard"'. 'So, what is the gold or golden standard? Inspired by the Olympic Games where the best athlete wins the gold medal, people who use "golden standard" think the term denotes the best standard in the world. Not bronze, not silver, but gold. Of course, this is incorrect'.

Claassen goes on to explain that 'gold standard' is a historical term borrowed from economists and signifies a monetary standard under which the basic unit of currency was defined by a stated quantity of gold. The value of each country's currency was weighed against the gold standard so that different currencies could be compared for international trading.

The term 'gold standard' first appeared in medicine in 1962 in the Lancet in an anonymous commentary, 'Toward gold standard' to plead for a set standard for the use of gold salts in patients with rheumatoid arthritis. From 1979 it took off in medicine and the number of publications using the term ballooned. Much to the dismay of a biochemist, Duggan (1992) who thought the term 'presumptuous' for a biological test since 'the subject is in perpetual evolution and gold standards are by definition never reached'. Duggan proposed abolishing the term 'because the phrase smacks of dogma . . . after all the financiers gave up on the idea of a "gold standard" decades ago'. Despite this, between 1995 and 2005, when the Claassen letter was published, over 10,000 publications mentioned 'gold standard'.

As Claassen points out, even in its glory days, the monetary gold standard was never considered perfect and, subject to endless debate, was dumped for a better system.

The history of the gold standard in economic terms makes for interesting reading. Once upon a time all trade imbalances were settled with gold and governments had a strong incentive to stockpile gold for more difficult times. The international gold standard emerged in 1871 in Germany with the majority of developed nations joining up, and the gold standard was at its pinnacle from 1871 to 1914 when near ideal political conditions existed amongst most countries. This came to an end with the outbreak of the Great War when political alliances changed, international indebtedness increased, and government finances deteriorated.

The gold standard is not currently used by any government. Britain stopped using it in 1931 and it was completely replaced by fiat money, which is a monetary system in which the value of a currency is instead allowed to fluctuate dynamically against other currencies on the foreign-exchange markets.

In reality the gold standard was rarely seen as a gold standard and was controversial for much of its history. Isaac Newton put Britain on a gold standard in 1717, formalised by the Royal Mint in 1816 with other countries following. After breaking down as a result of inflation during World War 1, a variant was restored in 1925, to be abandoned again in 1931. In the USA Richard Nixon removed its gold standard in 1971.

Even Cochrane reviews, considered to provide the best evidence for a range of medical questions in the human field, are subject to controversy. This is as it should be. Science and medicine are not fixed in stone or silver or gold but are subject to ongoing debate.

26.4 THE SPECTRUM OF CARE AND EVIDENCE-BASED VETERINARY MEDICINE

The use of the term 'gold standard' has led to some unintended and unfortunate consequences in veterinary medicine.

The concept of 'spectrum of care/contextualised care' has emerged over the last few years in veterinary medicine, perhaps as a way of explaining what the average general practitioner actually does, i.e. developing their treatment plans based on best evidence, owner's wishes and ability to pay, and the reality of practice. The emergence of spectrum of care seems to have been the result of a belated recognition that the gold standard doesn't exist, is not fit for purpose, and is unattainable.

It was pleasing to see that I am not the only practitioner with a concern about the so-called spectrum of care/contextualised care. As Tim Hutchinson notes in a letter to the Vet Record April 2024, 'contextualised care is nothing new. In fact 20 years ago, we used to call it simply being a vet and it was how we worked ... How did we go so wrong that we had to reinvent the wheel?'

Unlike the gold standard, the spectrum of care has been defined and looks very much the same as the definition of evidence-based medicine. A definition of 'spectrum of care' from Fingland 2021 is 'the ability to provide a variety of high quality evidence-based care options that meet the needs of both the patient and the client'. The Evidence-Based Veterinary Medicine Association (ebvma.org) defines EBVM as 'the formal strategy to integrate the best research evidence available combined with clinical expertise as well as the unique needs or wishes of each client in clinical practice'.

Members of Veterinary Humanities UK (vethumanitiesuk.org) argue that our profession 'should move away from using the term "gold standard care" and instead adopt "contextualised care"', which 'acknowledges that different treatment pathways are able to offer acceptable patient journeys in different contexts' (Skipper et al. 2021).

We now have spectrum of care, contextualised care, and also pragmatic care in the veterinary practice lexicon. Take your pick! To me they all describe my life as a veterinary practitioner, and I wonder if these terms are the result of an urge by human beings nowadays to stick labels on just about everything.

26.5 COSTS OF VETERINARY SERVICES

One reason for the emergence of the 'spectrum of care' concept appears to be a concern over costs of veterinary services and the inability to practise to the 'gold standard', which is assumed to be costly. As Collins (2020) points out in her letter mentioning the gold standard, veterinarians are becoming unaffordable.

The survey by Animal Medicines Australia (2022) shows that costs are an issue for avoiding a trip to the veterinarian in Australia and in the UK Google reported (2023) a 28% increase in searches for 'can I give my pet Panadol?' suggesting that pet owners are turning to home care of their pets because of veterinary costs, and there is ample evidence worldwide that as costs increase, veterinary visits decrease, and costs have been found associated with increasing abuse of veterinarians.

Stull et al. (2018) discuss the concept of a spectrum of care and the problem with gold standard care, and they quite rightly point out that effective care does not include unnecessary tests or procedures which are not in the best interests of the animal or its owner. They also point out that cost is a barrier to access to veterinary care and this can be detrimental to the pet's wellbeing with rises in veterinary costs associated with decreasing veterinary visits. Furthermore, the lack of affordable and accessible care 'poses a tremendous challenge for veterinarians attempting to provide health-care services to ensure the health and wellbeing of the pet population'.

They suggest some solutions to the problem of affordability.

1. Development, evaluation, and refinement of clinical guidelines. The use of guidelines in human medicine has been shown to be useful in avoiding the errors in medicine caused by cognitive bias especially commission bias where clinicians have the urge to do something, said to be the main reason for the overuse of antibiotics in human medicine.
2. Promotion of effective, evidence-based practices (Choosing Wisely) and suggesting that one way to improve veterinary care and control costs is to reduce the use of unnecessary tests and treatments and to raise awareness among pet owners and veterinarians about interventions that are ineffective to free up resources for evidence-based care. The Choosing Wisely initiative aims to identify ineffective diagnostic and therapeutic practices in human medicine and for clinicians and patients to think critically about the interventions they use or are offered.
3. Establishment of a veterinary practice research network. Data derived by private practice are important in guiding and evaluating treatments.

Guidelines need to be critically examined. The World Small Animal Veterinary Association 2022 guidelines, for example, should be viewed through an evidence-based lens. Some are unrealistic such as the need for all practices to use dental x-rays without references to support this as best evidence and my particular irritant, 'alternative' medicine, with the pain guidelines on the one hand stating the lack of evidence for acupuncture whilst at the same time stating that for neuropathic pain, 'acupuncture and medical massage . . . should be included in the analgesic regimen as soon as possible'.

Fingland et al. (2021) also write about spectrum of care and note that cost is a barrier to access to care and that there has been a steady increase in the proportion of owned pets in the USA that received no healthcare from a veterinarian coinciding with the costs of veterinary services rising more than inflation. They write that the concept of a spectrum of care 'aims to address the growing problem of affordability of veterinary care by providing a continuum of acceptable care that considers available evidence-based medicine while remaining responsive to client expectations and financial limitations, thereby successfully serving an economically diverse clientele'.

On the same topic, Grimm et al. (2018) discuss the findings of a working party set up by the European College of Veterinary Anaesthesia and Analgesia to discuss the ethics of clinical veterinary practice and without a single mention of a 'gold standard' came up with 'best interest principle' with an ethical question 'Where should the line on treatment be drawn?' replaced by 'How should the line be drawn?' They formulated a veterinary ethics tool, VET, to facilitate decision-making and stressed that interventions on companion animals should always be in the best interest of the patient.

26.6 HUMAN BEHAVIOUR AND EBVM

Whilst the use of best evidence and less of the gold standard is needed in veterinary practice, I believe there is one area that needs more attention and that is the impact of behaviour on clinical decision-making. We know that human behaviour change is important in improving animal welfare.

Cognitive biases are more likely to create error when our reasoning is automatic rather than deliberate, as it must be in a clinical setting and one of the major functions of EBVM is to provide tools and resources to make the knowledge base we employ more reliable.

It has been said that in human medicine most mistakes occur because of cognitive biases and not a lack of knowledge, and this is an area that could do with more focus in undergraduate veterinary degrees. An understanding of why humans act in certain ways can be useful when making clinical decisions. For example, a clinician may feel the urge to do something when they see a dog with kennel cough, not because the dog needs treatment but because the owner expects something. They may even think that the 'gold standard' demands some treatment. This is called commission bias.

We know from a systematic review that recovery time for dogs with kennel cough is the same whether they receive antibiotics or not. We are aware of the problem with antibiotic resistance and overuse of antibiotics; however, our biases may override this, and the pet owner expects you to treat their dog which has kept them up all night coughing. It is suggested that commission bias is the reason that medical practitioners overprescribe antibiotics. I understand that once upon a time, to deal with this bias, doctors could prescribe placebo pills in various colours with green being the most effective and that there may even have been coloured water for injection.

Then there is ambiguity bias where clinicians have no idea what is wrong with an animal and run a multitude of often unnecessary tests.

Knowledge may not be enough, and there can be a gap between what we know and what we do, and improving the design and implementation of evidence-based practice depends on successful behaviour change interventions, i.e. the capability to perform the function, the opportunity, and the motivation to perform it. An understanding of the Behaviour Change Wheel (Michie et al. 2011) and changing behaviours can be useful to improve clinical practice.

We need to bridge the gap between what we know and what we do by enablement (making it easier to do the right thing) and restrictions (imposing rules and consequences). Good guidelines are very useful in this situation.

26.7 BEST EVIDENCE IS BEST!

The mythical gold standard is definitely not best evidence or EBVM. It is most unfortunate to hear veterinarians state that they have to provide a lower level of care or euthanise an animal because they haven't been able to practise to the gold standard or the owner is unable to pay for referral to a specialist who can.

As a practitioner, I have never thought in terms of contextualised care, spectrum of care, pragmatic care, or advanced care (used in human medicine to determine end-of-life wishes thus misapplied in veterinary medicine), and I am concerned these could lead to some confusion and have unintended consequences if these words suggest an 'anything goes' approach.

In any case, it isn't just about costs of veterinary services. The concept of spectrum of care hinges on providing affordable care, but I contend that is the wrong way to look at the issue of affordability of veterinary services. Veterinarians shouldn't be suggesting that with spectrum of care, practitioners are providing an affordable service without the 'extras', but rather providing a service based on best evidence in which any pointless 'extras' were never needed in the first place. In other words, using EBVM.

Importantly, teaching EBVM is likely to result in changes to skills, attitudes, and behaviours as well as improving animal health and welfare, and using best evidence in decision-making is likely to improve veterinary health and welfare as well. The use of EBVM has the potential to improve the standing of veterinarians, prevent overdiagnosis and overservicing, and minimise cognitive bias.

As all veterinarians in practice are aware, it is sometimes the human animal who can be difficult and as animal owners become more knowledgeable and demanding veterinarians may be tempted to abrogate their professional responsibility onto the owner at the expense of the animal. This is a growing trend in human medicine where the public may believe that every medical problem needs a diagnosis and a treatment regardless of cost or efficacy. This invariably leads to overdiagnosis and overtreatment. In addition, greed, fear of legal action, and widespread commercial influences are contributing to a costly global trend towards unnecessary and potentially harmful medicine in the human field and increasingly in the veterinary world, with the huge growth in referral, specialist, and emergency practices.

The recent UK Competition and Markets Authority report into the veterinary sector supports this. It identified that there is often a focus on 'selling the most comprehensive, risk-averse or sophisticated treatment and testing options for a given condition, and therefore may not adequately encourage customers to consider simpler, lower cost options (including doing nothing)'.

It has been suggested that the current so-called cost of living crisis could lead to veterinarians adopting cost effective treatments that pet owners can afford, which would be a welcome move in ensuring the use of EBVM and avoidance of overtreatment and overdiagnosis, which erodes trust in the profession and impacts on animal health and welfare.

Veterinary professional ethics is about doing what is right and not what is asked for, and veterinarians should be focusing on using evidence-based medicine and good professional ethics that accept the reality of limitations of knowledge and aim to add to knowledge and improve the way we practise. All veterinary procedures should be based on good evidence, justifiable, and performed in the best interests of animals and their owners, keeping in mind that the first priority of the veterinarian is the animal and not the owner. Overdiagnosis and overservicing should be avoided at all costs. The public wants transparency and accountability and as a profession we should ensure that our actions maintain our standing and our social licence to operate.

Regardless of any debate over semantics, it definitely is time to ditch the gold standard.

REFERENCES

Animal Medicines Australia. *Pets in Australia: a national survey of pets and people.* 2022;40.

Claassen JAHR. The gold standard: not a golden standard. *BMJ*. 2005 May 14;330(7500):1121.

Clarke C, Knights D. Doubt, depression, anxiety – just some of the problems plaguing the veterinary profession. *The Conversation* 2018 May 18.

Collins L. Are we becoming unaffordable to owners? *Vet Rec*. 2020;187:278.

Duggan PF. Time to abolish 'gold standard'. *BMJ*. 1992 Jun 13;304(6841):1568–1569.

Fingland RB, Stone LR, Read EK, et al. Preparing veterinary students for excellence in general practice: building confidence and competence by focusing on spectrum of care. *JAVMA* 2021 Sept 1;259(5).

Grimm H, Bergadano A, Musk GC, et al. Drawing the line in clinical treatment of companion animals: recommendations from an ethics working party. *Vet Rec*. 2018 Jun 9;182(23):664.

Michie S, Van Stralen MM, West R. The behaviour change wheel: a new method for characterising and designing behaviour change interventions. *Implement Sci*. 2011;6:42.

Skipper A, Gray C, Serlin R, et al. 'Gold standard care' is an unhelpful term. *Vet Rec*. 2021 Oct;189(8):331.

Stephens T. It is time to ditch the 'gold standard'. *Vet Rec*. 2020 Nov 28;187(11):452–453.

Stull JW, Shelby JA, Bonnett BN, et al. Barriers and next steps to providing a spectrum of effective health care to companion animals. *JAVMA* 2018;253:1386–1389.

27 Informed Consent – In Whose Interests?

Carol A. Gray

27.1 INTRODUCTION – IF OUR PATIENTS COULD GIVE CONSENT . . .

The idea that our veterinary patients could give consent to their own treatment is appealing. We could then ensure that any decisions about treatment coincided with the patient's own ideas about what was in their 'best interests'. Dream on.

But wait a minute – where would this leave some of our preventative healthcare procedures? How many cats/dogs/horses/rabbits/etc. would agree to prophylactic neutering? We could explain to them, 'This procedure will prevent you from becoming frustrated if you are not given the chance to mate or reproduce; it will possibly lengthen your life and prevent some types of cancer, but it may also increase your risk of developing certain types of cancer; it will alter your behaviour, and it will stop you from experiencing any sexual encounters; it also removes part of your body'.

Even therapeutic procedures may be problematic: 'We would like to perform heroic surgery, to remove this cancerous growth; we are not sure how long the procedure will take or how you will feel when you recover from the surgery; it may not cure you, and you will need to be given several months of chemotherapy after the surgery, which may make you feel bad'.

Would many animal patients agree to either of these surgeries?

Of course, this is all fanciful, but the team involved in decisions about veterinary treatment should try to ensure that they prioritise the animal patient's best interests when making these decisions. In this chapter, I am going to suggest that the person who is best placed to advocate for the animal is the owner, but we need to remember that they are not a neutral party, and they may have their own ideas about what is best for their animal.

We will start with the fundamentals of decision-making on behalf of animal patients. In veterinary practice, we have handed this to their legal owners or their owner's appointed agent, but we have sometimes allowed these people to make decisions that are not always in the animal's best interests. Instead, we have embraced the concept of informed consent from medicine wholeheartedly, concentrating on making sure that we have given the owner/agent the required information to make an informed decision, and ensuring that they are aware of

Informed Consent – In Whose Interests?

their financial obligations. This has been done with the best of intentions – legally, to protect the veterinary professional from accusations of trespass and the animal owner from damage to their legal property, and ethically, to respect the autonomy of the animal owner. However, as a result of this (perhaps) reckless embrace, do the best interests of the animal enter the discussion at all?

In this chapter I will explore the ethical aspects of informed consent and will propose that we could use a 'shared decision-making' approach as a foundation for balancing owner autonomy with the best interests of the patient. I will introduce the term 'contextualised care', using this as a pivotal strategy to underpin decisions made about veterinary healthcare treatment. But first, we need to consider the contractual basis of veterinary healthcare.

27.2 WE NEED TO TALK ABOUT MONEY

As veterinary medicine is a private form of healthcare, requiring fees for service through either direct payment by the client or via insurance cover, an important part of the veterinary consent process involves disclosure of financial costs.

In addition to the contractual approach that the fee-for-service basis brings to consent, it also gives clients a form of autonomy over what happens to their animals. Owners can choose innovative and complicated surgery costing thousands of pounds for their pets, a decision that encompasses a debate about 'whether the expense of surgery is worth the companionship an animal brings' (Mills 2016). Indeed, overtreatment of animal patients may be a concern, as discussed by Grimm and others (2018) in their observation that 'the client's willingness to pay for treatment and an increase in treatment options for companion animal patients raise the question of which treatments are morally justified'.

Alternatively, owners can decide not to pay for any treatment for their animals.

The ability and willingness to pay for treatment are solely the owner's decision, with this aspect of decision-making for an animal regarded as a form of financial autonomy that must be respected. However, this is not an unrestrained autonomy. The veterinarian may refuse to carry out a specific treatment requested by the owner, especially if there is a welfare concern. Perhaps more importantly, if the veterinarian proposes a single treatment option for which the owner is unable to or refuses to pay, the veterinarian may need to suggest or agree with euthanasia of the animal patient. Therefore, it can be seen that animal patients are not entitled to equal treatment under the usual business terms of most veterinary practices. Any notion of justice for animals does not extend to equality of treatment when injured or sick. For the individual animal patient, the amount and availability of treatment depends on the owner, who retains financial autonomy over treatment decisions, sometimes resulting in a decision to end the animal's life on economic grounds. If we are genuinely to consider a 'shared decision-making' approach to veterinary healthcare, we need to factor in the part played by the owner's financial resources and willingness to spend these resources.

27.3 WE NEED TO TALK ABOUT BEST INTERESTS

Owners have legal obligations to provide for their animals' basic needs, and to prevent suffering, but they may be considered to have moral obligations to protect the interests of their animals, by virtue of the relationship that they have with them (Cooke 2011). Regardless of an animal's moral or legal status, it is the relationship between the animal and the caregiver (usually the animal's owner) that is fundamental to making decisions on a 'best interests' basis. One study found two main variations of the human–companion animal relationship, the first involving owners who see pets as 'loved family companions that are valued for who they innately are' and the second involving owners who consider pets as a 'self-project', for example, as toys, status symbols, or brands, thus contrasting those who consider pets as beings and those who see them as possessions (Beverland et al. 2008). Focusing on the former variation, Schicktanz (2006) describes one type of human-animal relationship as a 'friendship model', requiring that the human provides for basic needs and veterinary care while also defending an ethical basis for partiality towards these animals. If the relationship is based on a friendship model, the animal owner should be best placed to advocate for the animal's interests.

Protection of interests involves more than just prevention of harm or suffering. There is a difference between 'preference interests', which promote positive emotional states, and 'welfare interests', which provide for basic needs (Regan 2004, 87). It is challenging to provide for animals' preference interests. With current levels of knowledge about cognition in many animal species, it is difficult to ascertain their wishes or test their preferences. Nevertheless, Wise (2013) argues that many animals are capable of expressing what he calls 'practical autonomy', which consists of having desires, being able to act intentionally to try to fulfil these and having a sense of 'self'.

Moreover, animals can appear to react to any proposed treatment by showing aggression or fear-related behaviours, which could be regarded as a form of dissent. However, it is only in rare cases that the animal's preferences are taken into consideration; i.e. their assent or dissent is acknowledged. For example, in research, animal preferences are recognised in studies that are specifically designed to define these; in other studies, animals that are resistant to frequent handling and treatment may be excluded from participating on welfare grounds (Kantin & Wendler 2015). In veterinary practice, animals showing any dissent are often prescribed a program of behavioural modification. If urgent treatment is required, they are sedated or anaesthetised to enable treatment to be given, thus prioritising their health interests over other welfare interests (Gray et al. 2018).

This contrasts with the stated aim of 'best interests' calculations for human patients unable to consent. For such patients, 'best interests' no longer equates merely to 'best medical interests' (Coggon 2016). If the patient has had capacity in the past, then their previously expressed wishes or preferences must be prioritised.

It is much more difficult to protect the interests of patients who have never had capacity. A simple solution may be to employ an approach that prioritises the 'avoidance of harm'. Such an approach attempts to maximise the patient's

Informed Consent – In Whose Interests?

interests in remaining in good health, not being harmed and not suffering pain. However, this approach is reminiscent of the narrow 'welfarist' approach, which merely attends to providing for an animal's basic welfare needs. We know that best interests involve more than just avoiding pain and suffering. Although any living being's interest in not suffering is paramount, a focus solely on harm avoidance can result in animals leading unfulfilled lives, albeit free from pain. A more holistic understanding of interests is therefore required. Although preferences may be easily ascertained, a comprehensive calculation of best interests for animals is more difficult. One proposed list includes quality of life, the ability to function naturally, and the ability to participate in a mutually beneficial relationship with the owner (Schnobel 2017), which can be combined with individual lifestyle (proposed by the owner) and healthcare (proposed by the veterinarian) needs, but this approach highlights the difficulty of interpreting behaviour in another species. Another approach is to base a 'best interests' calculation on an existing formula, such as the one for children based on the United Nations Convention on the Rights of the Child. The list of criteria to be examined in this approach is as follows:

1. The animal's preferences (as interpreted by the owner)
2. Maintenance of relationships with humans and conspecifics
3. Ensuring wellbeing and protection from abuse, with special concerns for abused and stray animals
4. Advantages of treatment weighed against risks and side effects

(Gray & Fordyce 2020)

I propose here that although the calculation of the best interests of the animal is a joint enterprise between the veterinary professional (who can provide evidence of health-related benefits) and the owner, it is the latter who bears more responsibility for making the decision in those interests and who may be the most suitable candidate to decide on the animal's best interests if there is conflict. In most cases, it is the animal owner who knows and has a unique bond with the individual animal and, therefore, is best placed to interpret the animal's preferences and desires. It is the owner who will bear most of the emotional and relational burden resulting from any decision regarding veterinary healthcare. However, to qualify as the most suitable decision-maker for the animal patient, an owner must recognise the specific needs and interests of the animal, prioritising these as the basis for decision-making over the right to do as they wish with their property.

27.4 WE NEED TO TALK ABOUT SHARED DECISION-MAKING

Shared decision-making recognises that there are two (or more) experts in the room. The role of the veterinary professional in the consent discussion is to provide the owner with the information about proposed treatment options with a view to maintaining the ideal human-animal relationship but also to find out what the owner's concerns, hopes, and constraints may be. Instead of a single 'consent' conversation, the 'shared decision-making' approach comprises several steps (which can be conducted in a single consultation or over several days or weeks). First, the animal owner is told that there are several options. Then, each option is considered in depth. To enable a decision that also incorporates the wider interests of the animal requires the provision of information about the risks, benefits, side effects, costs, and long-term outcomes of each of the treatment options. The information provided by owners to widen the interests-based calculation might include the individual animal's behaviour, preferences (which could include, for example, being able to free range freely outside or mix with other animals of the same species), and dislikes; for example, a dislike of taking pills, having injections, or even visiting the veterinary practice at all may influence the choice of treatment.

Finally, a decision must be reached, and each decision will have more or less urgency. The health-related aspects of each option can be combined with the owner's knowledge of the individual animal's preferences to produce a genuinely best-interests-based shared decision, with each party involved to a greater or lesser extent in making that decision.

A 'shared decision-making' approach encourages the veterinary professional to match each proposed option with the owner's concerns and with the animal patient's interests, to hopefully allow a treatment choice that achieves the required outcome for all parties. A 'shared decision-making' protocol also usefully fulfils the requirements for informed consent.

27.5 WE NEED TO TALK ABOUT CONTEXTUALISED CARE

Achieving a balance in veterinary healthcare decision-making between client autonomy and patient best interests requires an unhurried discussion between the animal owner and the veterinary professional, with each option presented equally. This leads on to consideration of contextualised care. This term has been in use for several years now and has arisen from the requirement to offer alternatives to expensive and often unachievable 'gold standard' treatments (Skipper et al. 2021). In cases where an owner cannot or will not afford the most expensive (and strongly recommended) treatment, the client may feel that the only option may be euthanasia. But are there other options available?

Whether a client has insurance or not, respecting client financial autonomy should involve presenting all of the available treatment options, regardless of the presence or absence of insurance, and regardless of the latest equipment or expertise that the practice has invested in. Reasonable treatment options would include all treatments available at the practice, in view of current personnel and equipment, and the offer of referral to another practice if an alternative treatment, unavailable at the current practice, would be in the animal's best interests. It is then up to the humans involved to consider each option and balance the risks and benefits to the animal patient.

As an example, consider Taz, a one-year-old female entire Bengal cat. She is loved by a family who also wanted to breed from her. Unfortunately she escapes one evening, finds her way out on to the road, and is involved in a hit-and-run accident. She is found lying under a tree in a neighbour's garden the next day and rushed into her usual veterinary practice. The family does not have pet healthcare insurance. She has first aid treatment (pain relief and fluid therapy), and the results of diagnostic imaging show that her bladder is intact, but she has a badly smashed pelvis and open fractures to her right hind femur. There are several options:

1. Surgery to repair both the fractured pelvis and femur, but with a poor prognosis for the femoral repair
2. Surgery to repair the pelvis and to amputate the RH limb, with advice to neuter Taz when she recovers
3. Surgery to amputate the RH limb and allow the pelvis to heal with rest and pain relief, with advice to neuter Taz when she has recovered from the amputation
4. Surgery to try to salvage the RH limb, with conservative treatment of the pelvic fracture, with advice that Taz should be neutered

While this was discussed with the family, it becomes apparent that they are determined that Taz should have the chance to have kittens. They can find the money for the pelvic and femoral fracture repairs, and they are aware of the risks of infection and unsuccessful outcome, particularly for the femoral fracture. They decided that they will give the femoral repair two weeks, then if there are complications, they will opt for limb amputation. The veterinary team has agreed that this is a sensible option, and the surgery is booked for the following day.

Let's consider a different Taz. She has also suffered the pelvic and femoral injuries as a result of being hit by a car, but this time she belongs to an elderly owner and she is his much-loved companion. She is fully insured, and the same options are presented to her owner. This time, the option of amputating the limb and surgical repair of the pelvic fracture is chosen, with neutering when she has recovered from the pelvic surgery. The owner realises that Taz is likely to seek freedom when in season, and he does not want this to happen again. He had thought about having a litter of kittens, but it is much more important that Taz is comfortable and safe.

We have a final version of Taz. She belongs to a college student who has limited financial resources. In this case, she can find the money to pay for a limb amputation and will opt for conservative treatment of the pelvic fracture; she also does not have the time to bring Taz back for numerous repeat visits as she is working alongside her studies. She was intending to get Taz neutered anyway, as she did not want her to have kittens.

For our three versions of Taz, we have used a contextualised care approach that takes into account the best interests of the patient, the wishes and hopes of the owners, the financial resources available to the owners, and the unique circumstances of their lifestyles.

27.6 WE NEED TO COME BACK TO INFORMED CONSENT

How does contextualised care also satisfy the requirements of informed consent? Hopefully, it is apparent that it requires a truly 'shared decision-making' approach, where information is passed and received between veterinary and ownership teams.

In order to achieve the goals of protecting all three participants, informed consent must consist of an agreed and communicated balance between the autonomy of the client, the professionalism of the veterinarian or veterinary nurse, and the best interests of the animal patient. The tension between autonomy and beneficence has been more fully explored in a previous paper (Gray et al. 2018)

The veterinary professional can demonstrate respect for the autonomy of the animal owner through the following:

a. Presenting all reasonable treatment options
b. Providing scientific expertise and knowledge of the evidence of the risks and benefits of each treatment option
c. Presenting this information in a format that is understandable to the animal owner
d. Finding out what is important to the owner about their relationship with their animal
e. Soliciting the owner's idea of what would be in the animal's best interests
f. Supporting the owner to make the decision that fits best with their circumstances and prioritises the animal's best interests

The animal owner can demonstrate their knowledge of the best interests of the individual animal through the following:

a. Providing evidence of the animal's temperament, preferences, and lifestyle
b. Acting as the animal's advocate

However, the owner is also responsible for payment for treatment and for the provision of ongoing care, so they must contribute to the shared decision-making conversation through the following:

c. Identifying any individual constraints to the decision-making process, such as finances available, personal values and beliefs, and time and resources available for ongoing care
d. Considering each option in terms of its impact on the animal and on themselves in their particular circumstances, and sharing their thought processes with the veterinary professional

By moving the underpinning rationale for informed consent from the autonomy of the owner (or the autonomy of the veterinary professional) to the best interests of both the animal and the owner, decided jointly between the veterinary professional and the owner, informed consent becomes a means of protecting the three parties involved in the veterinarian-client-patient triadic relationship.

27.7 WE NEED TO CONSIDER THE PRACTICAL ASPECTS OF THE CONSENT PROCESS

Obviously, these conversations will take time. It is accepted as good practice that consent discussions should take place in advance of the planned treatment/surgery. For elective procedures, this could be several days before the animal's admission for treatment.

This is an ideal role for veterinary nurses who have had appropriate training in undertaking these types of consent conversation and can talk knowledgeably about the various options and the risks, benefits, and financial costs of each one.

In emergency situations, the focus is moved to provision of first aid to the animal patient, so a blanket consent for administration of any urgent treatment is required at first presentation, before a more in-depth discussion of next steps can be held. In these cases, the veterinarian in charge of the case is best placed to participate in these conversations, although a veterinary nurse could usefully step in to continue giving relevant information as the case progresses.

Finally, we need to recognise that informed consent is a process rather than an event. Things may change with our patients as we progress along the treatment path, and we need to maintain open communication with owners to ensure that consent is constantly being updated.

In summary, then, informed consent should be an ongoing process that ideally gives the animal owner plenty of time to consider options and make a decision, supported by veterinary professionals to make the decision that is right for them, their animal, and the veterinary team. By recognising contextualised care as a more suitable foundation for veterinary healthcare than 'gold standard' care, and by employing the principles of shared decision-making, we can ensure that consent is always informed and protective of everyone involved in the veterinary professional-client-patient relationship.

REFERENCES

Beverland MB, Farrelly F, Ching Lim EA. Exploring the dark side of pet ownership: status-and control-based pet consumption. *J Bus Res*. 2008;61(5):490–496.

Coggon J. Mental capacity law, autonomy, and best interests: an argument for conceptual and practical clarity in the court of protection. *Med Law Rev*. 2016;24(3):396–414.

Cooke S. Duties to companion animals. *Res Publica*. 2011;17(3):261–274.

Gray C, Fordyce P. Legal and ethical aspects of 'best interests' decision-making for medical treatment of companion animals in the UK. *Animals (Basel)*. 2020;10(6):1009.

Gray C, Fox M, Hobson-West P. Reconciling autonomy and beneficence in treatment decision-making for companion animal patients. *Liverpool Law Rev*. 2018;39(1–2):47–69.

Grimm, H, Bergadano A, Musk GC, et al. Drawing the line in clinical treatment of companion animals: recommendations from an ethics working party. *Vet Rec*. 2018;182(23):664.

Kantin H, Wendler D. Is there a role for assent or dissent in animal research? *Camb Q Healthc Ethics*. 2015;24(4):459–472.

Mills B. 'If this was a human ...': pets, vets and medicine. *Crit Stud Telev*. 2016:11(2): 244–256.

Regan T. *The case for animal rights*. 2nd ed. Berkeley: University of California Press; 2004.

Schicktanz S. Ethical considerations of the human-animal-relationship under conditions of asymmetry and ambivalence. *J Agric Environ Ethics*. 2006;19:7–16.

Schnobel S. Regulating the veterinary profession: taking seriously the best interests of the animal. *Prof Neglig*. 2017;33(4):239–261.

Skipper A, Gray C, Serlin R, et al. 'Gold standard care' is an unhelpful term. *Vet Rec*. 2021;189(8):331.

Wise S. The capacity of non-human animals for legal personhood and legal rights. In: Corbey R, Lanjouw A, editors. *The politics of species: reshaping our relationships with animals*. Cambridge: Cambridge University Press; 2013. p. 241–245.

28 The Death of Veterinary Euthanasia

R. Eddie Clutton

28.1 INTRODUCTION

Until recently, animal euthanasia seemed to be a relatively uncomplicated matter: the act was undertaken without much profound deliberation, and animals would be killed when vets and clients agreed that reasonably priced veterinary care was unlikely to improve the quality (QoL) nor, less importantly, the *quantity* of a sick and ageing animal's life. Reasons for killing animals would be implicitly understood by veterinarians and owners alike, and neither would seem to suffer undue psychological consequences once the act was complete and the animal buried. Euthanasia was a veterinary professional privilege which – regrettably – also solved problems *beyond* failing to maintain an animal's health and welfare. For example, animals would be euthanatised because they were no longer wanted, i.e. killed for convenience.

Things are no longer straightforward. Vets are more circumspect about euthanasia while companion animal owners are more likely to demand that more be done for their pets. Both changes support the impression that the previous usefulness of veterinary euthanasia is waning. This chapter does not re-examine the ethics of animal euthanasia (see Yeates 2010; Quain 2021; Cooney & Kipperman 2023) but because the demonisation of euthanasia as a veterinary therapeutic option has animal welfare implications, it attempts to (i) record euthanasia's changing role in veterinary practice, (ii) question the reasons for change, (iii) speculate on the possible outcomes for animals, owners, and veterinarians, and (iv) when these outcomes are undesirable, consider options for resolution.

28.2 CHANGING ATTITUDES TO ANIMAL EUTHANASIA

Singer's *Animal Liberation* (1975) ignited major changes in societal and cultural attitudes towards animals regarding their role in society, their intrinsic value, and their moral status. This elaboration of animal ethics and animal rights has coloured views on veterinary treatment and euthanasia at both societal and veterinary professional level. In more affluent societies, there is an increased emphasis on providing humane care for animals involving end-of-life considerations. Increased awareness about the importance of responsible pet ownership, preventive care, and the humane treatment of animals has also 'positively' influenced attitudes toward euthanasia (Mota-Rojas et al. 2021).

Attitudinal changes to animal euthanasia have probably been catalysed by the changing *expression* of anthropomorphism and its drift towards anthropocentrism. Humans have tended to the former for millennia, but the latter is a 21st century phenomena. Increasing numbers of companion animal owners now regard their animals as family members. One study found 6.9% of respondents reported ending relationships because their partners did not like their dog (Megna 2024). Anthropomorphism and an intensification of the human-animal bond has probably played a major role in raising owner circumspection on the subject of animal euthanasia (Wensley 2008).

The portrayal of veterinarians on TV may have given animal owners false expectations, i.e. that there are surgical solutions for animal conditions that euthanasia would previously have solved. A problem with these programmes that sensationalise 'new' breakthroughs and the people doing them is their failure to reveal the later demise of many animals when the breakthrough they enjoyed becomes a disaster they endured (Clutton et al. 2022).

The public debate on animal welfare following publication of *Animal Liberation* was not initially swamped by vets, and consequently, animal and veterinary ethics found themselves on divergent paths. Tannenbaum defined animal ethics as the moral obligations that people have for animals, and limited veterinary ethics to the provision of veterinary care (1995). This is helpful because veterinarians are frequently required to simultaneously serve conflicting human and animal interests, for example, in the case of tending farm stock, competition horses, or laboratory animals. Other areas examined in the analysis of the moral status of animals was their arbitrary killing. At one time many vets performed euthanasia without much in the way of questioning why, and for no better reason than the owner requested it. This was justified on the basis that if the vet didn't do it, the owner would either find someone else who would or simply abandon the animal. Nowadays this attitude seems to be far less common, and for numerous reasons, vets appear to be far less willing to kill pets 'on demand' (Yeates & Main 2011).

Changes in veterinary attitudes to euthanasia have probably also arisen from changes in the profession, specifically the greater proportion of female veterinarians. Women are more likely to disagree with convenience euthanasia (Hartnack et al. 2016), while male veterinary students tend to show a greater tolerance to killing animals (Ogden et al. 2012).

The result of these changes means that the often-unspoken consensus between owners and vets on the best time 'to put Fido to sleep' has become more difficult to agree upon. This has important implications for all involved. Clients mesmerised by the capabilities of 'supervets' may see their own general practitioners as less 'super', which is damaging to both the client-vet relationship, and the self-esteem of the practitioner (Lamb 2018). Other disagreements between the veterinary surgeon and client may lead to ill-feeling and a breakdown of trust especially with respect to costs (CMA 2024a). Most importantly, however, is the fact that the animal's welfare may be compromised (Clutton et al. 2022).

28.3 REASONS FOR ESCHEWING ANIMAL EUTHANASIA

Supporters of human euthanasia emphasise the importance of patient autonomy, i.e. the patient's right to make end-of-life decisions. Animals cannot make such decisions so human (owner and/or veterinary) advocacy is required. This must always ensure the animal's requirements are prioritised (Hiestand 2022). Consequently, reasons *not* to conduct euthanasia may be driven by the client with or without the vet's agreement.

On receiving news their pet has something which justifies euthanasia, many clients understandably ask, 'Is there nothing that can be done?' They ask this because they will have strong emotional bonds with their animals – who they may believe share their own fears of death and dying. In these circumstances, two options exist: palliation or further treatment.

28.4 PALLIATION AND HOSPICE

Previously, brief stays of termination gave time for grieving owners to accept the inevitable. However, new methods of QoL assessment, advances in animal pain management[1] and anthropomorphism mean that effective palliative care can now provide a suitable, though temporary alternative to euthanasia. However, there are challenges with animal palliative care. For example, QoL assessment is an imprecise science and leaves much scoring responsibility to subjective scaling and emotional clients. Second, some parts of the animal palliation industry appear to endorse practices that have a limited evidence base for efficacy, e.g. massage, therapeutic laser, chiropractic adjustment, and 'physical' therapy – whatever that might be.

Decision-making during palliation may be facilitated by pre-establishing humane endpoints (HEPs). In the United Kingdom (UK), HEPs are legal requirements for experimental animals and refer to predetermined physiological or behavioural signs that define the point at which an animal's pain, distress, or physical deterioration *must* be ended by euthanasia (Home Office 2017). In palliative veterinary medicine, endpoints could be established by the vet and owner before palliation begins and could form the contract identifying when euthanasia will be done without further discussion or delay. Applied expertly, palliative care is a suitable reason for withholding euthanasia – for just a *little bit* longer.

28.5 CLIENT-DRIVEN TREATMENT IN PREFERENCE TO PALLIATION, HOSPICE, OR EUTHANASIA

Not infrequently, a client's desire to continue treatment (rather than euthanasia or palliation) may run counter to the veterinarian's view that the animal should be killed because of poor welfare. This was considered 'most stressful' in one study evaluating the stress of ethical challenges amongst UK veterinarians (Batchelor & McKeegan 2012). Reasons for owners requesting further treatment include an inability to accept reality, naïve anthropomorphism, and false expectations raised by TV programs. Clients refusing to heed veterinary advice concerning their animal's welfare and euthanasia raise questions about pet ownership, veterinary care, and animal cruelty laws. In the UK, the Animal Welfare Act (2006) protects animal welfare and holds that any person with responsibility for an animal, i.e. the owner, commits an offence if an act, or failure to act, causes an animal to suffer unnecessarily. However, AWA (2006) contains no provisions that authorise vets to destroy suffering animals. In these circumstances, the Royal College of Veterinary Surgeons (RCVS) advises that vets should attempt resolution by advising the owner seeks a second opinion, ideally by phone (2024). Veterinary surgeons who are prevented from killing severely suffering animals by their owners may consider calling the police and having the client charged under the AWA (2006).

28.6 CLIENT-DRIVEN TREATMENT WITH VETERINARY CONCURRENCE

These days, insurance companies and/or crowdfunding will foot large veterinary bills encouraging anthropomorphic owners to request advanced 'last chance' or 'heroic' treatments rather than conduct euthanasia. Such clients will have little difficulty in finding vets agreeable to these requests because veterinarians have much to gain. Euthanasia-delaying options provide opportunities to conduct challenging diagnostic and interventional procedures during which they will gain clinical skills, experience, and advertisable kudos for their practice and take a professional fee even when treatments fail. Some may become famous (or infamous) by performing advanced techniques.

When non-euthanasia options become 'overtreatment'[2] or 'futile' or 'go too far', then the costs to the animal and client increase substantially and the veterinarian may find themselves on ethical thin ice. Therefore, when clients demand heroic interventions, the conscientious veterinary surgeon must ask whether the proposed treatment is (i) routine veterinary practice (RVP),[3] (ii) possible (i.e. do the skills and facilities exist?), and (iii) able to pass the 3Ps test. The latter asks three questions. First, how much pain (acute or chronic, physical or psychological) will treatment cause to the animal? Second, what price is paid by (i) the client in terms of financial cost, guilt, and caregiver burden and (ii) unwilling veterinary participants, e.g. nurses and students in terms of moral stress? Third, does the prognosis assure that the procedure will improve the pet's QoL for a period of sufficient duration to justify carrying it out in the first place? When answers to these questions indicate low pain and price with an acceptable prognosis, then foregoing euthanasia may be justified. When cases fail the 3Ps test, then palliation and hospice or euthanasia are the only options.

It seems paradoxical that modern owners appear to be permitting 'heroic' procedures on animals at a time when humans are voluntarily ending their own lives at unprecedented rates (Steck et al. 2018). Previously, humans complaining about the indignity of intensive medical treatment during terminal care would assert that 'this wouldn't happen to a dog'. Sadly, this is no longer the case. A reality injection,

The Death of Veterinary Euthanasia 269

formulated predominantly on the likely differences between how humans and animals view their own mortality, is possibly being underprescribed.

28.7 VETERINARIAN-DRIVEN TREATMENT WITH OWNER CONCERNS

An even more disagreeable situation arises when veterinarians prefer postponing euthanasia in favour of further diagnostic tests and/or treatment, despite the client expressing sincere reasons for wanting their pet terminated, e.g. a conviction that their companion has 'had enough', doubt over the proposed intervention's efficacy, and/or an inability to pay veterinary fees. Coercing owners with 'it's what their faithful companion deserves' is unprofessional. The Competition and Markets Authority's (CMA's) intimation that veterinary professionals might prey on an owners' desire to do the best for their pets by using the distress of an unwell pet or the need to make prompt decisions was rejected by the British Veterinary Association (BVA) and other veterinary professional organisations. However, the CMA's report (2024a) was based on nearly 45,000 client and over 11,000 veterinary professional responses, enough of whom thought that 'sophisticated and costly treatments' were of sufficient importance that the consultation document refers to it 25 times.

Clients who acquiesce to their veterinarian's wishes and find themselves suffering with guilt, dwindling financial resources, and caregiver burden (Spitznagel et al. 2017) should request a case re-valuation and/or a second opinion. If concerns are unheeded the client should raise a formal concern to the RCVS.

28.8 TOO EXPENSIVE TO DIE?

Owners may eschew euthanasia because they cannot afford the professional fee. In the UK, the CMA report identified problems with veterinary pricing structures relevant to euthanasia; i.e. most vet practices do not display prices on their website, pet owners might be overpaying for medicines, and practice conglomeration may have limited local competition (2024b).

Exorbitant veterinary euthanasia fees – real or imagined – are modest in comparison to those of the animal funereal industry that has recently flourished. In previous times a garden burial sufficed. These days, dead companion animals are mourned and cremated or buried in dedicated pet cemeteries. Pet urns and memorials are available including engravable ash containers which may be worn as jewellery. The charitable observer may see these as ways bereaved owners can uniquely commemorate their dead companion. Others may see it as ostentatious indulgence fuelled by gullibility, anthropocentrism, and too much disposable income. The end result, though, is that some owners may be disinclined to have their pet destroyed through fear of these unnecessary additional costs.[4]

A disinclination to pay veterinary fees for euthanasia which results in animal suffering puts the owner at risk under AWA (2006). Problems are avoided by referring owners to animal charities.

28.9 FEWER CONVENIENCE KILLINGS?

Increasing moral opposition to killing healthy animals amongst veterinarians may account for an apparent reduction in veterinary euthanasia. Moral stress was first highlighted as a veterinarians' problem in the 1980s and was related to killing shelter, unwanted, or 'surplus' animals (Rollin 1986). Since then, the specific relationship between ethical dilemmas in veterinary practice and workplace stress has been revealed (Batchelor & McKeegan 2012). This study revealed that vets regularly face two equally stressful scenarios: (i) the convenience euthanasia of healthy animals and (ii) financial limitations restricting treatment options.

Owners who do not share a veterinarian's distaste for convenience killing may find alternative less pleasant methods to solve inconveniences. When vets are asked but are disinclined to destroy animals enjoying a life worth living, they should scan the dog for a microchip and check associated databases to determine whether (i) the animal originated from a shelter with a 'return' policy or (ii) a named rehomer exists. Where euthanasia is required because clients are unable to pay, they should be apprised of the options, e.g. referral to a charity (RCVS 2024).

28.10 CONCERNS WITH COMPLEX ETHICAL QUESTIONS CONCERNING ANIMAL EUTHANASIA

The RCVS's Code of Professional Conduct (2024) and the BVA's recommendations (2016) on euthanasia are clear in directing veterinarians along paths of ethical decision-making. However, new graduates may feel inadequately experienced to make some decisions based on absolute uncertainty, e.g. 'Does this animal face a life not worth living?' or more complex ethical questions, e.g. 'Is euthanasia a welfare issue?' Under these circumstances, graduates may opt to postpone euthanasia, viewing this reversible option as the lesser of two evils. However, they may then experience guilt if the retrospectoscope reveals that the wrong decision was made and that the animal had subsequently suffered.

Such problems could be prevented by a more comprehensive coverage of the subject in the final year of vet school. In the clinic, the practice's euthanasia policy should be made available to the staff and clientele, as well as an experienced colleague able to provide a second opinion.

28.11 OVER-MORALISED VETS?

The role of moral evolution in 'the death of animal euthanasia' may have gone too far. In 2024, it became illegal in the UK to own without registration the American XL Bully, a dog breed disproportionately linked to 23 human deaths from dog attacks since 2021. A survey revealed that 60% of vets and 85% of nurses would refuse to comply with an order to euthanise a healthy XL Bully with no behavioural issues. So what responsibility is to be assumed by abstaining vets and nurses in the case where another human life is extinguished by a savage and illegally reprieved animal? Is the refusal to euthanise a protest against ill-conceived legislation rather than a sincere concern with the rights of a potentially lethal animal? Whatever the answer, withholding euthanasia for political purpose will not contribute significantly to a waning role of veterinary euthanasia.

28.12 GENUINE ADVANCES IN VETERINARY MEDICINE

An obvious reason for de-prioritising euthanasia as a veterinary therapeutic option is that considerable developments have occurred in the management of conditions which were previously considered terminal. Such developments are of proven benefit, affordable, and widely available and do not meet the criteria for overtreatment – for example, anaesthesia. In 2013, over 1000 readers of the *Veterinary Record* considered anaesthesia and analgesia to have been the most important innovation in the preceding 125 years, having had crucial effects on animal health and welfare (Taylor 2014). The veracity of this is obvious: animals which previously were considered too great an anaesthetic risk to undergo *any* form of procedure (and would be destroyed) can now undergo QoL improving procedures – and safely (providing they are cared for by proficient anaesthetists).

28.13 GOLD STANDARD CARE

The adoption of gold standard care (GSC) is probably a major cause for the 'death of euthanasia'. But what is GSC? One US pet insurance company states GSC is 'the highest quality veterinary care that all pets deserve to receive'. Their website explains, 'When your pet has gold-standard care, it means they have access to the best care possible, and are not limited nor excluded from exams, tests, procedures, or treatments that would benefit their quality of life' (Pawlicity Advisor 2024). The Veterinary Humanities Group UK is more circumspect and suggests the term GSC '*implies* that cutting edge technology and/or intensive intervention are, by default, the optimal and preferred options for veterinary case management' (Skipper et al. 2021). The insurance company concedes, 'Gold-standard care can be expensive, but pet insurance helps by providing a financial buffer so owners can prioritize their pet's health and wellbeing without fear of affordability'. Unsurprisingly, they then go on to sell various pet insurance packages for those who seek GSC for their pets. In contrast, Vet Humanities UK question whether GSC *always* equates to optimal care and opine that 'animal welfare is better served by active consideration of the most appropriate management options for each case', something they term 'contextualised care'. This agrees with Sackett's definition of evidence-based medicine (EBV) which gives equal emphasis to (1) the patient's situation, (2) the patient's goals, values, and wishes, (3) the best available research evidence, and (4) the clinical expertise of the practitioner (Luckmann 2001). When 'the patient's situation' is taken to mean the owner's wishes and willingness to pay and the animal's health and welfare, while 'the patient's goals, values and wishes' are McKeegan's unknowable 'what the animal wants' (Jarvis 2010), then Sackett's approach is probably more valuable in veterinary practice than GSC.

The ill-considered use of GSC can have adverse consequences for animals and clients. For example, when an idealised GSC is infeasible, both owners and vets may feel shame, guilt, anger, or dissatisfaction (Skipper et al. 2021). Arguably, vets trumpeting their GSC credentials may deter uninsured owners from engaging with veterinarians, in general, and compromise animal welfare by denying treatment to potentially treatable animals.

Neither Vet Humanities UK nor Sackett et al. offer explicit advice on euthanasia in the context of GSC or contextualised care, although it may be taken that the welfare of suffering animals facing a 'life not worth living' is ethically assured by that animal's humane destruction. Any 'standard of care' system that does not allow an animal a comfortable (and for its owner, affordable and guilt-free) escape from misery hardly meets any form of standard, and certainly not care.

28.14 SPECIALISATION AND CREDENTIALS

Whether GSC and its dismissal of euthanasia as a treatment for animal suffering arose in veterinary academic or a referral practice is an intriguing question. Both can expect to gain financially from GSC (and therefore buy the equipment and facilities to deliver it) while the staff in both are compelled to its practice (along with overtreatment) because their career progression will often depend on it.

Speciality residents seeking to sit board examinations must submit credentials based on clinical reports and logbooks. The former often take the form of case reports, the publication of which usually requires the description of previously unreported information. Therefore, residents striving for board eligibility would understandably prefer to carry out novel treatments in preference to euthanasia. Furthermore, 'breaking new ground' in an academic environment earns acclaim and accelerates career progression. For these and other reasons, some veterinary academics have come to regard euthanasia as an indicator of therapeutic failure rather than an act of mercy or clinical pragmatism. This belief not only promotes GSC and overtreatment, but when it prevails in teaching hospitals, it is likely to influence undergraduates' views before being propagated throughout successive generations of the veterinary profession.

There are various solutions to this. One might be to ensure undergraduates see enough grassroots general practice to be *au fait* with a world inhabited by uninsured animals and their less-than-affluent owners. Alternatively, vet schools might recruit adequately paid clinical demonstrators with experience at the coalface.

Speciality boards should restore euthanasia as an accepted therapy in specific cases. This could be achieved if case reports were allowed to follow the following format: 'Case X presented with severe Y and was diagnosed with Z. Despite various therapeutic options, e.g. A, B, C, and D (to be fully detailed and compared), the owner's unwillingness to proceed, coupled with the animal's rapid deterioration, meant that euthanasia was considered to be the best option to end its suffering'. Were such case reports marked similarly if not more generously than those describing innovative treatments, then the advantages of euthanasia might be rediscovered.

28.15 A TABOO SUBJECT?

Veterinary surgeons are at higher risk of suicide (approximately fourfold) compared with the general population (Bartram & Baldwin 2010), and studies have confirmed that conducting animal euthanasia alters a veterinarian's attitude to death and suicide. One study found destroying animals five times or more a week was associated with serious suicidal thoughts (Dalum et al. 2024), while another found an association between animal euthanasia and a lack of fear of death (Witte et al. 2013). Numerous questionnaire-based studies have examined the attitude of veterinarians to animal euthanasia, but one question that seems not to have been posed is whether fears (real or imagined) of an association between killing animals, and the risk of suicide leads to a deliberate or unconscious reticence to conduct euthanasia. If this were the case, then it would reveal another reason for the death of veterinary euthanasia.

28.16 CONCLUSION

Veterinarians who struggle with euthanasia-related decision-making may find the decision tree found in the BVA's 'Guide to Euthanasia' useful. The parallel use of a modified form of Sackett's definition of EBM (see previous) might also prove useful, although difficulty may be encountered interpreting point 2, i.e. the patient's (animal's) goals, values, and wishes. This is unfortunate because knowing this would probably dispel some guilt and self-recrimination felt by owners and vets when animals are destroyed. But how does one discover what an animal feels and wants? Questions such as 'Can animals (i) appreciate that their suffering might end, (ii) understand unpleasant treatments are for the best, and (iii) greatly value their own life, irrespective of its perceived quality, and therefore dread its extinction?' are similarly unanswerable, so they do not help. What can be assumed with confidence is that animals do feel pain and can suffer. That they are prepared to endure pain and suffering because they fear death more or can anticipate a time when they will feel better cannot be assumed with confidence. This balance of probabilities reinforces all ethical arguments for ending an animal's life humanely when death is in its best interests.

Euthanasia is the most effective and longest-lasting analgesic available to veterinarians and is 100% successful in curing animals of unmanageable pain and suffering. For this reason, its surreptitious retirement from the veterinary armamentarium must be resisted at all costs.

NOTES

1. Improved pain management is based on improvements in pain recognition, quantification, and treatment, using pre-emptive, polymodal, and prolonged analgesic strategies based on newer drugs with unique pharmacological properties and greater therapeutic indices.
2. Overtreatment: treatment that results in a poorer quality of life than no treatment or euthanasia, a treatment that is chosen in favour of a cheaper but equally effective treatment, or a treatment or test that makes no difference to the animal's condition or quality of life (Corr 2012).

3 Routine veterinary practice is defined by the RCVS as procedures and techniques performed on animals by veterinary surgeons in the course of their professional duties, which ensure the health and welfare of animals committed to their care. These can be thought of as the routine, established procedures undertaken on animals every day (RCVS 2024).
4 There is another paradox here. In a secular age, which rejects the divine origins of life, animals are enjoying internment with all the ritual trappings of a human burial (Serpell 2003). The Cartesian belief that only humans possess immortal souls seems to be under review.

REFERENCES

Animal Welfare Act 2006. *The National Archives* [Internet]. Up to date 2024 Sept 10. Available from: https://www.legislation.gov.uk/ukpga/2006/45/contents.

Bartram DJ, Baldwin DS. Veterinary surgeons and suicide: a structured review of possible influences on increased risk. *Vet Rec*. 2010;166(13):388–397.

Batchelor CE, McKeegan DE. Survey of the frequency and perceived stressfulness of ethical dilemmas encountered in UK veterinary practice. *Vet Rec*. 2012;170(1):19.

British Veterinary Association. Guide to euthanasia 2016. *BVA Resources & Guides* [Internet] [Downloaded 2024 Aug 23]. Available from: https://www.bva.co.uk/media/2981/bva_guide_to_euthanasia_2016.pdf.

Clutton E, Ware J, Murphy K, et al. Untested surgical procedures. *Vet Rec*. 2022;190(1):38.

Competitions and Markets Authority (CMA). CMA identifies multiple concerns in vets market. *GOV.UK* [Internet]. 2024a Mar 12. Available from: https://www.gov.uk/government/news/cma-identifies-multiple-concerns-in-vets-market.

Competitions and Markets Authority (CMA). Veterinary services for household pets in the UK. Decision to make a market investigation reference. *GOV.UK* [Internet]. 2024b Mar 12. Available from: https://assets.publishing.service.gov.uk/media/665052b-5c86b0c383ef64f51/__Final_report_of_the_consultation____.pdf.

Cooney K, Kipperman B. Ethical and practical considerations associated with companion animal euthanasia. *Animals (Basel)*. 2023;13(3):430.

Corr SA. Companion animals. In: Wathes CM, Corr S, May S, editors. *Veterinary and animal ethics: proceedings of the first international conference on veterinary and animal ethics, 2011 Sept*. Hoboken: Wiley-Blackwell; 2012. p. 188–200.

Dalum HS, Tyssen R, Moum T, et al. Euthanasia of animals-association with veterinarians' suicidal thoughts and attitudes towards assisted dying in humans: a nationwide cross-sectional survey (the NORVET study). *BMC Psych*. 2024;24(1):2.

Hartnack S, Springer S, Pittavino M, et al. Attitudes of Austrian veterinarians towards euthanasia in small animal practice: impacts of age and gender on views on euthanasia. *BMC Vet Res*. 2016;12:26.

Hiestand KM. The autonomy principle in companion veterinary medicine: a critique. *Front Vet Sci*. 2022;9:953925.

Home Office. Guidance on the operation of the animals (scientific procedures) act 1986 (ASPA). *GOV.UK* [Internet]. 2017 Dec 1. Available from: https://www.gov.uk/guidance/guidance-on-the-operation-of-the-animals-scientific-procedures-act-1986.

Jarvis S. Where do you draw the line on treatment? *Vet Rec*. 2010;167(17):636–637.

Lamb H. Are TV vets good or bad for the profession? *Vet Rec*. 2018;183(2):73.

Luckmann R. Evidence-based medicine: how to practice and teach EBM. 2nd ed. By David L. Sackett, Sharon E. Straus, W. Scott Richardson, William Rosenberg, and R. Brian Haynes, Churchill Livingstone, 2000. *J Int Care Med*. 2001;16(3):155–156.

Megna M. Pet ownership statistics 2024. *Forbes Advisor* [Internet]. 2024 Jan 25. Available from: https://www.forbes.com/advisor/pet-insurance/pet-ownership-statistics/#:~:text=As%20of%202022%2C%2044.5%25%20of,from%2025%25%20to%2029%25.

Mota-Rojas D, Mariti C, Zdeinert A, et al. Anthropomorphism and its adverse effects on the distress and welfare of companion animals. *Animals (Basel)*. 2021;11(11):3263.

Ogden U, Kinnison T, May SA. Attitudes to animal euthanasia do not correlate with acceptance of human euthanasia or suicide. *Vet Rec*. 2012;171(7):174.

Pawlicity Advisor. Gold standard care. *Pawlicity Advisory Dictionary* [Internet] [cited 2024 Aug 23]. Available from: https://www.pawlicy.com/dictionary/gold-standard-care/.

Quain A. The gift: ethically indicated euthanasia in companion animal practice. *Vet Sci*. 2021;8(8):141.

Rollin BE. Euthanasia and moral stress. *Loss Grief Care*. 1986;1(1–2):115–126.

Royal College of Veterinary Surgeons (RCVS). Code of professional conduct for veterinary surgeons. *RCVS Advice & Guidance* [Internet]. Undated [cited 2024 Aug 23]. Available from: https://www.rcvs.org.uk/setting-standards/advice-and-guidance/code-of-professional-conduct-for-veterinary-surgeons/pdf/.

Serpell JA. Anthropomorphism and anthropomorphic selection – beyond the 'cute response'. *Soc Anim J Hum-Anim Stud*. 2003;11(1):83–100.

Singer P. *Animal liberation: a new ethics for our treatment of animals*. 1st ed. New York: Random House; 1975.

Skipper A, Gray C, Serlin R, et al. 'Gold standard care' is an unhelpful term. *Vet Rec*. 2021;189(8):331.

Spitznagel MB, Jacobson DM, Cox MD, et al. Caregiver burden in owners of a sick companion animal: a cross-sectional observational study. *Vet Rec*. 2017;181(12):321.

Steck N, Junker C, Zwahlen M. Increase in assisted suicide in Switzerland: did the socioeconomic predictors change? Results from the Swiss National Cohort. *BMJ Open*. 2018;8(4):e020992.

Tannenbaum J. *Veterinary ethics: animal welfare, client relations, competition, and collegiality*. 2nd ed. St. Louis: Mosby; 1995.

Taylor P. Veterinary anaesthesia and analgesia: from chloroform to designer drugs. *Vet Rec*. 2014;174(13):318–321.

Wensley SP. Animal welfare and the human-animal bond: considerations for veterinary faculty, students, and practitioners. *J Vet Med Educ*. 2008;35(4):532–539.

Witte TK, Correia CJ, Angarano D. Experience with euthanasia is associated with fearlessness about death in veterinary students. *Suicide Life Threat Behav*. 2013;43(2):125–138.

Yeates J. Ethical aspects of euthanasia of owned animals. *In Pract*. 2010;32(2):70–73.

Yeates JW, Main DC. Veterinary opinions on refusing euthanasia: justifications and philosophical frameworks. *Vet Rec*. 2011;168(10):263.

29 Moral Stress, Emotional Labour, and Mental Health in the Veterinary Profession

Vanessa Ashall

29.1 INTRODUCTION

In this chapter I reflect on my experiences as a junior vet in mixed veterinary practice through the lens of my recent academic research in veterinary ethics and social science. My aim is to highlight the importance of attending to veterinary mental health through improved understanding of and support for the unique and complex ethical challenges faced by the profession. I introduce the concept of moral stress as a psychological consequence of the challenging ethical dimensions of veterinary work. I argue that the scientific roots of veterinary medicine and traditional veterinary ethical approaches continue to limit our engagements with important emotional, relational, and sensory aspects of veterinary ethics and wellbeing in the veterinary clinic.

Here I recount a personal experience of regularly attending a pig farm as a junior vet in a rural mixed practice. Referring back to this example I then go on to highlight aspects of veterinary labour which I believe are important for both veterinary ethics and veterinary wellbeing but which are not commonly foregrounded in traditional professional narratives.

29.2 SATURDAY MORNING

On a regular basis the local pig farm called the veterinary practice early on a Saturday morning to request a visit. The task to be undertaken is always the same – to replace and stitch in place a rectal prolapse in a breeding sow. As a junior vet, I was assigned this task, and it is interesting to recall that this job was in many ways less unpleasant than others, which might arise over a weekend on call. It was refreshing to leave the last of the busy morning surgery appointments to a colleague and to drive out to the farm which was scenic enough in good weather. The farmer himself was a pleasant man – respectful, talkative, and apparently interested in his animals and their wellbeing. I remember him being relatively responsible in that he dutifully made the call on a Saturday morning and spent his time and money dealing with the issue in this way rather than neglecting the problem entirely. There was also something comforting for a junior vet in dealing with a familiar problem on a familiar farm and it being considerably less of a life-and-death emergency than many other surgical tasks.

On arrival at the farm the task itself was relatively straightforward in a practical sense. It was always a different sow to be treated each week, not that this made any difference at all to me. The small area of their body that I came into contact with and the sheer number of sows on the farm meant that every case became the same swollen purplish-red protuberance of rectal mucosa emerging from a straining anus. The memories I have of this weekly ritual have thus become crystallised in my mind as the same event happening over and over again.

In my overarching recollection I can feel the pleasant sensation of sun on my back as I walk into the shed and stand behind the pig in question. The farmer is behind my left shoulder, keeping up a cheerful banter throughout and seemingly pleased to have my company at this point in his week. The anonymous rectal prolapse is presented between the metal bars of the farrowing crate which rather conveniently prevents the pig from moving whilst I stitch her anus closed. I have used a local anaesthetic to numb the surrounding tissues, and I insert a large, sharp needle with a wide tape like suture material to create a purse string suture. Each time I push the needle firmly into the pig's swollen skin, I wince slightly as a trickle of bright red blood runs down her rear end and drips into the pool of diarrhoea on the concrete floor in front of my feet. Finally, I tie the suture closed over my fingers and carefully adjust its diameter, and I feel pleased with the neatness of my work. As I carry my kit into the sunshine and back to the car, the farmer heads off in a different direction and waves a cheery goodbye. Neither of us look back again at the metal crate with its anonymous anus and its suture, the cropped curly tail, and the pool of blood-spattered diarrhoea. I remember thinking only that the best thing about these Saturday visits to the pig farm was the chance to call at the drive through McDonald's on my way back to the surgery.

What strikes me now about these visits is that I have remembered very specific tensions and contradictions in how I felt and what I did, but I had no way at the time of understanding or expressing them in meaningful ways, nor did they appear to play a major part in my clinical decisions and actions. Now, with the luxury of hindsight and considerable training in veterinary ethics and social sciences, this case appears to demonstrate a bewildering mix of desensitisation, intuition, disassociation, futility, guilt, personal relationships, power, and hierarchy in veterinary practice.

I now recognise that whilst I was well trained to perform specific surgery on individual animals I was not well equipped to deal with the realities of their existence as intensively farmed production animals. The reduction of an animal to a window of swollen flesh presented between bars, the sight of the bleeding caused by my needle and her permanent stream of diarrhoea intuitively pricked at my conscience. However, I was able to disassociate myself from everything surrounding the practical task at hand, and I did not even question the significance of this intervention, in spite of undertaking the same procedure on the same farm quite regularly. My friendly relationship with the farmer was all the more disorientating since he also kept his pigs this way and regularly paid for me to come and sew their anus closed. That I was able to move on, as I must, to enjoy the sunshine and anticipate a treat without thinking about her again has left a permanent residue of guilt that I was not even aware of at the time. Since the senior vets took charge of the presumably more pleasant and conveniently scheduled weekday herd health visits, addressing the causal mechanisms which underpinned this problem lay outside my junior sphere of influence. I recognise now that I was not empowered to help improve the pigs' welfare in any meaningful way beyond surgical damage limitation. Above all, I am struck by the fact that this was not even one of my most dreaded weekly tasks.

In the remainder of this chapter, I want to revisit some aspects of this case through sharing my understanding of moral stress and ethics in veterinary practice. I want to introduce some recent ideas and concepts which may allow us to understand and evaluate our experiences of veterinary labour in new ways. The first point I wish to reflect upon is the way that we think about and share our experiences of veterinary practice. I am aware that there could be criticisms of this honest account of my feelings and actions as a junior vet, and perhaps they would be justifiable. This I am prepared to risk to make the point that we are not accustomed to thinking about, much less talking about, our experiences of veterinary practice with honesty and self-reflection. There is little encouragement for vets to expose their doubts and difficulties and to be honest about the situations they have faced and the choices they have made. I have previously identified a need for us to embrace *'vulnerability with purpose'* (Ashall 2022) in our accounts of veterinary practice, for without risking our pride both as individuals and as a profession, we cannot hope to better understand what it really means to be a vet. We must move beyond sharing clinical and scientific accounts of success in veterinary medicine in our journals and in the media and make more visible the messy human realities of success, challenge, and failure in veterinary work. I suggest that the stories we have traditionally felt comfortable telling about ourselves and the veterinary profession do not help us to recognise and reflect upon the problematic aspects of our profession (Ashall 2022).

One way in which we are beginning to improve our understanding of the human aspects of veterinary work is through engaging with different research methods. Whereas contemporary veterinary medicine has been greatly influenced by a long history of scientific and clinical research, it is only very recently that social scientific research methods, particularly qualitative research, have become visible (May 2018). Veterinary social scientific research in the form of surveys, focus groups, interviews, and ethnographic observation has helped us begin to explore in more detail the realities of veterinary ethical decision-making and mental health within the veterinary profession. The relationship between veterinary ethical decision-making and mental health in the veterinary workforce was proposed as early as the 1980s (Rollin 1986) with the stressful effects of veterinary ethical dilemmas later demonstrated through survey work (Batchelor & McKeegan 2012). More recently, the specific concepts of veterinary moral stress, moral distress, and moral injury have been explored in more detail by several authors (Moses et al. 2018; Quain et al. 2022; Williamson et al. 2022; Gibson & Quain 2022; Ashall 2023), with current understanding being that moral stress lies at the lower end of a spectrum of psychological consequences associated with increasing intensities of moral discomfort (Quain et al. 2022; Ashall 2023). Moral stress has been defined as *'The feeling of not being able to do what you believe to be "the right thing" because of constraining personal, professional, organizational or client factors'* (Gibson & Quain 2022).

In my own work, I have shown that veterinary staff describe moral stress as a feeling of 'frustration' associated with not being able to do what they felt was right for animals in their care (Ashall 2023). Interestingly, most participants in my study reported that whilst they recognised this feeling, they had not previously been aware of the term moral stress (Ashall 2023). Furthermore, experiences of moral stress do not appear to relate necessarily to specific ethical dilemmas and decisions, which other authors have examined for their role in causing moral distress and moral injury (Moses et al. 2018; Quain et al. 2022; Williamson et al. 2022). My study highlights that moral stress can be caused by everyday monotonous and continual exposure to low level ethical challenge (Ashall 2023). A further crucial finding is that veterinary moral stress may be cumulative since study participants reported that the negative feelings associated with moral stress can build up over time and can even interact with other forms of workplace or personal stress (Ashall 2023). The possibility that much of the stress associated with veterinary work may be attributed to ethical dilemmas but that veterinary staff may not recognise this as the cause has also been previously raised (Moses et al. 2018). In my story, I describe some of the uncomfortable feelings associated with my visits to the pig farm, but it is also true that I was not aware, at the time, of the complex ethical underpinnings of my discomfort. In my case, the expectations of the farmer and my colleagues and the normalisation of the pig's condition created no opportunity for me to question my involvement on ethical grounds. That the specific details of this case and many others should stay fixed in my mind indicates that it did affect me at some level, in spite of the coping methods I employed through desensitisation and disassociation. These observations and the study findings I have referred to raise the possibility that vets may experience cumulative moral stress over time without even being aware of it, perhaps until or even beyond them choosing to leave the profession or experiencing mental health consequences.

In my story I describe the discomfort I felt as my needle caused the pig's skin to bleed, the sight of the blood mixing with soft faeces on the concrete floor and the disembodied way that the prolapse was presented to me through the bars of a farrowing crate. It has taken me a long time to find a way to understand why these things should matter and how the sights and smells and feelings that we encounter in our work are relevant to ethical veterinary practice. Much of the foundational academic work in veterinary ethics and the teaching of veterinary ethics to students, when it finally commenced, was based on a variety of traditional theoretical understandings of ethics which are by their very nature abstracted from the realities of our lived experiences in veterinary practice. I suggest that the traditional ethical language of 'right' and 'good' and the bioethical imperative to rank and balance the needs and preferences of different individuals do not help us to make sense of the morality of our lived experiences or to understand the ways in which we intuitively judge our own actions.

I have recently proposed that a feminist ethic of care approach is missing from traditional ethical analyses of the veterinary profession (Ashall 2022). Such an approach pays close attention to relationships in ethical decision-making and in particular to vulnerability, dependency, and the avoidance of harm (Gilligan 1993). If we reconsider for a moment my story, the language of vulnerability and dependency draws our ethical attention to the immobile pig and her living conditions but also to myself as a powerless junior vet and the farmer in his efforts to make a living. Furthermore, we may think differently about the actions of myself and the farmer in terms of an ethical imperative to prevent harm above the promotion of benefits. Of particular interest to me is the way that a care perspective connects with intuitive sensory and emotional responses; the blood, the diarrhoea, the swollen tissue, and the bars all felt significant to me, although they did not specifically feature in my decision-making. I have suggested that our feelings about and intuitive responses to our experiences in practice may be ethically relevant, not only because they affect our own wellbeing but because they may identify important aspects of an ethical problem which abstracted ethical reasoning fails to capture (Ashall 2022). Within a feminist ethic of care, these mundane, conflicting, and messy realities are central to both the way that we understand our ethical behaviour and the choices we might make through the lens of care. I believe that we will need to become better acquainted with emotional and sensory aspects of veterinary practice in order to be able to fully understand their psychological and ethical significance.

Whilst I experience negative feelings associated with the blood and the diarrhoea and the bars of the farrowing crate, they are remembered alongside my enjoyment of the farmer's cheerful banter, the sunshine, and the anticipation of a treat. Within the limited ethnographic studies of the veterinary profession, this frequent movement between positive and negative emotional states has been carefully observed (Morris 2012). I have proposed the term emotional juxtaposition to describe this experience and suggest that vets being required to move rapidly between positive and negative emotional states is a particularly difficult psychological aspect of many types of veterinary practice (Ashall 2022). A new focus on the emotional aspects of veterinary work also requires us to consider the ways in which we respond to and manage the emotions of our clients. I suggest that emotion management forms a critical part of veterinary labour and that *'Through kindness, professionalism and obligation vets appear to gather, supress and tidy away the messy human feelings which come into the clinic, alongside their animal patients. Vets must not only hide their responses to these negative emotions within their own professional personas, they must also hand out sympathy, compassion and other appropriate emotions, when required*' (Ashall 2022). I make the point that the veterinary profession may be viewed as an emotional sponge with regards to society's relationships with animals, absorbing and dispensing emotion as required, with consequent psychological and ethical implications. What do we know about the toll that this emotional sponge work takes on veterinary professionals and how does it implicate us in normalising some of the problematic aspects of society's relationships with animals?

Finally, I wish to show how a feminist ethic of care approach could alter both the scope and scale of veterinary ethical concern (Ashall 2022). In my story I describe my focus on the task at hand, replacing and securing the rectal prolapse, which may arguably be ethically justified since the sow would be in less discomfort and better able to pass faeces after this procedure. I have also described my resistance to sensory and emotional cues alerting me to the way the sows were confined to crates and their chronic diarrhoea, which likely contributed to the frequent prolapses. I was able to disassociate myself from the context surrounding my intervention and to view the procedure as beneficial in the circumstances. I believe that this decontextualising and individualising of veterinary ethical decision-making is very commonly practised by vets; indeed, it is perhaps an underpinning feature of veterinary practice since it permits us to intervene in standard ways with the aim of improving animal welfare across a bewildering spectrum of species and settings and according to the wishes and financial circumstances of the owner. For example, vets are charged with improving animal welfare in scientific research, intensive farming, animal sports, and animal-breeding programmes, but whether these scenarios are in themselves considered ethically justifiable is not a feature of everyday veterinary clinical decision-making. In my case there was something jarring about the fact that the sow's restraint within a farrowing crate made my task considerably easier because she was not able to move. I now recognise that my discomfort arose from the reality that by benefiting from the features of intensive farming practices, I had in some way become a part of the system.

Veterinary ethical decision-making has traditionally focused on the options available to vets when they are confronted with a clinical case or a specific health and welfare problem. Just as the farming practices and health status of the herd felt outside the scope of my influence during that visit, my research shows that vets can often feel they are working in scenarios where they can only choose between the least worst option for animals or where none of the outcomes which are possible feel ethical to them (Ashall 2023). This scenario precisely fits the definition of moral stress, where vets feel unable to do what they really believe is right; highlighting the context of veterinary ethical decision-making within a broader ethical terrain which may be considered beyond our scope of influence. Feminist scholars urge us to think in different ways about our ethical accountability, specifically to think in a linear sense about the ways that our relationships and responsibilities connect with those of others (Haraway 2016). In this way, my professional interaction with the sow undeniably brings me into an ethical relationship with the rest of the herd and with the pig farming industry. It also connects me with the farmer and their family, with the local and global environment, and with supermarkets, restaurants, meat eaters, and vegans, whether I like it or not. The profession must come to recognise and respond to veterinary decision-making as set against a backdrop of independently operating systems of animal ethics, research ethics, food ethics, and environmental ethics. If veterinary ethics merely restricts our concerns to those within a self-imposed and narrow sphere of professional responsibility, vets risk feeling further disempowered as ethical technicians within society's desired uses of animals.

In this chapter I have set out to draw attention to moral stress in the veterinary clinic and to argue for new ways of understanding and enacting ethical veterinary practice. The mental health of the veterinary profession is now an area of significant concern with the provision of mental health support being a contemporary priority for the Royal College of Veterinary Surgeons (e.g. Mind Matters Initiative). Recognising and responding to the role that moral stress plays within veterinary mental health concerns is of the utmost importance, and I have sought to show how this will depend upon us developing better models and methods for understanding and describing the complex realities of veterinary ethical decision-making. In particular, I have highlighted the need to develop more honest and reflexive narratives about our profession which make visible the most challenging aspects of veterinary labour. I have shown that emotional and sensory experiences of veterinary practice are underexplored for their psychological and ethical significance, for example, describing emotional sponge work as a difficult and largely unrecognised element of veterinary labour. Finally, if vets are to be truly empowered, we must broaden the scope and scale of veterinary ethical decision-making beyond individual case management in the veterinary clinic and attend more to our role in developing ethical relationships between humans and animals in broader society.

REFERENCES

Ashall V. A Feminist ethic of care for the veterinary profession. *Front Vet Sci.* 2022;9:795628.

Ashall V. Reducing moral stress in veterinary teams? Evaluating the use of ethical discussion groups in charity veterinary hospitals. *Animals (Basel).* 2023;13(10):1662.

Batchelor CE, McKeegan DE. Survey of the frequency and perceived stressfulness of ethical dilemmas encountered in UK veterinary practice. *Vet Rec.* 2012;170(1):19.

Gibson J, Quain A. Embracing clinical ethics support services in the UK veterinary profession. *In Pract.* 2022;44(7):421–425.

Gilligan C. *In a different voice: psychological theory and women's development.* 2nd ed. Cambridge: Harvard University Press; 1993.

Haraway D. *Staying with the trouble: making kin in the chthulucene.* London: Duke University Press; 2016.

May C. Discovering new areas of veterinary science through qualitative research interviews: introductory concepts for veterinarians. *Aust Vet J.* 2018;96(8):278–284.

Morris PM. *Blue juice: euthanasia in veterinary medicine.* Philadelphia, PA: Temple University Press; 2012.

Moses L, Malowney MJ, Boyd JW. Ethical conflict and moral distress in veterinary practice: a survey of North American veterinarians. *J Vet Intern Med*. 2018;32(6):2115–2122.

Quain A, Mullan S, Ward MP. There was a sense that our load had been lightened: evaluating outcomes of virtual ethics rounds for veterinary team members. *Front Vet Sci*. 2022;9:922049.

Rollin BE. Euthanasia and moral stress. *Loss Grief Care*. 1986;1:115–126.

Williamson V, Murphy D, Greenberg, N. Veterinary professionals' experiences of moral injury: a qualitative study. *Vet Rec*. 2022;192(2):e2181.

Part IIIC Veterinary Practice

30 The Customer Isn't Always Right
Why Business Ethics is not Professional Ethics

Tanya Stephens

Most veterinary practices in the past were independently owned, community centred and often small. This model has given way in some cases to a predominantly business model and increasingly the veterinary profession is referred to an an 'industry' despite the fact that veterinarians don't operate in factories!

At the same time, trust in the profession has been falling, at least in Australia, and perhaps this falling trust is related to some veterinary practices becoming first and foremost a business. The promotion of veterinary practice as a business can lead to a tension between the priorities of veterinary professionalism and those of a business agenda as the standards and ethics of a good business leader may not be the same as a good professional.

Business ethics, if indeed ethics exists in business, is not professional ethics and for the veterinarian the 'customer isn't always right' as providing a customer with what they want is at odds with what it means to be a professional which is to do what is right and not what is requested.

Whilst a professional can provide an ethical workplace to do business, veterinary ethics may conflict with a business agenda and the veterinary professional, where there is a conflict must ensure that the rights of the animal and the public take precedence over the rights of the business.

30.1 BACKGROUND

I am a small-animal practice owner and practitioner who very much enjoys practice, even the aspects that involve dealing with the human animal. At work every so often I flick through the increasing numbers of glossy magazines that come through the door. Mostly these contain multiple ads for new, often untested products and feel-good stories about amazing veterinarians and their wonderful practices. I'm envious if the images are of well-groomed and relaxed veterinarians in neat and tidy rooms, not at all like my practice. They all seem to have lovely smiles, nice hair, and clean shirts not covered in blood or hair with well-behaved dogs or cats sitting on tables beside them.

I usually toss these glossies in the recycling bin; however, one story caught my eye as it was written by a young veterinarian who stated that the way to grow a veterinary business was to give the customer what they want.

I realised that whilst I may have been distracted running my own practice, veterinary practice had become much more businesslike even to the extent of 'morphing' into an 'industry', an increasingly common term. Given that veterinarians generally don't operate in factories (industry: 'economic activity concerned with the processing of raw materials and manufacture of goods in factories'), I wondered what had happened to my profession.

At the same time as the promotion of our 'industry' as a business, trust in the veterinary profession in Australia has been falling for some time, and public trust in veterinarians is below that of nurses, firefighters, ambulance officers, pharmacists, general practitioners, preschool carers, and primary school teachers. Trust in veterinarians sits at 67, a fall from 71 a few years ago (Governance Institute of Australia. Ethics Index 2023). I suppose we should take some solace in the fact that we are above lawyers, real estate agents and politicians. I have no idea if falling trust is related to veterinary practice becoming businesslike, but it's a nice hypothesis.

I do, however, believe that the promotion of veterinary practice as a business can lead to a tension between the priorities of veterinary professionalism and those of a business agenda. (Stephens 2022).

'The standards and ethics of a good business leader may not be the same as those of a good professional. For example, finding a competitive advantage in the market may involve misleading the opposition, patenting trade secrets and skills and doing other things that may not be in the best interests of consumers and other businesses. Good professionals on the other hand will usually share specialist skills and knowledge with each other and will act in a way as to achieve what is in their clients' and patients' best interest' (Brennan 2008).

A professional has a special kind of calling. Professionals owe a special duty of care to those they serve; they have special duties to other professionals and responsibilities to society in general. Having specialist knowledge gives professionals an advantage over other members of society to whom they are giving advice. Society values professionals because of their perceived skill and knowledge in a given field of expertise and because of their codes of ethics. These moral codes compel professionals to behave better than members of other non-professional occupational groups and the rest of society. Society, for example, does not demand the same level of personal integrity from the dog groomer as the veterinarian.

While business often strives to provide customers with what they want, a profession will aim to provide what is right and appropriate not what is requested or demanded.

For veterinarians, who have as their first priority the care of the animal, this priority can bring them into conflict with economic interests or the interests of the animal's owner. Codes of professional conduct are often designed to ensure that when such conflicts occur, the interests of the patient and the safety of the public have priority over the needs of the business.

'It is certainly not always obvious how a veterinarian should act in a given situation. Each and every day veterinarians are faced with making ethical decisions and all of these decisions are potentially open to criticism by the owner, other veterinarians, society, professional veterinary boards, lawyers, insurers and others. In many ways the professional life of veterinarians is more complex and more likely to provide opportunities for conflict than the lives of other professionals' (Brennan 2008).

30.2 WHAT IS A PROFESSION?

> A Profession is a disciplined group of individuals who adhere to ethical standards and who hold themselves out as, and are accepted by the public as possessing special knowledge and skills in a widely recognised body of learning derived from research, education and training at a high level, and who are prepared to apply this knowledge and exercise these skills in the interest of others.
>
> It is inherent in the definition of a Profession that a code of ethics governs the activities of each Profession. Such codes require behaviour and practice beyond the personal moral obligations of an individual. They define and demand high standards of behaviour in respect to the services provided to the public and in dealing with professional colleagues. Often these codes are enforced by the Profession and are acknowledged and accepted by the community. (Australian Council of Professions 2024)

Furthermore, there is a body of evidence indicating that an individual draws on their profession for values, beliefs, standards of judgement, and intellectual stimulation, that the profession as an organisation has an impact on the ethics of its members and that the role of the profession is to provide 'what should be'. The requirement to provide statements of 'what should be' places a distinctly ethical responsibility on the profession as an organisation and requires that it have a distinctly ethical purpose (Harris 2015).

30.3 MORAL REASONING

There is significant agreement that a central feature of something being a matter of ethics is the recognition that there are appropriate interests other than one's own that should act as constraints on the unbridled pursuit of one's self interest and that there are times when one should allow one's pursuit of one's own interests to be constrained by the interests of others. Ethics is then concerned with exactly when, why, and how one's own interests should be constrained and to what effect and presumes that a moral judgement is principled, justifiable and has integrity (Cohen 2012).

30.4 VETERINARY PROFESSIONAL ETHICS

Veterinary ethics is concerned with how veterinarians make decisions and act as professionals for the provision of veterinary care. Animal ethics refers to the moral issues surrounding the use of animals. In the process of professional decision-making, veterinarians will frequently need to consider issues of animal ethics, but their professional ethics necessarily include and go beyond these concerns (Stephens 2012).

There are four branches of veterinary ethics (Tannenbaum 1989):

1. Descriptive veterinary ethics, which refers to the actual ethical views of members of the veterinary profession regarding professional behaviour and attitudes.
2. Official veterinary ethics refers to official veterinary standards adopted by veterinary professional organisations such as the Australian Veterinary Association.
3. Administrative veterinary ethics refers to the moral standards imposed on veterinarians by administrative governmental bodies, i.e. enshrined within and enforceable by law.
4. Normative veterinary ethics described as the 'activity of looking for correct norms for veterinary professional behaviour and attitudes'. Of the four branches this is of the greatest significance as it goes to the core of what it means to be a veterinarian because this branch of ethics requires the greatest level of autonomy and personal decision-making on the part of the veterinarian.

The law and codes of conduct relating to veterinarians provide an ethical framework to ensure that veterinarians work in an ethical environment and that the animal is the first priority. They are designed to ensure that where conflicts occur, the interests of the patient and the safety of the public have priority over the needs of the business.

A social contract is said to be at the heart of the professional relationship in that 'in exchange for the statutory restriction of certain acts to the profession members of the profession must act in the interests of society and its members' (Harris 2015).

Ethical problems are not confined to dilemmas where it is hard to discern the correct course of action. The engineers talk of balanced decision-making in the context of a social contract. Sometimes it is the action step or bringing oneself to do what is right that is the most difficult. Ethical action requires courage, fortitude, strength of will, and analytical discernment, which are best developed in the community with the professional organisation providing relevant examples

The views of professionalism by veterinarians may change over time. New students have been shown to have a 'naive view' of professionalism where attributes such as altruism and social justice are highly ranked. As they progress through their training and into the profession, these idealistic tendencies give way to 'more practical concepts' such as professional autonomy, commercialism, and lifestyle ethic. If the views of clients differ too much from practising veterinarians, this may ultimately lead the public to question if the veterinary profession is maintaining its side of the social contract (Roder et al. 2012).

30.5 ETHICAL ISSUES UNIQUE TO THE VETERINARY PROFESSION

This uniqueness is due primarily to the fact that veterinarians have as their first priority the care of the animal, a priority that may at times bring them into conflict with economic interests or the interests of the animal's owner. Ethical challenges exist as a result of the veterinarian's unique triangular relationship with the animal and its owner and veterinary decision-making attempts to balance all three, which can lead to conflicts of interest.

It is not always obvious how a veterinarian should act in a given situation. Each and every day, in practice, veterinarians are faced with making ethical decisions, and all of these decisions are potentially open to criticism by the owner, other veterinarians, society, professional veterinary boards, lawyers, insurers, and others.

Traditionally the veterinarian was a sole practitioner and therefore had only the relationships with client and society to consider. Today many veterinarians are employed by government, corporations, or large practices. This makes the 'balanced decision making in the context of a social contract' aspect of professional practice more complex and demanding. A profession-organisation conflict. An individual who is the member of a profession and an employee, director or manager in an organisation has an identity as a member of their profession and another identity as a member of the organisation. This complicates decisions as both organisation and profession may have expressed values and beliefs that are not congruent (Harris 2015).

30.6 BUSINESS ETHICS

The idea of business ethics is fairly recent, most likely in response to scandals. Some firms have adopted business ethics programs whilst others maintain that there is no distinct business ethics and that the ethical principles applied elsewhere in society should apply equally to business. For many, the purpose of business is seen to run counter to the principles of a healthy society. Protesters such as those who occupied Wall Street in 2011 have argued that much of business has lost sight of the societal perspective and that the purpose of business has become opposite to the purpose of society and society is worse off (Harris 2012).

Three views express the relationship between business and society and have held sway at different times in history.

1. Business and society are distinct realms. Business creates wealth and society (or government on its behalf) manages the distribution of wealth.
2. Business and society are competing worlds. Business is only able to prosper at the expense of society.
3. Business and society are intermingled, and neither can prosper without the other.

However, it has been argued that only the intermingled view is valid and that the aims of business and society are linked (Roder et al. 2012).

The relationship between ethical behaviour in business and profit has been well researched and the evidence is less than clear. Some studies show ethical companies doing better; others yield mixed results. Performance of the World's Most Ethical companies (http://www.ethisphere.com) gives an indication of how well ethical businesses perform or fail to perform.

So why might good ethics be good for business? Three reasons as to why ethics might pay is trust, focus, and culture. Ethical culture in a company is a reason people want to work there, buy from them, and have the respect of the community. This culture gives a competitive advantage.

One great pillar of ethics is the principle that requires respect for the humanity of fellow human beings and to treat them as unique and valuable individuals rather than solely as means through which to obtain things we want.

Unfortunately, we are all too aware of a lack of ethics in business, from tax avoidance to underpaying wages and aware that the public dislikes this lack of ethical behaviour. It's been well established that humans are inherently ethical and cooperative and prefer to work in an ethical environment.

30.7 'THE CUSTOMER IS ALWAYS RIGHT'

This term was originally coined in 1909 by Harry Gordon Selfridge, the founder of Selfridge's department store in London and is typically used by businesses to convince customers that they will get good service at this company and convince employees to give customers good service. However, from a purely business point of view, there are five good reasons why it's wrong.

1. It makes employees unhappy because it gives the customer more rights than an employee.
2. It gives difficult customers an unfair advantage. They receive better treatment than nice people.
3. Some customers are bad for business!
4. It results in worse customer service. Putting employees first rather than customers means employees who are happy give better customer service.
5. Some customers are wrong.

30.8 WHO IS THE CUSTOMER?

A customer is a person who buys goods or services from a shop or business. They generally lack loyalty and their needs are met by goods and services priced to sell. On the other hand, veterinarians and other professionals have clients, i.e. someone who receives professional services and to build long term professional relationships with.

30.9 PROFESSIONAL ETHICS VS BUSINESS ETHICS

In particular as companion ownership has increased in economic value and given the preponderance of veterinarians working in small practices, there has been a surge in the promotion of veterinary practice as a business. This has inevitably led to a tension between the priorities of veterinary professionalism and those of a business agenda.

The conflicts between the demands of running a business and acting in the interests of your patient can be explained in terms of a conflict of obligations. As a moral agent, I have a duty of care for my dependents so running a profitable business is a way of fulfilling this duty. However, on the other hand, I have a duty to the interests of clients and patients, and this may mean sacrificing easy profits from unnecessary interventions. The public expects that paying substantial fees for professional services is that such services are delivered in a way that prioritises the needs or interests of clients and patients rather than to the profit of the professional providing the service.

Codes of professional conduct are designed to ensure that where such conflicts occur, the interests of the patient or the safety of the public have priority over the needs of the business.

30.10 VETERINARY PRACTICE AS A BUSINESS

For any veterinarian running a business, there will inevitably be conflicts between commercial and professional duties.

The vast majority of veterinarians in Australia are in private practice operating in a business setting with no government subsidies. The need to maintain a financially viable practice creates unique ethical challenges for veterinarians faced with increasing demands from animal owners and the gulf between expectations and costs. In such a setting, veterinarians have a responsibility to ensure that professional ethics inform business decision-making and that the expenditure of their clients is well and effectively directed.

Although the notions of 'animal welfare' and 'appropriate' may not be agreed on, appropriate medical or surgical treatments can never mean 'treatments that maximise my profits' (Brennan 2008).

30.11 ETHICAL ISSUES ASSOCIATED WITH THE COSTS OF VETERINARY SERVICE

Increasingly companion animals are seen as members of the family (the rise of the 'fur baby') and there is an expectation from owners that their pets are entitled to the same level and affordability of healthcare as human members of the family. This gulf between expectations and costs can lead to ethical challenges for the veterinarian who must seek to strike a balance between providing an affordable service for animal owners with appropriate equipment and medicines whilst maintaining sufficient financial returns to ensure viability of the practice and a sufficient income for themselves.

The British Veterinary Association found in 2022 that 1 in 2 veterinarians in the UK have reported being exposed to online abuse, almost as common as abuse in person which stood at 82%. Past surveys have found that the costs of veterinary services are associated with increasing abuse. This has an impact on mental health and a reason to leave the profession.

The Animal Medicines Australia survey of pet owners 2022 (animalmedicinesaustralia.org.au) found that the cost of veterinary services is one of the main reasons 68% of pet owners gave for not going to the vet in the past year, up significantly from 55% in 2021. Although pet cats live in higher-income households, cat owners are more likely to exhibit higher financial vulnerability indicators and to have a household member who requires regular care.

Along with increasing costs of veterinary care has been the use of pay later services by veterinary practices. There is a concern that the use of these services allow owners to agree to more expensive or even unnecessary services. The Afterpay service VetPay had the dubious honour of being given a Shonky Award by Choice in 2022 (choice.com.au). VetPay is a quick-access loan product that markets itself as an 'affordable' service for caring animal owners who find themselves unable to cover the cost of vet bills.

All the animal owner has to do is pay 10% deposit and the rest in fortnightly payments, along with other costs which Choice said 'made it one of the most reprehensible credit products on the market'. Many online reviewers of the service accused it of preying on their emotional investment in their pets and owners ending up spending hundreds more than their original veterinary bill. Of particular concern is unsuitable loans to low-income earners and the ethics of using these services.

30.12 CONTEMPORARY FACTORS THAT CAN HAVE AN IMPACT ON VETERINARY PROFESSIONAL ETHICS

1. CORPORATISATION. This can result in ethical challenges because the ethics of the employed veterinarian may not align with those of the company management and shareholders who are expecting a return on their investment.
2. PAYING INCENTIVES. Paying incentives could risk overservicing, and in any case, there is good evidence that incentives are not as effective as satisfaction from doing a good job. The use of KPIs in the veterinary world could be seen as inappropriate and unethical and at odds with the professional imperative to do what is right (Main 2014).
3. PET INSURANCE. In Australia in 2022 around 17% of dog owners (down from 30% in 2019) and 12% of cat owners (down from 21% in 2019) had pet insurance, with costs being the main reason given for not having insurance. Pet insurance can give rise to its own ethical challenges (Awad & Stephens 2016). The problem with pet insurance may be that those who can afford veterinary care may not need insurance, whilst those who do may not be able to afford the insurance.
4. INCREASING SPECIALISATION? Impact on general practice income and abilities? Fragmentation of the profession with a loss of cohesion and collegiality?

The Customer Isn't Always Right 295

5. OVERDIAGNOSIS AND OVERSERVICING? 'The Australian veterinary industry is essentially unregulated from the standpoint of customer service' (choice.com.au). Choice found that the most consistent suspicion arose from the conflict between the idea of veterinary medicine as a healthcare profession vs a business.
6. NICHE MARKETS. E.g. Hospice care. Sports medicine and others may have an impact on general practice.
7. INEFFECTIVE THERAPIES. Concern that the use of ineffective therapies may lead to a loss of trust in the profession.
8. NEW TECHNOLOGY. New machines, e.g. CT and MRI. Expensive equipment can substantially add to the costs of veterinary services.
9. GIFTS FROM PHARMACEUTICAL COMPANIES. Do gifts lead to overservicing and conflicts of interest?

30.13 STRENGTHENING ETHICAL PRACTICES

There are five concepts underpinning the strengthening of ethical practices which provide a framework by which people who want to work and live in an ethical environment can ensure that they do so (Bowden 2012).

1. Distinguishing right from wrong: this is a fundamental requirement; can be submerged by our tendency to go with the majority.
2. Speaking out against wrong-doing: the most effective way of identifying and stopping wrongdoing in an organisation.
3. Establishing a code of ethics: need ownership to make these effective.
4. Institutionalising ethical behaviour and building an ethical culture.
5. Teaching and training in ethics.

30.14 SUMMARY

Business ethics, if indeed ethics exists in business, is not professional ethics and for the veterinarian the 'customer isn't always right' as providing a customer with what they want is at odds with what it means to be a professional.

Whilst a professional can provide an ethical workplace to do business, veterinary ethics may conflict with a business agenda, and the veterinary professional, where there is a conflict, must ensure that the rights of the animal and the public take precedence over the rights of the business.

Being a professional calls for self-reflection, and this need is particularly relevant for veterinarians in practice making clinical decisions. Any organisation where the entrenched professional response to a problem is to reflect on it, seek to understand it, and link it to knowledge, beliefs, practice, and values will often respond more effectively to challenges.

Generally, the cost of forming a profession is that the public expects enforcement of standards that protect animals from harm and give clear priority to the interests of patients and clients. This leaves plenty of scope for debate about what is in the interest of a particular animal, what animal welfare really means, and who is best able to represent animal interests in a given situation. There may in fact be no absolute right or wrong on any particular question but despite this, there can be agreement about general ethical aims and overall professional priorities.

Furthermore, professional organisations with a responsibility to state what 'should be done', influence ethics at personal and societal levels and contribute to the development of ethical capabilities among their members (Harris 2015).

Veterinarians have historically been good providers of role models for the placing of professional identity and values above those of employers or commercial interests and with a belief that welfare to animals is for the good of society.

It goes without saying that ethical decision-making and ethical behaviour are essential in upholding the integrity of the profession and maintaining relationships with the public. If trust in our profession falls, then we risk losing our position as the primary source of information on animal health and welfare.

REFERENCES

Australian Council of Professions. [Internet]. 2024[cited 2024 Jul 20]. Available from: https://professions.org.au/what-is-a-professional/.

Awad M, Stephens T. Ethical dilemma: what to do if a client asks you to change your records for a claim. *Aust Vet J*. 2016 Oct;94.

Bowden P, editor. *Applied ethics: strengthening ethical practices*. Tilde University Press; 2012.

Brennan A. *Competition, welfare and ethics in veterinary practice*. Proceedings of the Australian Veterinary Association Annual Conference, Perth; 2008.

Cohen S. The world of moral reasoning. In: *Applied ethics: strengthening ethical practices*. Chapter 1. Tilde University Press; 2012.

Governance Institute of Australia. Ethics index 2023. [Internet]. Undated [cited 2023 Oct 31]. Available from: https://www.governanceinstitute.com.au/news_media/ethics-index-2023-2/.

Harris H. Business ethics. In: *Applied ethics: strengthening ethical practices*. Bowden P. Chapter 11. Tilde University Press; 2012.

Harris H. The influence of professional associations on organisational ethics: the case of veterinarians. In: *Research in ethical issues in organisations*. Vol. 14. Emerald Group Publishing Limited; 2015. Leeds, UK.

Main D. Financial incentives. *In Pract*. 2014;36:262–263.

Roder C, Whittlestone KD, May SA. Views of professionalism: a veterinary institutional perspective. *Vet Rec*. 2012;171(23):595.

Stephens T. Veterinary ethics. In: *Applied ethics: strengthening ethical practices*. Chapter 19. Tilde University Press; 2012.

Stephens T. The customer isn't always right: why business ethics is not professional ethics. *Newsletter of the Australian Association for Professional and Applied Ethics*. Winter 2022.

Tannenbaum J. *Veterinary ethics*. Baltimore: Williams and Wilkins; 1989.

31 Corporatisation
Do Shareholders Care about Animal Welfare?

John Innes

31.1 INTRODUCTION

Veterinary practice has evolved and changed significantly over the last century. The books of Alf Wight (pseudonym: James Herriot) famously documented a fairy tale existence in a market town in the Yorkshire Dales region of northern England in the 1940s and 1950s, when vets were key players in the local community, supporting farmers, and tending to horses and family pets. During the 1960s to the 1990s, in many parts of the world, we saw a gradual growth of the small-animal sector as family pets moved from the backyard to the living room, and improvements in medicine and surgery allowed for the growth of small-animal practice in towns and cities. Clinics started to develop and enlarge, hospitals appeared, and more advanced referral centres opened. Instead of working in ones and twos, vets were now working in larger teams alongside increasingly well-qualified veterinary nurses and technicians.

In many territories around the world, ownership of veterinary practices was, on the face of it, restricted to registered veterinarians. However, we have seen that view challenged in many countries and the historical interpretation of various state laws has been questioned, or workarounds developed, to allow for non-veterinarians to engage in ownership.

Veterinary corporatisation began in the mid-1990s in the United States, specifically in 1994 when Mars Petcare acquired a stake in Banfield Pet Hospitals. On the other side of the Atlantic, the CVS group began consolidation of UK veterinary clinics at the end of the 1990s, but it was not until 2010 that corporate groups started to develop in other parts of the world.

In the United States, as of 2022, consolidator ownership of veterinary practices was estimated at 75% of specialty and emergency hospitals and 25% of general practices. Rules on who can own practices in the US are set at the state level. A number of states allow non-veterinarians to own veterinary practices outright, while others restrict ownership to licensed practitioners. Regardless, corporations can sidestep restrictions by setting up management companies that provide a host of services to businesses that technically remain owned by veterinarians (Kelly 2020).

In Europe, the current situation is rather different. On the one hand Sweden, Finland, Norway, Denmark, and the Netherlands are all at an advanced stage of the consolidation process: in these countries between one quarter and more than half of small-animal veterinarians work in groups. On the other hand, Spain, France, Germany, Austria, Ireland, Switzerland, Belgium, and Portugal are still just beginning the process, with groups employing less than 10% of small-animal veterinarians.

In the United Kingdom, 1999 was a landmark year. Prior to this, only qualified and registered veterinary surgeons could own a veterinary practice. The change in law was as a result of the Competition Act 1998. This act was a harmonisation with European competition policy because restricting ownership to vets would have been seen as an anti-competitive or a restrictive action. This seems strange in that some countries in the European Union still have restrictions in place. The Royal College of Veterinary Surgeons' Code of Conduct states that veterinary surgeons provide services through a variety of entities, including limited companies and partnerships, and may be managed by non-veterinary surgeons. Since 1999, we have seen rapid consolidation of the UK veterinary sector with an estimated 55% of practices owned by one of six large groups in 2024.

In Australia and New Zealand, consolidation is following trends in other parts of the world, with acceleration in recent years.

31.2 WHY DO CONSOLIDATORS EXIST?

This is a question that some non-commercial individuals can struggle to understand, but there are various motivators that drive the creation of consolidator groups, and this may be dependent on the business model. Consolidators might be private limited, private-equity-backed, or public companies. The majority of the large consolidators are funded through private equity groups. These groups are of different sizes and capabilities, but typically work to a 3-to-7-year cycle of 'buy, grow, and sell'. These groups are looking to add to the value of businesses through rapid growth and then selling on to a larger private equity group or ultimately moving to an initial purchase offering (IPO) and floating on the stock market. Such exit strategies are aimed at realising large returns on the initial investment – larger groups sell for greater multiples of existing operating profits compared to smaller groups. There have been many examples of smaller PE-backed veterinary practice groups being acquired by larger PE groups, and there has been some IPO activity (e.g. CVS Group has been on London's AIM listing since 2007).

Mergers and acquisitions (M&A) are a key way in which companies can drive growth. Throughout the last decade, in some countries or states, we have seen almost a frenzy of M&A activity. This was particularly the case in the United Kingdom when several groups were purchasing practices at a very rapid rate and competing with each other to do so. This competition drove up the multiples that these groups were prepared to pay and the heated activity created excitement and, no doubt, some fallout. Rapid purchasing of veterinary practices can occur as PE groups build towards an exit – 'stuffing the pipeline' with new practices or even 'deals in progress' can be seen as valuable to the next buyer. What receives less attention in the media is the 'wake' of such activity as companies struggle to integrate so many practices in such a short space of time.

Private companies, or listed companies, may have different behaviours to PE-backed groups. Mars Petcare, for example, is a private, family-owned business. Mars is involved in multiple territories around the world but also has a long track-record in pet nutrition. Such 'synergy' between business activities is another factor that drives consolidation – having lots of veterinary clinics through which to sell pet food is an obvious driver, although it can be argued that this is a threat to competition because the veterinary clinics have no choice but to sell the business owners' pet food.

Publicly owned companies are beholden to their shareholders, and these may be private individuals but, more importantly, institutional investors. Such investors have significant power to influence company behaviour. Shareholders need a return on their investment and this may come through an increase in share price and/or dividends. Investors will gauge companies on various financial metrics such as earnings per share (EPS). EPS is a measure of a company's profitability that indicates how much profit each outstanding share of common stock has earned, and it is calculated by dividing the company's net income by the total number of outstanding shares. Growth is an important driver of share price and publicly owned veterinary companies will look to grow through acquisition of veterinary practices but also through acquisition or start-up of other allied businesses with synergies and which assist with 'vertical integration'. Such integration involves buying up supply chains to veterinary practices such as diagnostic laboratories, crematoria, referral practices, equipment suppliers, and even white-label pharmaceuticals. Such activities can drive significant profits for the company, but there are concerns that this behaviour is a threat to competition because veterinary practices have no choice for their suppliers. In theory, there may also be a threat to clinical freedom, or clinical choice. Whilst publicly owned companies will engage in acquisitions of veterinary practices, they tend not to be as aggressive as private-equity-backed groups because they are more beholden to their shareholders and also to stock market regulators; this will often limit the 'multiples' that such companies will pay for practices compared to private equity.

Buying power is another factor that drives consolidation. Large practice groups have huge buying power and this may result in the negotiation of large rebates from manufacturers. Such rebates are typically not seen by the individual veterinary practices but benefit the parent company's bottom line.

31.3 HOW DO FUNDING MODELS INFLUENCE COMPANY BEHAVIOUR?

When a corporate group is formed, it is typically initially financed by bank borrowing. If it begins to grow, it may become necessary to finance the group with equity, usually by bringing in a private equity fund to provide capital. Private-equity-backed companies tend to aim for quick external growth (e.g. by increasing the number of clinics owned by the group) in order to increase the value of the company over a relatively short period of time, generally a 3-to-7-year cycle. It is commonplace for a private equity fund to take profits after a few years, and for another fund to take its place. After several investment cycles, the corporate group may become part of a multinational group, or go public and make an initial purchase offering (IPO) to become listed on a stock market. From this point, rapid external growth is no longer the sole priority; acquisition of new sites is still important, but internal growth by increasing revenue and profit from each of the group's clinics becomes a major objective.

It is clear from these observations that veterinary clinics, and the veterinary teams within, are vehicles for company growth and private equity profit. The following discussion will explore how this search for profit can create a tension with the fundamental priorities of veterinary professionals which are to champion the health and welfare of animals committed to their care.

31.4 COLLATERAL EFFECTS OF CONSOLIDATION

Consolidation brings economies of scale. Centralising business support functions such as HR and finance can obviously reduce costs for practices and increase profits for the parent company. Such moves do not directly affect animal welfare but they can have a significant impact on veterinary teams. If such services are good and efficient, this can help veterinary teams concentrate on their primary endeavours, but if such services are poor, it can lead to distractions and stress for veterinary teams. Physical and mental distance between these support functions and the veterinary practices can often cause frustration and a feeling of 'us' and 'them'; local leaders can feel disempowered. Such feelings have a negative impact on morale and reduce wellbeing of veterinary practice teams. Low morale in the workplace is unlikely to improve the quality of veterinary care.

Another common change following acquisition is that companies will typically move all their clinics on to a single practice management system which will allow for corporate-level data and reporting. Again, such changes can cause stress within veterinary teams and the change may not be seen locally as 'positive', particularly if users feel that the new PMS is not as good as the previous one (of course, the opposite is also possible). It is likely that such important changes do have effects on veterinary care, even if this is only temporary, as clinical teams cope with the disruption and adapt to new ways of working. As in other sectors, large companies are at risk of cyber attacks because they are attractive to cyber criminals, and we have seen examples of this in the veterinary sector (BBC 2024). Such attacks can paralyse operational activity and will undoubtedly have an impact on clinical care during such a crisis.

Consolidators will often look to centralise purchasing activity and use the power of bulk purchasing to reduce the costs of sales. Such negotiating with suppliers often leads to restrictions on the choice of drugs and consumables in the company's clinics. Whilst most companies will have clinical committees that discuss such decisions, there is a clear commercial pressure in many instances and compromises are often made. Whilst this does not itself threaten animal welfare, it may reduce choice for clinicians and clients.

Vertical integration is a business strategy that is undertaken by some large groups. This is where a company may develop or acquire businesses that serve the veterinary clinics, such as diagnostic laboratories, equipment suppliers, out-of-hours clinics, referral clinics, and crematoria. Company clinics will often be forced to use the company-owned suppliers, which obviously reduces choice and reduces competition; it is likely that such strategies have increased prices to clients because competition for those business-to-business services has been removed.

The acquisition of a veterinary practice brings many changes to the practice. There is the emotional impact on practice teams. The author has witnessed this first-hand as the purchaser tells the practice team that their clinic has been acquired and they now have a new employer. Understandably, members of practice teams can be shocked by such news, and this can cause significant stress. It is quite common for an acquisition to disrupt a practice team in the short to medium term as individuals come to terms with new ownership, new ways of working, and perhaps the loss of expectations and future plans. If the parent company is stretched, this stress to a practice can be even worse because they can struggle to find support and guidance at an already stressful time. This can have a marked negative impact on wellbeing of team members, although some team members will see new opportunity for themselves and embrace the change. Either way, ownership change is disruptive and will distract team members, and there are likely downstream consequences for client and patient care, at least in the short term. Acquisition can also result in personnel changes, and in a tight labour market, this can result in loss of service provision and quality of care.

At a macro level, consolidation has affected the structure and power of the veterinary professions. Veterinary associations, open to all members of the professions, often have been very active in promoting clinical standards but we have seen that consolidation can weaken the traditional associations. Large companies tend to turn inwards on matters that would once would be the preserve of the large associations. Large companies may or may not support membership of professional or clinical associations and they tend to stage their own 'conferences' rather than encourage participation at industry-wide events. Another important effect of the consolidation of buying power is that the commercial exhibitions at veterinary conferences have sometimes shrunk as the number of decision-makers has reduced. Suddenly, manufacturers see less return on a presence at a commercial exhibition and may reduce or withdraw their investment. A reduction in such sponsorship reduces revenue for veterinary associations. We have seen this effect starkly in the UK, most notably at BSAVA Congress which has shrunk in size and sponsorship since the halcyon days of the 1990s.

31.5 BENEFITS OF CONSOLIDATION

The traditional structure of veterinary practice had undoubtedly led to a very fragmented and diverse landscape. Each practice, or a small group of practices, would develop its own culture and values, and these influenced clinical practice and standards. Regulators have traditionally had only 'light touch' powers regarding practice standards and, although standards schemes exist, they are typically voluntary.

Many of the large groups have clinical committees and 'quality improvement' structures. The scale of large groups provides powerful, large datasets and the employment of vets and others in full-time quality improvement activity is a welcome development. Such groups can have a positive impact on clinical standards and clinical audit practices and can help support clinicians to develop. The veterinary profession has traditionally not had access to such large datasets, and these provide new opportunities for benchmarking and impactful clinical research. In the author's opinion, whilst it may not be the sole responsibility of a chief executive officer (CEO) to lead this, it is the responsibility of a CEO to ensure that corporate clinical governance structures are in place and given appropriate priority.

The large groups are obviously keen to recruit and retain veterinarians and veterinary nurses, in what can be a tight labour market. New graduate programmes, run at scale, are a relatively new phenomenon in our sector but are generally welcomed by new graduates because they receive dedicated support, support from peers, and formal training and mentorship.

Beyond new graduate programmes, some groups also have continuing education and training units that provide *ad hoc* and modular training programmes. The benefits of such units are obvious and may have helped to reduce the costs of postgraduate training.

Whilst many regret the loss of veterinary ownership of veterinary practices, there are many professionals who are quite happy not to be involved in ownership and are very content to do a clinical job without the distractions of business ownership. One can argue that being able to focus on clinical service provision is a positive drive for animal welfare. For such individuals, consolidation can provide an opportunity and may open up career pathways, other than ownership, that did not exist before.

31.6 FUTURE PERSPECTIVES

The rapid consolidation of the veterinary sector has perhaps surprised the professions, regulators, and the public. In many territories, regulations were written in a different era, and it is time for legislation to catch up with the times. In the United Kingdom, at the time of writing, the Competition and Markets Authority (CMA) has consulted on a proposal to make a market investigation reference into the veterinary services market for household pets in the UK. The CMA, a non-ministerial government department, exists to help people, businesses, and the UK economy by promoting competitive markets and tackling unfair behaviour. Clearly, to announce such a potential action, the CMA has sufficient concern regarding a substantial lessening of competition in the sector. These signals suggest that public and government opinions are moving towards renewed regulation of the sector to protect consumers and, hopefully, animal welfare. It is vital that veterinary practices, including those owned by large corporations, are regulated to protect competition and to protect animal welfare such that profits are not prioritised over and above other important aspects of a thriving and successful veterinary sector. Clinical corporate governance needs to be given equal footing to other aspects of corporate governance.

Veterinary professionals have, historically, been some of the most trusted in society; Alf Wight knew this very well. It would be very serious indeed if that trust were to be lost.

REFERENCES

BBC. Vet firm CVS hit by cyber-attack. *BBC News* [Internet]. 2024 Apr 8. Available from: https://www.bbc.co.uk/news/articles/cmjm2v5660xo.

Kelly R. Ireland: stronghold for independent veterinarians no more? *VIN News* [Internet]. 2020 Apr 23. Available from: https://news.vin.com/default.aspx?pid=210&Id=9609207&f5=1.

32 Costs of Veterinary Services as an Animal Welfare Issue

Nigel R. Taylor

The CMA (Competition and Markets Authority) have announced a proposal for a Full Market Investigation of the veterinary sector. An initial request for public submissions resulted in 56,000 responses (11,000 from the vet profession), an historic number of replies, highlighting the strength of feeling about the cost of veterinary care in the United Kingdom.

I tell you this, James, there are great days ahead!

That sunny afternoon, in the garden of Britain's sunniest veterinary practice, Skeldale House, Siegfried Farnon could not have imagined how right his cheerfully optimistic forecast would be. Wonderful advances in therapeutics, medical technology and surgical procedures would revolutionise the veterinary world he and James Herriot knew, totally transforming and changing it for ever. Siegfried would have been amazed by the many remarkable discoveries and advances we have made – and not a little surprised, I expect, at how lucrative it has all become!

Today it's been estimated that the UK's veterinary industry is worth £2 billion annually. No wonder then that in recent years we've seen the unrelenting growth of corporate practices, frequently backed by private equity finance, each seeking their own slice of the veterinary cake. Couple that with the recorded large increase in pet ownership, particularly dogs, since COVID-19 and its consequent lockdowns, and it's not surprising that veterinary practice profits are at an all-time high. So high that one major corporate group, CVS, were able to report a 50% jump in pre-tax profits to £53.9 million in the financial year 2022–2023. But it's not only the corporates who are consistently upping the cost of veterinary care, after all some 45% of UK veterinary practices are registered as independent. No, veterinary pricing is rising rapidly in every UK practice, and it would seem this is causing the profession more than a little reputational harm.

Criticism of our care is everywhere – from the National Press, Television, Radio to right across the broad spectrum of social media. We've gone from 'Herriot Heroes' to 'Not so Supervets' almost in the blink of an eye. Young vets, in particular, are finding social media criticism of them and their professional care highly

Costs of Veterinary Services as an Animal Welfare Issue 305

demotivating, making many question their professional future. And this is by no means only a UK phenomenon, Australia, the USA, and many other countries are reporting similar client dissatisfaction with veterinarians and the care we offer.

In the modern era the majority of veterinary practitioners are engaged in companion animal practice, so, unsurprisingly, this is where most veterinary criticism is coming from. It's easy to see why. Put simply, veterinary care, for many, is rapidly becoming unaffordable. Owning a pet will always be a choice which brings with it the responsibility of an animal's lifetime care – that'll never be inexpensive, easily running into many thousands of pounds for cats and dogs. As there's no National Health Service for pets, owners need an increasingly more realistic awareness of their full financial commitment to the animals they welcome into their families. VAT at 20% on veterinary fees in the UK automatically inflates care costs by a fifth, but it's the way even most basic care has escalated in cost that's causing the most concern.

Try a simple Internet search and you'll find initial consultations come in at £50–60 plus VAT per animal. Add on fees for potential clinical tests, like blood screens, and medication and you're quickly paying three figure sums for a ten-minute consultation. For most breeds, routine surgical procedures, like spaying, coupled with pre-operative blood tests, are comfortably into the hundreds of pounds. A fee of £500 for a standard bitch spay isn't uncommon. Whilst should you opt for laparoscopic surgery, which is becoming increasingly available, particularly for the larger breeds of dog like Great Danes, you won't get much change, if any, out of £1000.

If your pet is unfortunate enough to need a referral to a specialist, then hopefully you'll either have pet insurance or a robust credit card. Pricing in the veterinary referral sector can be eye-wateringly high. In 2022, a tibial plateau levelling osteotomy (TPLO) started at about £2200, a hemilaminectomy came in at £6400 plus, whilst a single lumbosacral epidural injection was listed by one referral centre at £630. Since 2022 we have been living through a period of increased economic inflation, which, naturally, is being reflected in all veterinary care costs, especially in the specialist referral sector. Highly specialised surgery will always, rightly, command premium pricing, but it's easy to see how easily orthopaedic enthusiasms, for example, can run away with costs, making many procedures appear unaffordable to the ordinary client. So lucrative have these specialised surgical services become that glossy adverts, many featuring caring surgeons at work, aimed at the pet market have started appearing online and elsewhere offering surgical package deals. A fixed price to fix your pet! North West Referrals (NWR) offer BOAS (brachycephalic obstructive airway syndrome) referrals, nares and soft palate correction, for breeds like pugs and French Bulldogs at a fixed price of £1500 (plus VAT), including meds and consult, whilst another NWR advert offers TPLO for cruciate repair at a fixed price of £2195 (plus VAT). We've come a long way since Siegfried and James' only allowed advertising was their brass plates on the wall at Skeldale – their small size regulated fiercely by the RCVS! Such is the competition in the orthopaedic referral world that at least one specialist practice now offers a 12-month surgical guarantee for all work they undertake. A good move perhaps, as high fees definitely deserve high rates of satisfactory outcomes.

Away from the rarified world of veterinary specialists, a common cause of financial concern for the pet owner is the out-of-hours emergency call. More than anywhere else, this is where fees charged and profits generated collide face-to-face, often in highly charged emotional situations, with the welfare needs of the animals in our care. It's not unusual to find a call-out fee is over £200 (plus VAT) – a not inconsiderable amount, even before a pet's illness or emergency condition is diagnosed and treated. So we shouldn't be surprised that clients are now thinking more than twice in many potentially life-threatening conditions before they consider making that call for urgent help. But, surely, acute conditions like gastric torsion seen early, can only benefit from urgent, timely care. Delay, even for a few hours, shifts the clinical odds profoundly towards the animal's disadvantage.

It's worth remembering, though, that client hesitation caused by financial concern isn't restricted to life-or-death emergency out-of-hours calls. Far more prosaically, it's the general care that animals deserve throughout their lives that may be suffering more in an era of high veterinary fees. So concerning are the increasing costs of veterinary care that in 2023 the PDSA reported that 17% of owners it surveyed had not registered their pet with a veterinary practice, believing it to be too expensive for them. Inevitably, this has many potential health and welfare consequences. Young animals who don't receive initial health checks may well have underlying conditions which often lead to ongoing debility and ill health. Early diagnosis, which often leads to resolution of their problems, is denied them because of perceived cost implications. A pet that hasn't seen a vet will not have received its primary vaccinations, leading it potentially vulnerable and at risk of infection from all too preventable illnesses, such as distemper and parvovirus. It's also worth remembering that the fewer animals vaccinated, the easier it is for viruses to spread amongst local pet populations putting many more pets at risk of disease. Preventive healthcare by vaccination is one of the most valuable health interventions we make. If pets aren't receiving their initial vaccine protection, it's highly unlikely we'll ever see them for any vaccination, including boosters, during their lifetime. As vaccine take-up drops due to cost, the risk of widespread infections amongst pets may well increase alarmingly. Those of us who remember when distemper and parvovirus were frighteningly common will never forget the canine patients we treated and those we often lost because of these twin killers. Vaccination has been extraordinarily successful at reducing their occurrence, perhaps leading to a sense of complacency amongst pet owners. Viruses never really go away, so it would be sad if cost induced vaccine hesitation undid so much that has been achieved in dealing with these eminently preventable infections.

The PDSA also reported that 10% of pet owners they surveyed could not afford to have their pets neutered at current prices. Behavioural and health consequences for the majority of female animals in particular which remain unneutered are well known to the profession. So, generally, we encourage neutering as a beneficial procedure, but if our costs are causing owners to hesitate, then it's highly likely we'll be seeing many more related conditions, such as pyometra and mammary tumours, in the not-too-distant future. All of which will obviously have a less-than-beneficial effect on canine patients in our care. There's also likely to be an increase in unplanned canine and feline births, adding to yet more welfare issues as puppy and kitten numbers increase. Perhaps, of all the surgical procedures we perform, this has to be one of the most affordable, and we need to ensure its cost does not escalate until neutering becomes a luxury choice for owners rather than the routine choice it should be.

All healthcare is holistic. Away from the clinical dramas of particular illnesses and diseases there are many general conditions that each, in its own subtle way, affects the health and general longevity of patients in our care. This is where routine examinations, especially when animals are presented for vaccination, prove so helpful to the clinician. Top amongst common conditions which affect animal health more than we might imagine is dental disease. Almost every dog or cat over the age of five has a degree of dental disease. It's relatively easy to diagnose and, caught early, can be quite effectively treated. In fact it's highly likely that most pets will need a few sessions of dental treatment during their lives. However, what should be a routine part of healthcare has become dramatically expensive. Veterinary dental care will always be relatively expensive as our patients require general anaesthesia for it to be undertaken. Currently, though, it's costing several hundred pounds per treatment, often far more than fees charged for comparatively complex human dental care. Practices typically request pre-operative blood tests which will cost the client £60 plus before they proceed to the full general anaesthesia animal dentistry requires. These, particularly in elderly cats, often highlight underlying raised liver or kidney parameters, so frequently these patients will receive intravenous therapy during their dental anaesthesia. Again, whilst this is a more than useful supplement for an anaesthetised patient, it would appear that many practices charge relatively high fees for intravenous fluid therapy. This runs the risk of compromising animal welfare when a client, already faced with a large fee for a routine dental procedure, opts out of fluids on the grounds of avoiding extra cost without fully appreciating the benefits their pet receives from having intravenous fluid support during anaesthesia. Most veterinary dental work is fairly straightforward – a combination of scaling and polishing the teeth with the occasional extraction. Specialist dental care, such as orthodontics and root canal treatments, is not common. However, the fees for routine necessary and beneficial care can be very high. A close acquaintance, owning two older cats with the usual feline teeth issues encountered with age, was recently quoted £600 for each cat's dental procedure after an initial consultation fee of £100. Unsurprisingly, perhaps, both cats have yet to receive any dental care because she considers the fees quoted way above affordable. Locally though, she is unable to receive lower quotes for the dental work as her town practices are all owned by the same corporate veterinary group. This is becoming a common occurrence in many parts of the UK and may well be contributing to less dental care for animals with concomitant health and welfare concerns. Dentistry is a particularly contentious area for pet owners as they are often aware of the many health implications of poor oral health but find the costs required for treatment increasingly prohibitive. And if they turn to pet insurance, they find little or no comfort as most veterinary health insurance policies specifically exclude dental care from their cover. This isn't altogether surprising as most pets require ongoing dental procedures during their lifetime, particularly as they age. Repeated care triggers repeated claims, which, from an actuarial point of view, are probably best avoided.

But, probably, amongst the most contentious areas of concern in the vet-client relationship are the fees attracted by animals that have ongoing, chronic conditions such as diabetes, hyperthyroidism, arthritis, or heart disorders. Once past the initial phase of examination, investigation, and diagnosis, most animals are fortunate to be offered regular treatment – often for life. It's become the practice, backed by enforceable legal protocols, for pets to be subject to check-up examinations before regular medication is dispensed to owners. This, of course, is highly sensible and responsible practice, but the cost of these check-ups can, in themselves, appear prohibitive, especially if they're frequent. A fee of £25–30 plus VAT once or twice a year is probably manageable, but some conditions require checks on a monthly basis for medicines to be dispensed. Once you've paid the check-up fee, there's still the medication to be paid for. It's easy to see why, in the Internet age, many clients feel that veterinary medicines are disproportionately overpriced when supplied by veterinary practices. A simple search of many online pharmacies reveals quite quickly much lower fees for common veterinary pharmaceuticals. Why, many clients ask, is there such a discrepancy between on line prices and those charged by my own vet? No wonder then that many, despite having to pay a prescription fee (£25–30) first, turn to online pharmacies to access lower prices for the medications their pets need. Some are turning to overseas online pharmacies, many of which supply medicines with no prescription requirement. There may well be quality control implications here, but of even more concern, I suspect, are those owners who are now turning to treating their animals with human medication, such as over-the-counter eye preparations, with their only clinical advice coming from Dr Google MRCVS and his associates via web-based forums. Such care is not only not in the best interests of pets, it may well be illegal. Anti-parasitic treatments, preventive and otherwise, are now largely a POM-V exercise, requiring a clinical examination before their supply. Again, the costs on line are considerably less than an in-practice purchase. Most clients pay for the necessary prescription check, despite the cost, before purchasing flea, tick, and worm control products online, but there are many who don't, regarding such consultations as an unnecessary expense. They will source such products from suppliers happy to supply with no veterinary checks at all. It's worth remembering that dispensing veterinary medication can have unforeseen consequences, not only for the patient in our care. Increasingly, for example, the scientific community is becoming aware of the environmental impact of anti-parasiticides, especially drop-ons, so added to the many potential animal welfare effects of unregulated supply, we also need to consider loss of opportunity to discuss with an owner the most appropriate anti-parasitic treatment frequency for their pet. Reducing overtreatment reduces potential environmental impact.

Having the time to discuss in a holistic way the health and welfare of an animal with its owner during a consultation is the primary foundation for any relationship between a veterinarian and his or her clients. It's our communication with clients at this time that demonstrates not only our clinical understanding of their animal's needs but, perhaps as importantly, that we care. But in the ever busier atmosphere of many veterinary clinics today, it's not surprising that empathy burnout is not at all uncommon, leading to client dissatisfaction as clients feel shortchanged on veterinary compassion despite being asked to pay high fees for their interaction with the vet. The ten-minute consultation, resulting in high client turnover, is common to most veterinary practices. Controlled by computer, these ten-minute windows for diagnosis and treatment planning can work relatively well. But, all too often, the clinician's time is eaten up by the practice's desire to maximise sales in wormers, flea treatments, and selling the current Pet Club offer, leaving little chance to discuss their patient's real needs.

Emergency consultations can disrupt in a moment the smooth running of ten-minute routine consults. I once encountered a young Dalmatian puppy with a luxated lens in one eye, the result of a dog attack. If its sight was to be saved, the puppy required urgent treatment. So I took to the phone to arrange surgical intervention from a local ophthalmic specialist. They weren't available, so I had to ring around to seek help elsewhere. It didn't take long for all planned ten-minute appointments to be thrown into disarray, so I found myself being rebuked by the receptionist for keeping clients waiting. There are, sometimes, priorities in veterinary care – priorities all clinicians recognise – and saving sight is one of them.

At another practice, a recently opened corporate, I was presented late one day with a tiny kitten whose owner had fallen on to it after tripping in his home. Although the young cat was subdued and looked uncomfortable, an examination didn't reveal any major problems, like fractures, so I treated it with a suitable analgesic and sent the client home somewhat relieved. Next morning, the kitten was much better. The owner was relieved, but as I examined his cat, he suddenly burst into tears, inconsolable with guilt at the pain he'd caused his pet. So I did what hopefully any veterinary surgeon would do – I reassured him the kitten was well and explained that unfortunately accidents do happen, and I told him not to upset himself unduly as things had turned out well. This took time but gradually his tears subsided and he regained his composure. There was then a knock at the consulting room door. A dressing down from the practice manager was on its way. 'Have you forgotten you're only booked for a ten-minute consult? We have clients waiting, you know'. Now I might be wrong, but I've always taken the view that veterinary medicine is very much a people profession as much as it is an animal one. Showing empathy and compassion for owners is every bit a part of our role as our understanding of animal health and disease. Showing you care shouldn't be subject to a profit-driven ten-minute rule.

This is never more evident than when it comes to the final stages of an animal's life. Of all the services we offer pets and their owners, this is perhaps one of the most important and certainly the one that our reputation as a caring profession is frequently judged by. How caring we are was severely called into question during the COVID-19 crisis. Strict social distancing rules, obviously well intentioned, severely restricted veterinary interaction with clients. This was never more evident than in the way we had to modify our approach to euthanasia. No longer could pet owners and their family members be present when a much-loved pet was being put to sleep. Instead, pets were handed over to clinic staff, often in outside car parks, and taken away to be euthanised. That often much wanted final contact was lost, leading perhaps inevitably, to a loss in client confidence too. Some saw us as very uncaring, particularly as euthanasia charges remained high and have continued to escalate, leading to a still stubbornly present opinion that we care more for profit than for people and their pets.

How clients perceive us has a direct impact on animal welfare. If we are seen as chasing profit from animal care, then we run the risk of animals not being presented for the treatment they need and deserve, with many implications for their welfare. Many pet owners are turning to the major animal charities, such as RSPCA, PDSA, and Blue Cross, for help as veterinary care becomes ever more unaffordable. As a result, the animal charities are increasingly under more and more financial pressure themselves as they try to offer assistance. Partnerships between the major charities in many parts of the United Kingdom (UK) are currently being set up in an attempt to ensure that many animals, especially in socially deprived areas, have some access to veterinary health support. Many provide vouchers to aid payment for veterinary fees. Dependence on charities shows no sign of going away and is likely to increase as financial uncertainty continues to prevail for many.

Meanwhile the corporate sector of veterinary practice continues its acquisition of independent practices, increasingly restricting the choice potential clients have for sourcing veterinary interventions. My own nearby city now has only one independent practice – every other veterinary outlet belonging to one of two major corporates. This may be changing as creeping veterinary corporatisation has attracted the attention of the Competition and Markets Authority (CMA) – the UK competition regulator. A review is currently underway of how veterinary services are bought and sold amid concerns that pet owners may not be getting a good deal or receiving the information they need to make good choices. The CMA have appealed to pet owners to contact them – such is the level of public discontent with vets' fees, and there's every sign their postbag will be full!

It's not only the UK that's concerned about the corporate takeover of veterinary medicine. France, concerned that the ownership structure of veterinary practices by corporates undermined veterinarians' professional independence, is considering legislation that restricts practice ownership to veterinary surgeons only. This was the situation in the UK for many years until rules on practice ownership were relaxed by the RCVS. This change of practice regulation has been the open door for the rapid rise of corporatisation in the veterinary profession.

As the public have become increasingly dissatisfied with the profession as they have found fees escalate and reach unaffordable levels, some innovation in practice structure has arrived, particularly in the independent sector. Most notable of these are the practices now operating on a subscription model. A variation on the Pet Club schemes that offer discounts on vaccinations, deworming, and flea treatment, these subscription practices offer a more complete veterinary service for pets to subscribers. One of the most notable of these is a private practice attached to, and acting as a teaching hospital for, a new UK veterinary school. Garden Vets at Keele aim to change the face of pet care by offering a comprehensive range of subscriptions for pet owners. For £54 a month, dog owners are offered unlimited consultations, medications, referrals if needed, routine boosters, surgeries, and more. Similar subscription deals for all pets, including cats, rabbits, and animals with complex needs (£128 monthly), are part of the Garden Vet offer.

Such subscription offers, where available, might well provide not only a more affordable alternative to more common veterinary practice care but also a possible better deal for owners than pet insurance, which is currently not the panacea it promises to be. It will be interesting to see how this novel business model performs. At least one recently launched membership practice with initial aims to provide a nationwide network – largely in supermarket car parks – has closed a Cheshire outlet after two years of operation, citing challenges such as a shortage of qualified vets and nurses, amongst others. A second outlet planned by the company is reported as being 'on hold'.

The costs of running any veterinary practice are undoubtedly very challenging. Quite clearly, a corporate model has many advantages when it comes to purchasing medicines and consumables, as well as recruiting staff with attractive salary packages and the potential of well-defined career progression. So it's highly likely the corporate model is here to stay – albeit with some restriction on future acquisitions. How much the independent sector will decline or the 'subscription model' succeed is anybody's guess – the pet-owning public will decide.

It's clear the profession would do well to review its fee structures and their control in all areas of veterinary activity. Our clients' perception – real or imagined – of our increasing unaffordability is doing little for vets' professional reputation and, more importantly, less for the welfare of the animals in our care who will be denied veterinary help they need and deserve.

I tell you this, James – if we're not careful, there could be grim days ahead!

32.1 ADDENDUM

In September 2023, the CMA launched an initial review of the veterinary sector in the UK. This prompted 56.000 responses from the public and the veterinary industry. Some 11,000 responses came from those working in the veterinary profession – approximately one-fifth of UK vets and vet nurses, many reporting the pressures they face including acute staff shortages which are having a deleterious effect on their wellbeing. This level of response was unprecedented in the CMA's history. Pet owners were concerned about their inability to access price lists, the costs of veterinary prescriptions, and potentially overpaying for medicines.

The CMA further reported their concern that, in some areas, clients have little choice of veterinary care provider for their animals, as large corporate groups are acting in ways which may reduce competition and choice. The CMA was further concerned that clients were less able to access simpler, lower cost treatments which they might prefer, as, due to significant investment in advanced equipment, large corporate groups may concentrate on providing more sophisticated, higher-cost treatments. It was also suggested that pet owners may be overpaying for medicines and prescriptions in part because current regulatory regimes restrict practices' ability to source less expensive medication online. Attention was also drawn to the current Veterinary Surgeons Act, which dates from 1966 before non-vets were unable to own practices. Its antiquity limits leverage the RCVS has over commercial and consumer facing aspects of veterinary businesses, for example, how prices are communicated and whether there is transparency about the ownership of practices and other veterinary services. It was noted that nearly a third of the veterinary practices have not signed up to the RCVS Practice Standards scheme, which applies to vet practices rather than individual vets. The CMA have taken a provisional view that outcomes for consumers could be improved if regulatory requirements and/or elements of best practice were monitored or enforced more effectively.

In March 2024, the CMA launched a four-week consultation seeking the veterinary sector's views on the proposal to launch a full market investigation. RCVS, BVA, BSAVA, BVNA, and other veterinary organisations submitted their considered responses to the CMA's provisional investigation. The main UK veterinary corporates have also submitted their responses to the CMA. All have stressed ongoing current efforts within the industry which aim to address the issues the CMA initial investigation have raised. The effects on veterinary staff likely to be caused by a prolonged formal market investigation have been drawn to the CMA's attention. Many practice teams have been receiving an increase in client abuse since the CMA process began in 23 September and its activities highlighted regularly by television, radio, social media, and newspaper reports often quite critical of current veterinary professional activity. It's thought that a prolonged formal market investigation will exacerbate the level of abuse veterinary teams may receive.

As of 22 April 2024 no decision had been announced by the CMA as to whether a formal Market Investigation will be taking place. However, given the strength of feeling noted by the CMA in the historically large number of replies it has received to its initial call for responses from the public to a proposed investigation, it would be reasonable to suppose a formal market investigation into the UK veterinary profession is a highly likely prospect.

Part IIID Veterinary Clients

33 Anthropomorphism in Veterinary Practice

R. Eddie Clutton

33.1 INTRODUCTION

Anthropomorphism – the attribution of human traits, feelings, qualities, etc. to non-human animals, inanimate objects, natural forces, etc. – has been an innate characteristic of the human psyche for about 40,000 years. In veterinary practice, the most likely foci of anthropomorphism are the companion animal subjects of veterinary care. Used intelligently by conscientious veterinarians, anthropomorphism has potential for increasing client understanding, improving communication, and facilitating informed decision-making. However, its cynical misuse can be used to mislead clients for goals other than ensuring the health and welfare of animals, when it becomes unprofessional and contemptible. Applied uncompromisingly by less-than-thoughtful owners, uncritical anthropomorphism might force conscientious veterinarians to do things they'd prefer not to, causing moral stress. That anthropomorphism is regarded in some quarters as fundamentally unscientific means conscientious veterinarians may find themselves sailing between the Scylla of evidence-free practice and the Charybdis of the veterinary art. Understanding the nature of anthropomorphism may help veterinarians navigate safe passage between six-headed monsters and voracious whirlpools, while benefitting debates on animal euthanasia, veterinary overtreatment, veterinary ethics, and animal rights.

33.2 HISTORY

Authorities appear to agree that anthropomorphic tendencies appeared in the Upper Palaeolithic Period (50,000 – 12,000 years ago) when human behaviours began elaborating: people started forming more complex social groups that ritually buried their dead, and technological innovations, e.g. boats, bows, and arrows, allowed the development of more systematic fishing and hunting methods. A growing preoccupation with animal habits and behaviours probably permitted more complex and successful hunting strategies based on forward planning and the ability to accurately predict the movements and behaviour of the species hunted (Mithen 1998).

Early Indo-European cultures promoted anthropomorphism in the form of fables, i.e. short stories based on animal stereotypes which illustrated principles of life and/or attempted to morally educate children. The Western tradition is typified by Aesop (sixth century BC) who originated, amongst others, 'The Hare and the Tortoise' and 'The Boy Who Cried Wolf'. These fables have not only endured, but some of Aesop's animal stereotypes are recognisable today, e.g. the wise owl and the cunning fox.

The anthropomorphism, which flourished in the 19th century when cleverly illustrated children's books became widely available, e.g. Carroll's *Alice's Adventures in Wonderland* (1865), Sewell's *Black Beauty* (1877), Kipling's *The Jungle Book* (1894), Potter's *The Tale of Peter Rabbit* (1902), Graham's *The Wind in the Willows* (1908), and A.A. Milne's *Winnie-the-Pooh* (1925), differed from C.S. Lewis's *The Lion, the Witch, and the Wardrobe* (1950) in using anthropomorphised animals to entertain rather than morally educate the young. In contrast, Orwell's *Animal Farm* (1945) used anthropomorphic farm animals to send a political rather than a moral message to adult readers. Richard Adams raised political and societal awareness using anthropomorphised rabbits and dogs in *Watership Down* (1972) and *The Plague Dogs* (1977), respectively.

Developments in media technology carried anthropomorphism through the 20th and into the 21st century. Since Disney's earliest animated film (which featured Oswald the Lucky Rabbit [1927] and whose ironic lucklessness gave rise to Mickey Mouse [1928]) over a third of the films flying the Disney banner, including *Bambi* (1942) and *101 Dalmatians* (1961) have featured anthropomorphic animal characters. However, not all animated anthropomorphisms have been morally educational: Hanna and Barbera's *Tom and Jerry* portrayed an early form of 'punk anthropomorphism' in which a cat and a mouse continuously attempted to kill each other using inconceivably cruel (though imaginative) methods. More recently, animals have entertained children as anthropomorphised protagonists in computer games. In *Crash Bandicoot* and *Sonic the Hedgehog*, the animal characters are player-controlled, behave like humans, talk, and appear to possess human levels of self-awareness.

Unsurprisingly, anthropomorphism's societal values have shifted from the educational to the commercial, and whilst animals have been used for some time in advertising to define brand image, companion animals are now the indirect targets of anthropomorphic merchandising. Evidence for this can be found by entering 'Birthday presents for dogs' into the Google search engine, which on 26 April 2024 resulted in just over 41 million results. This indicates a worrying drift towards anthropocentricism, whereby an animal's reality is *only* viewed in terms of human values and experience. It also has important implications for animal welfare because such unnecessary merchandise may not only directly harm animals (see the following), but some may have been tested on experimental animals (Park et al. 2020).

The human tendency to anthropomorphism has evolved over approximately 40,000 years and in becoming a major element of children's learning and entertainment ensures its entrenchment in the human psyche is profound and widespread. While this varies amongst individuals and cultures (Waytz et al. 2010) anthropomorphism probably represents the 'default position' for most human adults (Guthrie 1997) – including animal owners. In these, convictions that their animals can think and emote like humans may be near-impossible to expunge and may affect their ability to make sound judgments with respect to veterinary treatment. Anthropomorphism is also likely to compromise animal welfare when it affects the judgement of veterinary surgeons who fail to identify its limitations or who capitalise upon it for purposes other than optimising animal health and welfare.

33.3 SCIENCE AND ANTHROPOMORPHISM

Anthropomorphism is generally regarded as scientific anathema (Kennedy 1992), and using the term in veterinary contexts often prompts unease. Yet its relationship with scientific thinking has been undulant and continues to undergo revision; there is no absolute consensus on its overall scientific utility.

A Cartesian interpretation prevailed before 1859; animals were automata reacting only by instinct and habit. In contrast, humans possessed an immortal soul that elevated them above the brute creation and conferred language, rationality, intelligence, and consciousness. The publication of Darwin's *On the Origin of Species* (1859), which held that living things were inter related undermined this position. Darwin's own anthropomorphism is clear: 'the lower animals, like man, manifestly feel pleasure and pain, happiness and misery'. This opinion, while initially accepted, faced increasing challenges as psychology, comparative psychology, and ethology grew as independent scientific disciplines. Arising in the 1930s, ethology, i.e. the objective study of spontaneous species-typical behaviours of animals in their natural habitats, erased residual scientific support for anthropomorphism – but only for three decades. Re-establishing the 'mind' in experimental psychology in the 1960s saw scientific attitudes shifting again (Miller 2003), and throughout the 1970s animal behaviourists *au fait* with cognitive approaches developed new fields of enquiry, e.g. cognitive ethology and animal cognition, which were less dismissive of anthropomorphism. In 1976, Griffin wrote, 'Ethologists and comparative psychologists have discovered increasing complexities in animal behaviour during the past few decades. The flexibility and appropriateness of such behaviour suggest not only that complex processes occur within animal brains, but that these events may have much in common with our own mental experiences' (Griffin 1976). Since then, there have been attempts to reintroduce anthropomorphism as a respectable branch of psychology (Wynne 2007), for example, critical anthropomorphism (Burghardt 1991), biocentric anthropomorphism (Bekoff 2000), and animal-centred anthropomorphism (de Waal 1999). Of perhaps greater veterinary relevance is theriomorphism (Timberlake 1999) (discussed later). Despite differences between these approaches, they share the belief that projecting oneself into the situation of an individual of another species can lead to the production of useful hypotheses for further scientific study, i.e. anthropomorphism is no longer scientifically sinful. The contentiousness of anthropomorphism remains, therefore, greatest amongst ethologists and comparative psychologists and its potential to derail scientific advancement is most likely when testing hypotheses in animal behavioural science. Its threat to the scientific basis of those parts of clinical veterinary practice that are unrelated to ethology is probably minimal. Perhaps then, the question of greater concern to veterinarians, their clients, and to veterinary medical educators, is the significance of making false anthropomorphic assumptions about an individual animal's behaviour in veterinary practice. A case may be made that if anthropomorphism *per se* does not harm individual animals then why not indulge it? The counter-case is that naive anthropomorphism can be harmful when applied to large companion animal populations and is tacitly supported by a veterinary profession which should know better. The counter-case is important because the numbers of dogs and cats being kept for companionship is rapidly increasing throughout the Western world. Companion animal (particularly dog) ownership in the United States (US) has increased 56% since 1988; as of 2023, 66% of US households own a companion animal (Megna 2024).

33.4 CHANGES IN THE HUMAN–COMPANION ANIMAL BOND

Animals are becoming 'humanised' in numerous ways and for numerous reasons – not least financial gain. Dogs, which previously had names reflecting personal attributes, e.g. Fido (from *fidus* [Latin] meaning 'faithful') and were fed table scraps, are becoming almost indistinguishable from human family members. Animals called Luna and Charles are now fed products which are visually appetising to humans and being made from human-grade meat that is hypoallergenic and free from artificial colourings, flavourings, and preservatives. Such products are also commonly available in organic and vegan options. About half of American dog owners have now celebrated their dog's birthday at which their pets appear dressed in the designer-label fashions their owners feel their pet should wear (Serpell 2015). In a recent UK psychological report, 76% of 1,000 people questioned allowed their dog to sleep with them and 'let them feel the love' – whatever that means (Velez 2024). While such interactions may strengthen the human-animal bond and accentuate the owner's care and interest in their animal's wellbeing (Mota-Rojas et al. 2021), welfare problems arise when humanisation is excessive yet remains unrecognised because an owner considers their pet to be near-human.

That 85–97% of dog owners currently consider their pets as family members (Megna 2024; Brown 2023) explains an increasing tendency for owners to make personal sacrifices for their animals. One study found that 14% of US dog owners had moved from an apartment to a house so their dog would have a yard (Megna 2024). That said, regarding pets as family members is not to surrender reason: in the eyes of some owners, animal family members remain animals; i.e. the relationship is unfettered by anthropomorphism. In these circumstances, owner sacrifices are a matter of personal choice and indulgences are inconsequential, providing they do not adversely affect the animal's physical and mental health (which they frequently do – see the following). There is evidence that animals admitted to the family unit are allowed to exercise their conferred human characteristics to the detriment of other human family members: 51% of US animal owners consider their pets to be as much a part of their family as a human member (Brown 2023).

33.5 ANTHROPOMORPHISM IN VETERINARY PRACTICE

Anthropomorphism has at least five important ramifications for veterinarians: they may create public health problems; animals (and owners) can benefit when pets are sensibly treated as family members; projecting human needs onto animals may lead to misinterpretation of the actual intentions underlying animal behaviour and cause human-animal conflicts; extreme expressions of anthropomorphism can cause physical and psychological harms to animals that may require veterinary treatment; opinion differences between veterinarians and owners concerning the extent to which animals can become 'humanised' can compromise animal welfare, challenge the client-physician relationship, and lead to stress-related disorders in either human party.

33.6 ANTHROPOMORPHISM AND PUBLIC HEALTH

Humans frequently demonstrate interspecific affection by kissing, but knowing that dogs (and some cats) (i) taste and eat unsavoury material, e.g. vomit, faeces, putrescent animal carcasses; (ii) communicate intraspecifically through naso-anal exploration; and (iii) enjoy poor dental hygiene makes kissing one's quadrupedal companions highly questionable. Hygiene aside, kissing dogs and cats risks contracting diseases. Dogs commonly carry *Capnocytophaga* in their mouths and saliva, which, while normally innocuous, can compromise the health of the immunosuppressed. Cat-associated zoonoses travelling the faecal-oral route include giardiasis, campylobacteriosis, salmonellosis, and toxoplasmosis. Knowing that the mouth, nose, and perineum are the primary locations of methicillin-resistant *Staphylococcus aureus* colonisation in dogs and cats (Khairullah et al. 2023) should deter those humans inclined to kiss their pets in such places.

33.7 ANTHROPOMORPHISM AND ANIMAL BENEFITS

Anthropomorphism probably encourages animal welfare by raising interest in animal rights and positive thinking towards pro-animal movements, while sensitising owners to their animal's pain may prompt earlier veterinary consultation (Butterfield et al. 2012). While this may apply generally, its consequences at individual animal level depends on the enthusiasm with which anthropomorphism is applied; its imprudent and excessive application can be harmful. There appears to be no consensus concerning the effects of anthropomorphism on companion dogs' psychological wellbeing (Mota-Rojas et al. 2021), but the physical consequences are real enough (*vide infra*).

Ignoring some of the human-like characteristics of animals, i.e. 'anthropodenial', is likely to compromise their welfare in obvious ways (de Waal 1999). Consequently, unless there are clear reasons not to do so, many believe it reasonable to give animals the 'benefit of the doubt' when questions concerning their capacity to experience simple emotions, both positive and negative, arise (Bekoff 2000). Such an attitude has been a major factor in fuelling advances seen in animal pain management over the last five decades.

33.8 THE HUMAN BENEFITS OF ANTHROPOMORPHISM

It is widely held and experimentally supported, that human-animal bonds (HABs) improve physical and mental health in people (Engel 1981). In providing social support, HABs improve mental health, e.g. reduced anxiety, depression, and stress (Friedmann et al. 2015) which consequently improves physical health (Oosthuizen et al. 2023). Perhaps less widely appreciated is that anthropomorphism *per se* is critically important in this. Attributing human social motivations to animals facilitates the formation of HABs in the first instance and from which emotional and physical benefits later arise (Serpell 1991).

33.9 ANTHROPOCENTRICISM AND ANIMAL HARMS

Anthropocentrism interprets reality only in terms of human values and experience. Its application, i.e. projecting human needs onto animals, may lead to misinterpretation of the actual intentions, motivations, and emotions underlying animal behaviour and lead to human-animal conflicts (Sueur et al. 2020). This occurs when anthropocentricism ignores Von Uexkull's *umwelt* – the 'sensory world' particular to individuals of each species (Schroer 2021). And while there is overlap in the human and companion animal *umwelten* (which facilitates interspecific communication) (Bradshaw & Casey 2007), major differences can lead to the human misinterpretation of animal needs. For example, a dog's ability to hear higher frequencies than humans (Bradshaw 1992) means that noise levels in veterinary hospitals containing metal cages may cause considerable auditory distress in dogs (Sales et al. 1997). When such kennels are cleaned with strong-smelling disinfectants, canine olfactory sensitivities may be similarly assaulted (Sommerville & Broom 1998). An appreciation of the *umwelt* is also important in theriomorphism (see later).

33.10 ANTHROPOMORPHIC OWNERS AND ANIMAL HARMS

Anthropomorphism provides an opportunity to make money in ways that frequently compromise animal health and welfare. Numerous items are now available that satisfy the questionable needs of owners rather than the biological needs of the animal (Forbes et al. 2018). In addition to the traditional squeaky toy, one can now buy strollers and prams (difference unclear), breath-freshening foods, jewellery (for dogs, not owners), fragrances (from the Pawfume ShopTM), designer clothes (including design-your-own bandanas), nappies (washable or disposable), nail polish (from PawdicureTM), coat dyes (12 colours available from OpawzTM Permanent Pet Hair Dyes), birthday cakes (with or without squeaks), and shoes (with or without socks). Those adversely affecting an animal's physical health have been extensively detailed (Mota-Rojas et al. 2021), so only four notable examples are reviewed here. First, carrying dogs (or using strollers) for prolonged periods causes physical harms, e.g. muscle atrophy, and psychological injury. Restricting a dog's freedom of movement limits natural inclinations to explore, interact, and control interesting environmental features, and can lead to emotional disorders, including phobias and anxiety (Mota-Rojas et al. 2021). Second, differences between the digestive function and nutritional requirements of dogs and humans are so great (and obvious) that warnings against feeding animals human diets should be unnecessary. Feeding dogs junk food, e.g. sweeties, chocolate, ice cream, etc., which are universally condemned by human nutritionists, are unlikely to be good for companion animals – even those forced to consume the dairy-free, vegetarian, or vegan options. Third, in discussing cosmetics and coat dyes, Mota-Rojas et al. raise questions on human behaviour, asking why some humans apply such products on their pets, while others are vehemently opposed to testing cosmetics on animals in general (De Lapuente et al. 2014). Finally, the article expresses concerns about clothing animals (in contrast to putting warm waterproof jackets on whippets in cold, wet, and windy Scotland) warning that animals encumbered by unnecessary clothing may be unable to avoid hazards, e.g. aggressive dogs, motor vehicles, etc. (On a related point, the psychological effects of being made to wear Dracula costumes at Hallowe'en are speculative, but one struggles to see this as a meaningful refinement of the companion-animal bond and raises the question of whether treating one's animals as objects of hilarity reflects thoughtful animal ownership).

33.11 ANTHROPOMORPHISM AND THE VETERINARIAN-CLIENT RELATIONSHIP

Different anthropomorphic tendencies between owners and veterinarians can lead to disagreements and adverse consequences for both human parties and the animals involved. The greatest animal harms occur when an owner's belief that their pet deserves human standards of care are exploited by veterinarians.

33.12 ANTHROPOMORPHIC OWNERS

Vets are commonly expected by anthropomorphic owners to 'do everything possible'. When fully aware of the welfare costs to the animal and the futility of treatment, such vets frequently suffer moral stress (Batchelor & McKeegan 2012).

33.13 ANTHROPOMORPHIC VETS

Vets who genuinely or disingenuously promote the belief that animals are small humans and should be treated accordingly may cause feelings of guilt in owners who do not or cannot afford to share that view. Owners, who ultimately pay for treatment, may suffer 'caregiver burden' when coerced by vets to accept treatment which – for reasons of their own – they would prefer their animal did not receive (Spitznagel et al. 2017). Pragmatic owners may also be made to feel guilty for rejecting the recommendations of vets who they believe are offering well-meant advice.

33.14 THE PERFECT (ANTHROPOCENTRIC) STORM

A companion animal's welfare is likely to be optimised when vets and owners share a common anthropomorphism tempered by their shared perception of 'what the animal wants' (Jarvis 2010). In contrast, animal suffering is likely to be greatest when vets and owners share a common anthropocentricism. Vets who genuinely or, more reprehensibly, claim to believe that an animal's reality exists only in terms of human values and experience, and who convinces or deals with owners of similar persuasion, will be comfortable conducting major surgical or oncological procedures on animals irrespective of what the animal wants or whether it may be causing considerable suffering. Procedures conducted under these conditions are often unproven, unauthorised, unregulated, and impermissible under the professional guidelines and so are fundamentally unethical. Often touted under the terms 'innovative' and/or 'last chance', such procedures achieve wide acceptability because their unpleasant features tend not to be disclosed (Clutton et al. 2022). In the final analysis, the veterinarian(s) involved benefit financially and reputationally and irrespective of case outcome. Clients suffer financially and often emotionally. Animals which survive such procedures often just suffer.

33.15 ANTHROPOMORPHISM, ANTHROPOCENTRICISM, AND DEATH

The moral justification for allowing any physical and psychological suffering that arises when animals are treated as human or near-human patients depends on a significant unknown – the animal's cognitive-evaluative capabilities. Answers to some questions are required: Do animals recognise that noxious veterinary procedures may be in their own long-term interest? Does an animal value its own life and desire its prolongation irrespective of circumstances? Do animals fear death? An ability to answer such questions would go far in directing the ethical prolongation (and termination) of an animal's life. Until then, guidance might be taken by rationalising that animals do feel pain and can suffer and probably don't understand death. In this case euthanasia is a legitimate and ethical way to end an animal's suffering when other options are likely to fail.

33.16 CONCLUSIONS

The most important problem arising from anthropomorphism is that it may cause animals to suffer. This might be prevented if the following nine propositions were accepted by both veterinarians and owners. First, there are many psychological and physiological differences between companion animals and humans. Second, animals are unable to appreciate the significance of their disease and will probably regard all well-meant therapeutic interventions as unpleasant, i.e. animals undergoing veterinary treatment always experience some degree of psychological suffering, even when treatments are innocuous (Hiestand 2022). Third, animals undergoing noxious treatment will always experience pain and distress and suffer physically and psychologically, transiently or permanently. Fourth, animals appreciate pain and suffering in real time, and have limited capacity to remember, or anticipate a time when the pain has or will not exist. Fifth, compared with humans, companion animals probably have a limited capacity for self-awareness and the ability to place a value on their own lives – irrespective of its quality. Sixth, animals probably have a limited capacity to countenance (and fear) their own or the death of others. Seventh, the degree to which vets prioritise their sworn commitment to the health and welfare of animals in their care varies considerably. Eighth, veterinarians have much to gain beyond improving the health and welfare of animals by promoting anthropomorphism. Ninth, the client will almost always be financially and emotionally liable for treatment irrespective of its success, or whether the animal lives, suffers, or dies.

Finally, veterinarians attempting safe passage between six-headed monsters and voracious whirlpools may be tempted by theriomorphism, a form of tamed anthropomorphism that recognises umwelt. The concept, proposed by Timberlake, involves putting oneself into a position based on an animal's specific physiological capabilities (Timberlake 1999) – and with which veterinarians should be reasonably familiar. In an example cited by Wynne (2007), the theriomorph is asked to adopt the umwelt of a lioness stalking zebra, i.e. feeling the brush of cover, the sun's heat, interpreting the posture and body language of other pride members, feeling hungry, recognising zebra as food, etc. Theriomorphism, i.e. adopting the umwelten of companion animals undergoing painful veterinary procedures, might offer one way to reconcile anthropomorphism with humane and evidence-based practice.

REFERENCES

Batchelor CE, McKeegan DE. Survey of the frequency and perceived stressfulness of ethical dilemmas encountered in UK veterinary practice. *Vet Rec.* 2012;170(1):19.

Bekoff M. Animal emotions: exploring passionate natures: current interdisciplinary research provides compelling evidence that many animals experience such emotions as joy, fear, love, despair, and grief – we are not alone. *BioScience.* 2000;50(10):861–870.

Bradshaw JWS. *Behavioural biology*. Thorne C, editor. Oxford: Pergamon Press; 1992.

Bradshaw JWS, Casey RA. Anthropomorphism and anthropocentrism as influences in the quality of life of companion animals. *Anim Welf.* 2007;16(S1):149–154.

Brown A. About half of U.S. pet owners say their pets are as much a part of their family as a human member. *Pew Research Center* [Internet]. 2023 Jul 7. Available from: https://www.pewresearch.org/short-reads/2023/07/07/about-half-us-of-pet-owners-say-their-pets-are-as-much-a-part-of-their-family-as-a-human-member/.

Burghardt GM. Cognitive ethology and critical anthropomorphism: a snake with two heads and hognose snakes that play dead. In: Ristau CA, Marler P, editors. *Cognitive ethology: essays in honor of Donald R. Griffin*. Hillsdale, NJ: Lawrence Erlbaum Associates, Inc.; 1991. p. 53–90.

Butterfield ME, Hill SE, Lord CG. Mangy mutt or furry friend? Anthropomorphism promotes animal welfare. *J Exptl Soc Psychol*. 2012;48(4):957–960.

Clutton E, Ware J, Murphy K, et al. Untested surgical procedures. *Vet Rec*. 2022;190(1):38.

De Lapuente J, Borras M, González-Linares J, et al. Los métodos alternativos en el estudio de la seguridad de cosméticos. *Rev Toxicol*. 2014;31:140–148.

de Waal FBM. Anthropomorphism and anthropodenial: consistency in our thinking about humans and other animals. *Philos Topics*. 1999;27(1):255–280.

Engel GL. The clinical application of the biopsychosocial model. *J Med Philos*. 1981;6(2):101–123.

Forbes SL, Trafford S, Surie M. Pet humanisation: what is it and does it influence purchasing behaviour? *Dairy Vet Sci J*. 2018;5(2):1–5.

Friedmann E, Son H, Saleem M. The animal-human bond: health and wellness. In: Fine AH, editor. *Handbook on animal-assisted therapy*. San Diego: Academic Press; 2015. p. 73–88.

Griffin DR. *The question of animal awareness: evolutionary continuity of mental experience*. 1st ed. Oxford: Rockefeller University Press; 1976.

Guthrie SE. Anthropomorphism: a definition and a theory. In: Mitchell R, Thompson NS, Miles HL, editors. *Anthropomorphism, anecdotes, and animals*. New York: Suny Press; 1997. p. 50–58.

Hiestand KM. The autonomy principle in companion veterinary medicine: a critique. *Front Vet Sci*. 2022;9:953925.

Jarvis S. Where do you draw the line on treatment? *Vet Rec*. 2010;167(17):636–637.

Kennedy JS. *The new anthropomorphism*. 1st ed. Cambridge: Cambridge University Press; 1992.

Khairullah AR, Sudjarwo SA, Effendi MH, et al. Pet animals as reservoirs for spreading methicillin-resistant staphylococcus aureus to human health. *J Adv Vet Anim Res*. 2023;10(1):1–13.

Megna M. Pet ownership statistics 2024. *Forbes Advisor* [Internet]. 2024 Jan 25. Available from: https://www.forbes.com/advisor/pet-insurance/pet-ownership-statistics/#:~:text=As%20of%202022%2C%2044.5%25%20of,from%2025%25%20to%2029%25.

Miller GA. The cognitive revolution: a historical perspective. *Trends Cogn Sci*. 2003;7(3):141–144.

Mithen SJ. *The prehistory of the mind: a search for the origins of art, religion and science*. 1st ed. London: Thames and Hudson Ltd; 1998.

Mota-Rojas D, Mariti C, Zdeinert A, et al. Anthropomorphism and its adverse effects on the distress and welfare of companion animals. *Animals (Basel)*. 2021;11(11):3263.

Oosthuizen K, Haase B, Ravulo J, et al. The role of human-animal bonds for people experiencing crisis situations. *Animals (Basel)*. 2023;13(5):941.

Park SY, An JH, Kwon H, et al. Custom-made artificial eyes using 3D printing for dogs: a preliminary study. *PLoS One*. 2020;15(11):e0242274.

Sales G, Hubrecht R, Peyvandi A, et al. Noise in dog kennelling: is barking a welfare problem for dogs? *Appl Anim Behav Sci*. 1997;52(3):321–329.

Schroer SA. Jakob von Uexküll: the concept of umwelt and its potentials for an anthropology beyond the human. *Ethnos*. 2021;86(1):132–152.

Serpell J. Beneficial effects of pet ownership on some aspects of human health and behaviour. *J R Soc Med*. 1991;84(12):717–720.

Serpell JA. History of companion animals and the companion animal sector. In: Corr S, Sandøe P, Palmer C, editors. *Companion animal ethics (UFAW animal welfare series)*. West Sussex: Wiley Blackwell; 2015. p. 8–23.

Sommerville BA, Broom DM. Olfactory awareness. *Appl Anim Behav Sci*. 1998;57:269–286.

Spitznagel MB, Jacobson DM, Cox MD, et al. Caregiver burden in owners of a sick companion animal: a cross-sectional observational study. *Vet Rec*. 2017;181(12):321.

Sueur C, Forin-Wiart MA, Pelé M. Are they really trying to save their buddy? The anthropomorphism of animal epimeletic behaviours. *Animals (Basel)*. 2020;10(12):2323.

Timberlake W. Biological behaviorism. In: O'Donohue W, Kitchener R, editors. *Handbook of behaviorism*. San Diego: Academic Press; 1999. p. 243–284.

Velez L. Should dogs sleep on your bed? *OneVet Special Reports* [Internet]. 2024 May 18. Available from: https://www.onevet.ai/should-dogs-sleep-on-your-bed/.

Waytz A, Cacioppo J, Epley N. Who sees human? The stability and importance of individual differences in anthropomorphism. *Perspect Psychol Sci*. 2010;5(3):219–232.

Wynne CDL. What are animals? Why anthropomorphism is still not a scientific approach to behavior. *Comp Cogn Behav Rev*. 2007;2:125–135.

34 Going to Extremes
High Financial Cost, Overtreatment and Palliative Care

Polly Taylor

The United Kingdom's (UK's) Competitions and Markets Authority (CMA) has recently embarked on an investigation into the veterinary sector (CMA 2024) as a result of reports highlighting the current high cost of veterinary treatment for pets. The response of the British Veterinary Association was that advances in veterinary treatment are beneficial to animals and owners alike and that such new developments are inevitably expensive.

34.1 FUNDING ADVANCED VETERINARY TREATMENT

There is no question that advanced treatments are expensive. This is all too clear in the medical world where astonishing life-changing developments in treatment are not universally available due simply to the high cost (Alexander 2024). It is quite understandable that advanced diagnostic imaging such as magnetic resonance imaging (MRI) is costly whatever the species (although people do not usually need to be anaesthetised as animals do). Complex surgery requiring specialised equipment and prolonged anaesthesia is equally pricey, and new drugs reflect decades of development leading to eye-watering price tags.

Many pets are now regarded as surrogate human members of the family and deemed worthy of the same treatments as would be given to their human counterparts. This has led to some desperate funding of extreme veterinary treatment. Such cutting-edge treatment often lacks evidence of efficacy and benefit, but this does not appear to be a deterrent and can engender huge costs for advanced diagnostics and treatments. It is not uncommon for these sums – which can be upwards of tens of thousands of dollars – to be met by veterinary insurance, crowdfunding, and/or lines of credit.

Let's take, for example, a 10-year-old Labrador retriever diagnosed with terminal cancer. Advanced veterinary care could involve the following:

- Initial laboratory assays, potentially including early cancer diagnostics
- Advanced imaging under anaesthesia, for workup and staging, not to mention restaging during the clinical course

- Surgery, ranging from biopsies to large resections to (at the extreme) endoprostheses
- Radiation therapy, possibly involving stereotactic delivery
- Systemic antineoplastic therapy, ranging from steroids to conventional chemotherapy to targeted agents to immunotherapy

Each of these can cost thousands of dollars alone, may not result in prolonged survival, and could result in poorer quality of life. But hope is a very convincing motivator. Healthcare advances in humans have been translated to animals, without necessarily proving that the benefits outweigh the harms. Advanced veterinary care can be funded without the degree of necessary evidence generally required in human healthcare, leading to the potential for unlimited pursuit of futile and cruel treatment.

34.1.1 INSURANCE

In the UK, pet insurance is said to be carried on approximately half of pets. In the United States (US) it is a smaller but growing proportion. Pet insurance enables extremes that might otherwise be cost prohibitive; however, the system is beginning to falter and premiums are escalating well beyond increases in the cost of living (Morgenson et al. 2023). For example, one annual health insurance premium in the US for a young healthy Labrador increased from around $750 in 2017 to almost $2000 in 2022. Insurance companies would insure for any treatment prescribed by a licensed veterinarian, even without evidence of efficacy. This led to some enormous payments, particularly if the procedure failed and remedial treatment was also required. Insurance companies were thus funding unsubstantiated and potentially harmful treatments – and footing the bill when things went wrong, which was passed down to the policyholder in subsequent years. Conflicts of interest can also come into play. Some veterinary professionals promote pet insurance from which they benefit financially, if not directly as paid spokespersons, then via remuneration for veterinary care. Professor Noel Fitzpatrick (the UK's *Supervet*) is quoted on pet insurance provider PetPlan's website as saying, 'As a vet I always want to do the best I can for all my patients and Petplan really help me to do that' (Petplan Experts 2023). In the US, Trupanion came under scrutiny for incentivising veterinary clinics that promoted its insurance policies (Lau 2018). Increasingly, veterinary corporate chains are buying into pet insurance. Furthermore, Banfield and VCA (divisions of Mars) offer Optimum and CareClub 'wellness plans', which, to be fair, they carefully distinguish from insurance (Banfield 2023; VCA Animal Hospitals 2023). JAB, which is a holding company for several veterinary corporate chains around the globe, has garnered the attention of the US Federal Trade Commission (FTC 2022). JAB has also been acquiring pet insurance companies. In May 2023, it expanded its global pet insurance reach by acquiring a majority of Zoetis-launched Pumpkin pet insurance. During the associated press release, JAB boasted that it expected to have more than four million pets insured under its platform by the end of 2024 (Business Wire 2023).

34.1.2 Crowdfunding

Like pet insurance, crowdfunding also enables extreme treatment. It is particularly worrying as it often raises money via social media where there is no peer review or assessment of the veracity of the claim or likelihood of success. One example that comes to mind is a chicken named Huey, hatched with a backward leg (ABC13 2017). Huey was transferred to a Texas rescue home that consulted with a celebrity veterinary surgeon and fundraised approximately $4,000 to pay for surgery, which was meant to be broadcast on the surgeon's reality show. The first attempt at surgery was halted after a complication, but it was subsequently reported that Huey had a successful second surgery but died within hours due to a complication. Huey never featured on the television show. Another celebrity veterinary surgeon who is well known for surgical extremes has a media and fundraising policy in which clients must agree to refrain from referencing names related to his practice in fundraising campaigns (Fitzpatrick Referrals 2024).

Crowdfunding for what is essentially a lost cause also destroys quality of life. An English mother of a daughter dying of breast cancer ran a crowdfunding Internet site to enable her daughter to receive a new lauded but untested treatment abroad. The treatment was unpleasant, required much travelling away from home and was unsuccessful in either saving or prolonging the woman's life. The mother regretted forever after that she had spent the little time left with her daughter travelling to the foreign clinic and administering the crowdfunding.

34.1.3 Lines of Credit

If all else fails, lines of credit are also an option, if not through conventional credit cards then via lenders like CareCredit or ScratchPay (Whittenburg 2023), which have potential for very high interest rates. Late payments and/or failure to pay off in the prescribed period can result in additional costs. When faced with veterinary bills, particularly for sick or injured pets, distressed owners may make hasty decisions that can result in significant debt. This is not unique to veterinary healthcare; however, the much shorter lifespan of an animal, lack of evidence and patient welfare are vital to consider before treatment, particularly with extreme measures. Ideally, the conversations and paperwork surrounding large lines of credit should involve a careful discussion (not just electronic processing on handheld devices, now so common in executing contracts) and, if time permits as for elective procedures, breathing space to permit time to consider.

34.2 OVERTREATMENT

In spite of the escalating cost, advances and developments in veterinary treatment have undoubtedly led to better veterinary care of animals in many cases. However, particularly as a result of specialisation, the concept of 'gold standard treatment' has led to inappropriate overtreatment in a number of scenarios.

34.2.1 GOLD STANDARD TREATMENT

Research into specific medical and surgical diseases has led to considerable in-depth knowledge of these conditions. Applying appropriate treatment for each aspect of the disease is seen to be the correct course of action – 'gold standard'. This has itself led to a wide range of treatment options with varying degrees of evidence for their effect. In many cases the effect on one particular body system is examined in isolation. Combining all treatments shown to have some effect in a particular disease does not always result in an overall improvement in the animal's quality of life (QOL). Niessen (2018) cited the case of Mrs Tibbles' cat: this cat, we shall call Smokey, was old and had compensated chronic kidney disease (CKD) and osteoarthritis (OA). The OA pain was managed with oral meloxicam syrup, and he drank enough water to prevent uraemic malaise and ate ordinary grocery store tinned cat food. On presentation for routine vaccination – no mean feat as Smokey hated travelling anywhere by car, let alone to the veterinary clinic – he underwent a 'health check', and the following was diagnosed and treatment recommended. The meloxicam should be discontinued due to concern about his CKD. His blood pressure was high, so daily treatment with two sets of oral tablets was prescribed. A prescription diet formulated for cats with CKD was recommended and a monthly blood test to monitor his health proposed. Smokey would not take the tablets and bit his owner in the process of being dosed. He hated the food and stopped eating. Without the meloxicam he was in pain and stopped going out or moving round the house. Visits to the veterinary clinic became a nightmare: in short, Smokey was in pain and miserable, and the relationship with his owner broke down. The treatments offered for each aspect of his comorbidities were 'gold standard' for that condition. However, applied in real life, particularly when all were combined, destroyed the cat's quality of life (and his owner's) with no perceivable benefit. So maybe his life expectancy would have been extended a few months if he ate the kidney diet and took the tablets. But if taking the tablets and eating the diet made life miserable, what was the point of those few extra months?

Another feature of 'gold standard' treatment and humanised pets is the incentive to apply all the recommended treatment options regardless of the pet's age and the family context. Henry is a 12-year-old Labrador, already towards the end of his expected lifespan, who, when 11 years old, developed a mast cell tumour between the digits of one hind paw. He was otherwise well, and his lifestyle was entirely unaffected by the tumour. Relatively noninvasive local treatment with Stelfonta® plus chemotherapy produced 12 months remission. However, the tumour returned at the same site 12 months later – detected by a routine post-treatment bimonthly examination. Henry was not lame and appeared unaffected by the tumour. At this point the recommended – gold standard? – treatment was staging with a CT scan of thorax and abdomen, followed by ultrasound scan of abdomen and fine-needle aspiration of regional lymph node(s), liver, and spleen, all requiring general anaesthesia and costing between £2,000 and £3,000 (any subsequent treatment would be in addition to this). The owners were less concerned by the cost, which was not unreasonable for the procedures proposed, but by the question of need for this degree of intervention. This dog's current QOL was excellent, he was towards the end of his expected lifespan and, if metastatic disease were to be detected, what was to be done about it? Henry was not showing any signs of ill health. Any treatment proposed, such as chemotherapy, would negatively impact his QOL. In addition to any unpleasant side effects, he would find frequent visits to the clinic for treatment distressing: treatment had the potential to harm his remaining years. Henry himself could not understand that the unpleasant interventions might be of any benefit; and indeed, since his life expectancy was already almost reached, even prolonging life, for which he had no concept, would be of little importance. On top of all this, carer burden comes into play (Spitznagel et al. 2017). Caring for a dog under treatment for a potentially life-ending condition takes its toll on the family and may damage the relationship with the dog. The option not to undertake the diagnostic procedures and any resulting recommended chemotherapy was likely to give Henry the happiest remaining life. Fortunately for Henry, his GP was prepared simply to repeat the Stelfonta® injections; the paw lesion has resolved, and with no additional clinic appointments, investigations or chemotherapy Henry has continued to enjoy his untroubled life.

Taking the ultimate treatment for a diagnosed condition out of the context of the animal's situation in life, and those of its owners, can lead to further unquestionably detrimental overtreatment. Consider the case of Elsa, a 14-year-old cross-bred bitch. She has chronic renal failure, OA and insulin-controlled diabetes, all of which are under control through diligent owner management. Elsa developed a cough and decreased exercise tolerance, which on investigation was diagnosed as a result of a large thoracic tumour. Surgery to undertake an exploratory thoracotomy and tumour excision was proposed. Both anaesthesia and surgery were challenging, lung lobes were removed and the tumour debulked, but complete resection was impossible. Elsa was allowed to recover from anaesthesia and remained under intensive care for several days but was never well enough to return home. She died after spending a week in intensive care. Thoracic surgery to remove a life-threatening tumour is a well-accepted treatment for a thoracic mass. However, in the context of an old dog with serious comorbidities, such an approach cannot be regarded as the best option for the patient. Pragmatic, contextualised – call it what you will– treatment would have served Elsa rather better. The cough and exercise tolerance could have been managed with medical (palliative) care until such time it was deemed her QOL had deteriorated too far when euthanasia would provide a dignified and peaceful end – in familiar surroundings, not in the unfamiliar context of the intensive care ward with numerous tubes still attached.

34.3 END OF LIFE AND PALLIATIVE CARE

How should veterinary care of old animals be mastered? Should the life of an old animal be drawn out when body systems are failing? The ability to apply advanced veterinary care and to prolong life has led to a dilemma in treating these pets. There may be advanced interventions that could be applied, but will they lead to good QOL – a life worth living? Palliative care is specialised medical care that focuses on providing relief from the pain and other symptoms of a serious illness, it does not aim to cure the disease. Palliative care may be the most appropriate treatment for an old animal such as Elsa, where treating the symptoms of the respiratory disease would make life more comfortable but not attempt to stem the disease progression. As long as some sort of decision point is identified before QOL starts to deteriorate, this approach can lead to the animal having a good life until the disease progresses too far and euthanasia takes place. Palliative care is now a full-blown specialty in the human medical world. Hospice, simply defined, is palliative care at the end of life (Goldberg 2016). End-of-life care treats symptoms and enables the patient to live as well as possible until death and to die with dignity. Hospice is the philosophy of care that regards death as a natural process, prioritising comfort and quality over quantity of life as death draws near.

Even in the veterinary world, palliative care is becoming a specialty; we must beware of treating animals as people. Their lives are much shorter than ours, they do not have any concept of the future, and they do not understand why they hurt and feel ill – but animals do have the option of euthanasia. We should not be keeping incurably sick and unhappy animals alive, simply because we have the means of so doing; this is particularly important when it is, in fact, for the owner's benefit, not the animal's.

The concept of keeping animals alive beyond good QOL is not limited to dogs, cats and other small animals. How happy (or not) are those horses and ponies, kept alive for 'just one more summer' with daily pergolide to manage their Cushing's syndrome (PPID) but feed restricted to prevent laminitis? What about pet farm animals 'rescued' from the meat trade? They are herd animals, often kept alone, becoming obese, some even undergoing difficult neutering surgery because they have become aggressive. What life have they been rescued for?

According to the National Council for Palliative Care (2024), palliative care has been defined by the National Institute for Clinical Excellence (NICE) as follows: 'Palliative care is the active holistic care of patients with advanced progressive illness. Management of pain and other symptoms and provision of psychological, social and spiritual support is paramount. The goal of palliative care is achievement of the best quality of life for patients and their families. Many aspects of palliative care are also applicable earlier in the course of the illness in conjunction with other treatments'. Hence, true palliative care for an animal must provide the best quality of life for that animal and its carers. Most important: this is a dog, cat, horse – not a human. The best QOL that is provided must be for the species concerned, not from a human perspective. Euthanasia is an option to end suffering that can be applied to an animal when the palliative care is no longer able to provide that good life. Euthanasia is not failure – it is a real option to provide excellent animal welfare. Miserable animals do not have to be kept alive as do humans where euthanasia is illegal. The old saying 'a day too early is better than a day too late' was never more applicable than in this context, or even more appropriate, 'it's better to be a week too early than a minute too late' (Vogelsang 2015).

REFERENCES

ABC13. Nearly $4K needed to help chicken with backwards foot. *ABC13 Houston* [Internet]. 2017 Feb 10. Available from: https://abc13.com/1748925.

Alexander C. What's the cost of sickle cell anemia treatment? *GoodRx Health* [Internet]. 2024 Jan 30. Available from: https://www.goodrx.com/conditions/sickle-cell-disease/sickle-cell-anemia-treatment-costs.

Banfield. Optimum Wellness Plans®. *Banfield Pet Hospital* [Internet]. 2023 [cited 2023 Oct 19]. Available from: https://www.banfield.com/en/products/optimum-wellness-plan.

Business Wire. Jab's pet insurance platform acquires pumpkin, expanding its global leadership in the fast-growing pet insurance industry. *Business Wire* [Internet]. 2023 May 16. Available from: https://www.businesswire.com/news/home/20230515005814/en/JAB%E2%80%99s-Pet-Insurance-Platform-Acquires-Pumpkin-Expanding-its-Global-Leadership-in-the-Fast-Growing-Pet-Insurance-Industry.

Competitions and Markets Authority. CMA presses ahead with full investigation into vets market. *GOV.UK* [Internet]. 2024 May 23. Available from: https://www.gov.uk/government/news/cma-presses-ahead-with-full-investigation-into-vets-market.

Fitzpatrick Referrals. Fitzpatrick Referrals Ltd terms and conditions of business. *Fitzpatrick Referrals Pet Owners Payment Options* [Internet]. 2024 [cited 2024 Aug 29]. Available from: https://www.fitzpatrickreferrals.co.uk/app/uploads/2024/08/Fitzpatrick-Referrals-terms-and-conditions-web-8.2024.pdf.

FTC. FTC takes second action against JAB consumer partners to protect pet owners from private equity firm's rollup of veterinary services clinics. *Federal Trade Commission* [Internet]. 2022 Jun 29. Available from: https://www.ftc.gov/news-events/news/press-releases/2022/06/ftc-takes-second-action-against-jab-consumer-partners-protect-pet-owners-private-equity-firms-rollup-of-veterinary-services-clinics.

Goldberg KJ. Veterinary hospice and palliative care: a comprehensive review of the literature. *Vet Rec*. 2016;178:369–374.

Lau E. Trupanion relationships with veterinarians under scrutiny. *VIN News* [Internet]. 2018 Nov 1. Available from: https://news.vin.com/default.aspx?pid=210&Id=8781533&f5=1#:~:text=Washington%20state%20regulators%20are%20looking,the%20company%20to%20prospective%20customers.

Morgenson G, Paredes D, Nguyen V. As pet insurance becomes more popular, pet owners fret about rising prices, denied claims and long waits for reimbursement. *NBC News* [Internet]. 2023 Aug 16. Available from: https://www.nbcnews.com/business/personal-finance/pet-insurance-dogs-cats-rising-prices-denied-claims-rcna93933.

National Council for Palliative Care. Palliative care explained. *NCPC* [Internet]. 2024 [cited 2024 Aug 29]. Available from: https://www.ncpc.org.uk/palliative-care-explained/.

Niessen S. How should quality of life assessments for pets and owners guide clinical treatment decisions for patients with chronic disease? *Proc London Vet Show*. 2018;1:91–93.

Petplan Experts. Professor Noel Fitzpatrick. *Petplan* [Internet]. 2023 [cited 2023 Oct 19]. Available from: https://www.petplan.co.uk/pet-information/experts/supervet-noel-fitzpatrick/#:~:text=Professor%20Noel%20Fitzpatrick%20%2D%20Veterinary%20Surgeon%20%2D%20Petplan%20%7C%20Petplan.

Spitznagel MB, Jacobson DM, Cox MD, et al. Caregiver burden in owners of a sick companion animal: a cross-sectional observational study. *Vet Rec*. 2017;181:381–387.

VCA Animal Hospitals. VCA CareClub. *VCA CareClub Pet Wellness Plan* [Internet]. 2023 [cited 2023 Oct 19]. Available from: https://vcahospitals.com/careclub.

Vogelsang J. The biggest mistake pet owners make at the end. *Huffpost* [Internet]. 2015 Sept 21. Available from: https://www.huffpost.com/entry/the-biggest-mistake-pet-o_b_8166102.

Whittenburg J. What is CareCredit for pets? *USA Today* [Internet] 2023 Mar 3. Available from: https://www.usatoday.com/money/blueprint/pet-insurance/what-is-carecredit.

35 Give the Dog a Bone

Tanya Stephens

This old man, he played one,
He played knick-knack on my thumb,
With a knick-knack paddywack,
Give the dog a bone,
This old man came rolling home.

This nursery rhyme, first published in 1906, most likely originated from the time of the Irish Potato Famine in 1845. It is said that people who would see the Irish (Paddy) starve would happily give a bone to a dog (learnarhyme.com).

Nowadays, the saying 'give the dog a bone' appears to have a number of meanings in the UK, including giving a person what they want and it seemed an appropriate sentence to describe the situation where giving a dog a bone, which we assume they would prefer to having a carrot, could lead into a discussion around pets, climate change, sustainability, and an increased interest in veganism.

The world's population currently sits at 8 billion but is predicted to reach 9.7 billion by 2050 (UN's 2022 report). The FAO estimated that between 691 and 783 million people in the world faced hunger in 2022, an increase of 122 million from 2019. The IPBES Global Assessment Report on Biodiversity and Ecosystem Services paints a grim picture of a rapid decline in ecosystem health associated with increased food production and in Australia the Australian Government State of the Environment Report 2021 demonstrates that our environment is under extreme pressure.

With increasing hunger in the human population and food production impacting on ecosystem health, should society be questioning increasing pet ownership as a luxury we can't afford?

35.1 PETS ARE PLENTIFUL

Whilst people in high-income countries have always kept pets, pet ownership has surged in low- and middle-income countries due to demographic changes, an expanding middle class, rising income levels and the COVID-19 pandemic. Millennials are leading the trend as they are likely to have children later in life if at all, having replaced children with pets, have higher incomes and are better educated. In China, a relaxation of pet ownership regulations and a falling birth rate have likely contributed to the increase in pet ownership which surged by 113%

between 2014 and 2019. It has been estimated that China will in future have the most pets in the world.

The Global State of Pet Care (healthforanimals.org) 2022 states that there are likely over a billion pets worldwide. Families in the US, Brazil, the EU, and China alone account for over half a billion pet dogs and cats while more than half the world is estimated to have a pet at home. The EU has an estimated 92 million dogs and 113 million cats, China has an estimated 74 million dogs and 67 million cats, and the US has 85 million dogs and 65 million cats.

Currently, America is the number one pet-owning country, with 70% of households having a pet, with pet ownership tripling since the 1970s, and China is the second largest pet-owning country. It might look like the UK has a dog on every corner but it has only around 13 million. The USA also has the most domestic cats, again followed by China and India has the fastest growing dog population in the world. The dog is the most popular pet worldwide but over a quarter of pet owners have a cat.

The COVID-19 pandemic has had a significant impact on pet ownership in Australia and the number of Australian households owning pets increased from 61% in 2019 to 69% in 2021. The total number of pets in Australia has increased from 28.5 million in 2019 to 30.4 million in 2021 (Animal Medicines Australia 2021). Nearly 2 in 5 dogs in Australia have been acquired since the onset of the pandemic, and a quarter of all pet dogs today are two years or younger, and over 2 in 5 are small dogs with so-called designer breeds remaining popular.

In the UK more than two million people adopted a pet during the pandemic.

The Animal Medicines Australia report, Pets in Australia (2022), has dogs as the most popular pet, with almost half of Australian households having at least one dog, 48% – up from 40% in 2019. Cats are the second most popular with a third of all households housing at least one cat, 33% – up from 27% in 2019. There are over 6 million pet dogs and over 5 million pet cats in Australia. Also, 2 in 5 have only one pet, and the rest have more, up from 22% in 2019 to 28% in 2022. Finally, 25% of dog owners have more than one dog and 33% of cat owners have more than one cat.

Of the 31% of Australian households currently without a pet 60% are interested in getting a pet, with an estimated 3.5 million households actively considering new pets in the next 12 months and a further 4.4 million are broadly interested.

The Animal Medicines Australia survey of pet ownership 2022 makes for fascinating reading. In 2022 17% of pet owners bought or made outfits and costumes for their pets vs 13% in 2019. Among those pet owners, 8% set up social media accounts for their pets vs 5% in 2019, and 6% admitted wearing matching outfits and accessories with their pets vs 3% in 2019. In 2022, 7% threw a birthday party. Additionally, 20% had given them premium/expensive human food, 9% video-called them when away from home, 27% left on the heating/cooling, lights, or TV/radio for them, 31% had given them gifts for special occasions, 31% referred to themselves as the 'parent', and 43% allowed them to sleep in/on the same bed (guilty of this one).

Australians are estimated to be spending over $33 billion annually to keep their pets fed, healthy and well-accessorised with food representing 51% of all expenditure followed by veterinarians at 14%, products and accessories at 9%, and pet healthcare products at 9%. Australians spend $17.1 billion a year on pet food and $3.0 billion on products or accessories. Around 89% of this total is on dogs and cats.

35.2 THE CARBON PAWPRINT

The carbon pawprint is a term that has arisen to quantify the environmental impact of pet ownership. Not surprisingly, as pets have increasingly become members of the family, owners, or, should I say, 'pet parents', are wanting the best for them which includes high quality, human grade food and not table scraps. The ecological paw print of companion dogs and cats (Martens et al. 2019) is a useful tool to measure the environmental impacts of companion animals and argues that an assessment should be made as to whether and how the pet food system can sustainably support the health and nutrition of the growing numbers of companion animals.

In 2016 in the USA there were 163 million dogs and cats and it was estimated that what they eat is responsible for the release of up to 64 ± 16 million tons CO^2 equivalent methane and nitrous oxide and their diet is estimated to constitute around 25–30% of the environmental impacts from animal production – land, water, fossil fuel, etc. – and they produce $30\% \pm 13\%$ by mass as much faeces as Americans. Increasing pet ownership in countries such as China and trends towards higher quality meat is suggested as adding to the environmental impacts of human dietary choices. In the USA dogs and cats consume as much dietary energy as 62 million Americans or one-fifth of the population Okin (2017).

The global production of dry cat and dog food is estimated to emit greenhouse gases each year equivalent to total emissions from countries such as Mozambique or the Philippines. The pet food industry is undoubtedly a big contributor to carbon emissions according to Alexander et al. (2020).

A concern around the environmental impact of pet ownership is not new. In 2009 a book, *Time to Eat the Dog: The Real Guide to Sustainable Living*, by Robert and Brenda Vale, compared owning a big dog as equivalent to having a large petrol guzzling car in the garage.

There is no doubt that pets are important (otherwise, we wouldn't keep so many), and there is a suggestion that the beneficial effects on mental health actually lowers the human carbon footprint, although it may be difficult to quantify this. Companionship is the main reason given for pet ownership, and the benefits of the human-animal bond are highlighted even though there are at times mixed results from pet ownership. The bond may not always be in the animal's best interests if a dog is left alone all day, and whilst pet owners report they are happier and healthier, they also report anxiety, insomnia, depression, obesity, ulcers, and panic attacks. Cats don't care so much, but for the dog it's a mixed bag. So-called village dogs may in fact have a better life than mollycoddled 'designer dogs', suggests Meyer et al. (2022).

According to the Animals Medicines Australia survey, despite 85% of owners saying their pets have positively impacted their lives, 79% of current owners acknowledge experiencing at least some difficulty, up from 66% in 2019. This is mostly to do with cleaning up from pets.

It's not just what cats eat out of a tin either. In Australia, feral cats and domestic ones as well have led to the mass extinction of native wildlife. It has been estimated that cats have played a leading role in most of Australia's mammal extinctions since 1788 and continue to have an impact on 123 other threatened species with cats likely to be killing more than three billion animals per year (Legge et al. 2020). Even dogs can have an impact on wildlife, such as shorebirds, as birds are particularly sensitised to dogs and vast numbers of dogs let loose at beaches can have a significant impact.

In addition, dog waste with its high nitrogen and phosphorus content has an environmental impact as do large numbers of 'doggy poo bags', and let's not forget the impact of various diseases spread from dogs and cats to wildlife, such as distemper, and the possible impact of various companion animal parasiticides on aquatic organisms and the environment.

Whilst there is an argument that commercial pet food is made from the leftover cuts of meat, mostly offal, that humans don't and won't eat and therefore save it from landfill, there is a suggestion that humans should eat at least some of this instead and it could be used elsewhere, e.g. as biofuel. However, there is definitely a move to feed pets better food, including high-quality fresh meat. In addition, the raw feeding movement has gained some momentum in the 'dog eat dog' world of pet feeding.

Alternative proteins, such as insects, could play a role to feed dogs and cats (and humans), and in Australia, there is an abundance of low methane emitting kangaroo (estimated 46–50 million and counting) that is sustainably harvested for people as well as pets (Stephens 2021).

There are other environmental impacts of pet ownership. The fancy beds, the special toys, the Halloween costumes and all the special treats much of which are destined to landfill and even kitty litter has an environmental impact, especially clay-based products.

35.3 SHOULD DOGS AND CATS BE VEGAN?

There has been an increased interest in vegan diets for pets which no doubt mirrors society's interest in veganism around concerns to do with animal welfare and sustainability. It makes sense that those who choose a vegan diet will also want to do this for their dogs and cats, somewhat overlooking the ongoing problem of the environmental impacts of vast amounts of dog and cat waste or cats eating native birds and possums or dogs chasing shorebirds.

According to the Vegan Society, Veganism is a growing trend in society with between 2 and 3% of people adopting veganism in the UK, and 46% of UK residents between 16 and 75 years are considering reducing their intake of animal products. In 2023 3.4% of people in the EU followed a vegan diet. In Australia 2%

of the population say they are vegans (vegansociety.com). Demand for plant-based products has increased worldwide, and there has been a decrease in meat consumption in high-income countries, although this decrease is offset by the increase in meat consumption in low- and middle-income economies.

It follows that there is an interest by vegans in vegan cat and dog foods with a number now on the market. Dominguez-Oliva et al. (2023) undertook a systematic review of vegan diets for pets and determined that although there was no convincing evidence of major impacts of vegan diets on dog and cat health, high-quality studies are needed and a cautious approach should be taken and that commercially produced diets formulated especially for the target species be sourced if feeding a vegan diet.

Knight (2023) outlines the environmental impact of pet ownership and maintains that implementing nutritionally sound vegan diets for pets would spare from slaughter vast numbers of livestock and free up vast amounts of land thereby feeding additional people. However, I'm not quite sure what the plans would be for existing livestock or livestock farmers for that matter or even what should be done about pest animals which impact crops, such as mice if the main aim is to avoid killing animals.

Knight et al. (2023) undertook a survey of 1,242 cats fed a meat-based diet and 127 a vegan diet for about a year and determined that cats fed the vegan diet were healthier than the meat fed ones. Cat owners (or guardians as they are called in this paper) reported the outcomes. There were limitations to the study which Knight noted, including the fact that some cats were fed treats, some offered dietary supplements, and some vegan fed cats were not always confined and so could have supplemented their vegan diet with rats. In addition, the study authors admit 'we acknowledge the reliance on guardians limits the reliability of our results, for example due to lapses of memory'. The author also emphasises the need to ensure the diet is nutritionally adequate and to check labels.

Despite the author noting these limitations, the paper generated loads of publicity with headlines such as 'Vegan diet healthier for cats than meat according to a new survey' and 'Vegan cat food beneficial, study finds' in the *Vet Practice Magazine*. There was even an article in *The Guardian* (2023) 'Knight noted that large scale studies had already shown that dogs and cats can be just as healthy, or even more, on a vegan diet, so long as they eat pet food that is specially formulated with additional vitamins, amino acids and minerals to ensure it is nutritionally sound'. The British Veterinary Association and Blue Cross were also quoted to advise against feeding animals a vegan diet as it can be difficult to get the balance of nutrients right.

It seems to me that if there is a need to add to vegan pet foods (which are already highly processed) vast quantities of essential supplements, is it as sustainable as claimed? We know that the production of omega-3 supplements has led to devastating overfishing and that younger vegans are eating significantly more ultra-processed plant-based convenience foods than their predecessors, and this may be less environmentally sustainable (MacDiarmid 2022).

The Knight study has some glaring limitations, such as the lack of detail of actual ingredients of the diet, any objective veterinary assessment, laboratory data, comparison of diets with and without supplements, and information on how many tasty rats the 'vegan cats' ate. The author had stated, 'We did not further inquire about details of diets, including nutritional soundness indicators such as packaging claims of compliance with the nutritional guidelines of the European Pet Food Industry Federation or the Association of American Feed Control Officials'.

You could postulate that the cats in the study appeared to do 'well' because of the supplements and not the food. Supplement manufacturers are certainly doing well with the market booming. The global pet supplement market was worth AUD 2.8 billion in 2022 and predicted to grow to AUD 4.6 billion by 2030, especially as animals age and owners buy supplements for animals with old age ailments, which incidentally mostly lack evidence of efficacy and impact on sustainability.

I wasn't the only one to be concerned with this study. Veterinarians Alexandra Whittaker from the University of Adelaide and Andrea Harvey, a feline specialist at the University of Technology Sydney, also expressed their concern (the Conversation 2023) and stated that in fact the evidence that cats fed a vegan diet tend to be healthier based on this study is far from conclusive. That it was not possible to confirm exactly what the vegan cats ate, what treats and supplements were added, and, being outdoors, what animals they may have eaten. It is also not clear how long they were on the diet.

Finally, owners made subjective observations, and owners who had reduced meat in their diet were overrepresented in the vegan category cohort, which would no doubt have coloured their observations. Harvey also noted that the study was funded by ProVeg International, a food awareness organisation that promotes plant-based products raising significant conflicts of interest.

Harvey goes on to say that plant-based diets lack a range of nutrients cats need and that cats on vegan diets can develop severe deficiency disorders. Supplements can be added, of course, but the average cat owner is not going to be an expert in cat nutrition, and cats have never lost their hunting instinct and so probably prefer the taste of meat. Whittaker points out that a concern with vegan diets is a lack of taurine, which is essential for cats, and taurine deficiency can cause retinal degeneration and cardiac problems.

Knight et al. (2022) also undertook a survey of dog owners and vegan dog foods and found that those fed a raw diet were slightly healthier but described limitations to this study as well, such as the feeding of treats and subjective assessment by pet guardians. Despite this, Knight asserts that 'when jointly considering health outcomes and dietary hazards, our results and those of other studies indicate that the healthiest and least hazardous dietary choices for dogs are nutritionally sound vegan diets'. Knight later issued a correction to this story pointing out that in fact ProVeg International funded the study.

The health claims of this diet have been challenged by Richard Barrett-Jolly and Alex German (2024) of the University of Liverpool who analysed Knight's results and concluded that the claim the authors made in favour of vegan diets was not backed up by the data and that it was not accurate to conclude that 'nutritionally-sound vegan diets are the healthiest and least hazardous choices for owners to feed their pet dogs'.

Josh Loeb (2020) raised concerns about vegan dogs and cats and posed the question 'Would you feed your rabbit meat?' 'A carnivorous rabbit is something out of a Monty Python film but is it any weirder than a vegan dog? How about a vegan cat?' Loeb points out that animals should not be forced to share our values, and in fact, feeding a pet a vegan diet may mean owners are neglecting their pet under the Animal Welfare Act. Furthermore, he notes, dogs need vitamin D, which can only be sourced from animal products when included as an ingredient in pet food, which means that 'complete vegan' dog food is a legal oxymoron.

There is a risk that the 'research' and headlines around pet foods may not be taken seriously if the research is flawed, and this would be a shame as dog and cat nutrition has a significant environmental impact mainly because of the dependence on meat.

It is therefore pleasing to see the current discussion around feeding pets with the BVA (BVA 2024) launching a new policy position which encourages veterinarians to have conversations about nutrition with pet owners. As the BVA President Anna Judson points out, there is a surge in alternative approaches to pet food and choices play a pivotal role in the health of the animal and have a wider impact on human health and environmental sustainability. There is also a lack of long-term evidence-based research, and there should be better labelling of pet food and better labelling and traceability of the animal by products that make up one of the major sources of protein in many cat and dog foods. Lack of regulation around pet foods is an ongoing problem worldwide.

Continuing discussion around pet feeding is essential and veterinarians need to be well informed about public perceptions and new developments in this field. To this end, Ward et al. (2020) have produced a thoroughly researched, scientific, and exhaustive overview of new technologies and emerging alternative approaches to pet feeding aimed at reducing the environmental and animal welfare impacts.

35.4 ROBOTIC PETS

Forget about pets! Could technologies allow us to replace companion animals? Should we in fact be keeping robots instead? Rault (2015) asks if pet ownership in its current form is unsustainable in a growing urbanised population, and whether new technologies represent the future of pet ownership, helping tackle its sustainability while solving animal welfare issues. Can new technologies represent the future of pet ownership? What will be the place of pets in a digitally driven human society?

There are now a huge number and variety of digital 'pets' on the market, and some so realistic they have been shown to reduce medication use in dementia wards. According to Melson et al. (2009), the fact that robotic pets appear to give rise to similar responses as live pets suggests that the human-animal bond is only dependent on us, and does it matter if the benefits of robotic pets outweigh the risks, sparing animal welfare issues, or could artificial pets make us humans insensitive to the treatment of live animals (Kahn et al. 2006)?

Could the emergence of AI and technological advancement change the way we view animals and pet ownership? A robot may be enough companionship in this era of social connection. Whilst it may seem feasible to program a doggy robot to fetch slippers, it is difficult to imagine a robot keeping you warm in bed at night.

35.5 IS IT TIME TO 'EAT THE DOG'?

It is difficult to predict if pet ownership will continue to surge. The 'pet honeymoon' or 'COVID-19 pet spending spree' may be over, at least in Australia, with natural disasters, increasing living costs, and lack of affordable pet-friendly housing now placing pressure on pet owners.

We need to ask if an estimated 9.6 billion people in 2050 can keep pets at the same rate we do now and feed themselves, or will pets become a luxury we can't afford? As the impacts of climate change and feeding a burgeoning human population impinge on public consciousness, the public may in fact decide that it really is time to 'eat the dog'.

It is a discussion we need to have, and veterinarians are at the forefront of ensuring that if pet ownership is to continue at its present rate and if companion animal veterinarians want to keep their jobs, we need to do all we can to ensure that pet ownership is sustainable. Veterinary input is essential in any discussion around environmental sustainability and sustainable veterinary practice.

REFERENCES

Alexander P, Berri A, Moran D, et al. The global environmental paw print of pet food. *Glob Environ Change.* 2020;65:102–153.

Animal Medicines Australia. Pets and the pandemic: a social research snapshot of pets and people in the COVID-19 era. 16 August 2021.

Barrett-Jolley R, German AJ. Variables associated with owner perceptions of the health of their dog: further analysis of data from a large international study. *PLoS One* 2024 May 15. Available from: https://doi.org/10.1371/journal.pone.0280173.

British Veterinary Association (BVA) policy position on diet choices for cats and dogs. 2024. [Internet]. 24 July 2024 [cited 2024 Oct 31]. Available from: https://www.bva.co.uk/media/5997/bva-policy-position-on-diet-choices-for-cats-and-dogs.pdf.

Dominguez-Oliva A, Mota-Rojas D, Semendric I, Whittaker A. The impacts of vegan diets on indicators of health in dogs and cats: a systematic review. *Vet Sci.* 2023;10(1):52.

Kahn PH, Friedman B, Perez-Granados DR. Robotic pets in the lives of preschool children. *Interact Stud.* Jan 2006;7(3):405–436.

Knight A. The relative benefits for environmental sustainability of vegan diets for dogs, cats and people. *PLoS One* 2023. Available from: https://journals.plos.org/plosone/article?id=10.1371/journal.pone.0291791.

Knight A, Bauer A, Brown H. Vegan versus meat-based cat food: guardian reported health outcomes in 1,369 cats after controlling for feline demographic factors. *PLoS One* 2023;18(9). Available from: https://doi.org/10.1371/journal.pone.0284132.

Knight A, Huang E, Rai N, Brown H. Vegan versus meat-based dog food: guardian reported indicators of health. *PLoS One* 2022 Apr 13;17(4). Available from: https://journals.plos.org/plosone/article?id=10.1371/journal.pone.0291214.

Legge S, Woinarski J, Dickman C, et al. We need to worry about Bella and Charlie: the impacts of pet cats on Australian wildlife. *Wildl Res*. 2020;47:523–539.

Loeb J. The trouble with vegan cats and dogs. *Vet Rec*. 2020;186(7):197. Available from: https://doi.org/10.1136/vr.m663.

MacDiarmid JI. The food system and climate change: are plant-based diets becoming unhealthy and less environmentally sustainable? *Proc Nutr Soc*. 2022 May;81(2):162–167.

Martens P, Su B, Deblomme S. The ecological paw print of companion dogs and cats. *Biosci*. 2019 Jun;69(6):467–474.

Melson GF, Beck A, Friedman B. Robotic pets in human lives: implications for the human-animal bond and for human relationships with personified technologies. *J Soc Sci*. 2009;65(3):545–567.

Meyer I, Forkman B, Fredholm M, et al. Pampered pets or poor bastards? The welfare of dogs kept as companion animals. *Appl Anim Behav Sci*. 2022;251. Available from: https://www.sciencedirect.com/science/article/pii/S0168159122000983.

Okin GS. Environmental impacts of food consumption by dogs and cats. *PLoS One*. 2017. Available from: https://doi.org/10.1371/journal.pone.0181301.

Rault J-L. Pets in the digital age: live, robot, or virtual? *Front Vet Sci*. 2015;2. Available from: https://doi.org/10.3389/fvets.2015.00011.

Stephens T. Kangaroo management and animal welfare. *Ecol Manag Anim Welf*. 2021 Nov;22(S1):71–74. Special issue: *Optimum Management of Overabundant Macropods*.

The Guardian. Worlds dogs going vegan would save more emissions than UK produces. 4 October 2023. Available from: https://www.theguardian.com/lifeandstyle/2023/oct/04/worlds-dogs-going-vegan-would-save-more-emissions-than-uk-produces.

Ward E, Oven A, Bethencourt R. *The clean pet food revolution: how better pet food will change the world*. Lantern Books; 2020.

Whittaker A, Harvey A. Is it really safe to feed your cat a vegan diet? *The Conversation*. 2023 Sept 14.

Part IIIE Vets in Society

36 Is the Veterinary Profession Encouraging Exploitation of Horses in Sport?

Sue Dyson

This essay is based as far as possible on current evidence, but it obviously has a personal flavour.

36.1 A PERSONAL EXPERIENCE

I was involved in the investigation of a chronic, major decline in performance in a professionally produced, well-ridden 5* level event horse with a relatively high insured value. The horse had very poor development of the 'topline' and pelvic musculature, reflecting how the horse's movement patterns had adapted to chronic discomfort. The final diagnosis was bilateral front foot pain associated with osteoarthritis of the distal interphalangeal (DIP) joints and deep digital flexor tendinopathy, bilateral hindlimb proximal suspensory desmopathy, with adhesions of the suspensory ligaments to the adjacent soft tissues, and a substantial component of lumbosacroiliac joint region pain. The Ridden Horse Pain Ethogram (RHpE) score was 12/24, which was reduced to 2/24 after diagnostic anaesthesia had alleviated the majority of pain (Dyson 2022). Based on previous experience of management of this type of case, and the treatments that had already been performed, I considered that even with extensive veterinary interventions and a team approach to management the prognosis for the horse to return to its former athletic activity at 5* level was extremely poor. The horse was insured for permanent incapacity as a 5* level event horse, and I was prepared to support an insurance claim. The experienced, well-respected veterinarian advising the insurance company had a different opinion and insisted that the horse underwent medication of the forelimb DIP joints and the sacroiliac joints and repeated extracorporeal shockwave treatments of the hindlimb suspensory ligaments. The horse deteriorated and the insurance company was provided with photographic and videographic evidence. The veterinarian advising the insurance company insisted that the horse underwent a further round of treatment, with further deterioration of the horse's condition, manifest as additional postural and movement changes, with the horse being reluctant to lie down. The RHpE score was now 15/24. Despite being provided with extensive evidence of the horse's progressive decline in level of comfort a third round of treatment was proposed, however, I refused to undertake this and insisted that the horse's welfare must be considered first and foremost, not the insured value of the horse. In my opinion decisions were being made with complete disregard of the horse's wellbeing. The claim was finally accepted.

36.2 CONFLICTING PRESSURES

Veterinarians working in the sports horse industry are placed under enormous and sometimes conflicting pressures to 'keep horses on the road' or to facilitate return to athletic function as soon as possible after injury, without thinking about the longer-term consequences for the horse; or to use a medication that is not licensed for use in the horse or is not of proven safety or efficacy in the horse, but the rider or trainer considers that it may not be a detectable substance and may 'fix' the horse. It appears to have become fashionable in the sports world to use 'maintenance injections' or so-called 'prophylactic medication' when no preexisting problems have been identified and there is no proven efficacy of such treatments. There is also unrelenting pressure to treat without an appropriate investigation and a specific diagnosis. Moreover, a veterinarian may be put under the pressure that if they do not carry out the treatments advocated by the rider or trainer then they will engage someone else to perform the treatment. Clients may be using two or more veterinarians, playing one off against another, and discouraging transparency, so that a veterinarian may be requested to treat without knowledge of what has been done before. The mantra 'buyer beware' reflects the lack of transparency and honesty in some of the professional horse world.

36.3 ESTABLISHING MORAL AND ETHICAL BOUNDARIES

As a veterinarian treating sports horses, one needs to establish your own moral boundaries, to inform and lead clients and to educate both the public and the rule makers. The profession should also set some ethical guidelines. People need to be aware that there is a difference between performance enhancement versus enabling a horse to return to function after injury, and to fulfil its potential. It has apparently been accepted by the public and rule makers that removal of a chip fracture is a perfectly acceptable method of treatment – it is the logical treatment to prevent further joint injury – and to restore the joint to more normal function. Yet there has been controversy about the management of hindlimb proximal suspensory desmopathy by neurectomy of the deep branch of the lateral plantar nerve and plantar fasciotomy. There is evidence-based information that horses with hindlimb proximal suspensory desmopathy have a guarded prognosis for return to full function as a non-lame sports horse with conservative management, or by local treatments of any form, yet surgical management of appropriately selected horses results in a 78% chance of long-term return to full function. The surgery does not alter limb function, other than allow a horse to work pain-free, and post-operatively, in the majority of horses, the treated ligaments appear to improve in infrastructure based on ultrasonographic evaluation. Just as with chip fracture removal the procedure allows a horse to work pain-free and potentially progress in its performance to fulfil its natural potential. Moreover, the sooner such problems are identified and managed appropriately, the less likely it is that the horse will develop other secondary problems. Veterinarians need to be able to argue confidently, coherently, and with an evidence base to protect their social licence to treat horses morally.

Veterinarians need to be seen to be acting morally and not experimenting with novel treatments unless there is some basic scientific rationale for the use of any particular treatment. Likewise, a veterinarian needs to know when to stop continued treatment being performed, at a client's request, despite no evidence of clinical improvement. The veterinarian should be leading treatment based on the knowledge of an accurate diagnosis, and knowledge of the treatment options, their likelihood of success and any potential deleterious consequences.

Consider a showjumper jumping at 1 m 40 cm, which has a foot-related lameness and underwent magnetic resonance imaging to determine the presence or absence of a severe deep digital flexor tendon (DDFT) injury. A substantial lesion was identified, and a veterinary surgeon recommended palmar neurectomy, despite this not being permitted under the competitive rules, and a major DDFT lesion being a contraindication for neurectomy. The owner elected to proceed with surgical treatment. This resulted in improvement in lameness, and with repeated intra-thecal medication of the navicular bursa, the horse returned to competitive showjumping for >12 months before sustaining rupture of the DDFT and subluxation of the DIP joint, a career-ending injury, severely jeopardising the horse's quality of life. This was clearly both contravening rules and predictably not in the best interests of the horse's long-term welfare.

In most sports disciplines horses are required to undergo vaccination, at least against equine influenza, at mandated intervals. If an owner missed a scheduled vaccination by as little as a day, there may be pressure to back date the horse's passport to fulfil competition requirements. The efficacy of vaccination and the welfare of the horse are not in jeopardy, but this reflects the pressures placed on a sports horse veterinarian, who again should be the leader and not jeopardise their own professional integrity.

What should a veterinarian advise about the management of a horse that windsucks, especially when we know that such horses may be quicker learners than those that do not windsuck and can be highly successful athletes? A rider may consider the horse's behaviour unacceptable, but do they understand the horse's physiological needs? Is it legitimate, with our current knowledge about neurotransmitters and mental wellbeing, that the 'problem' is addressed by the use of a collar or surgical management, as I recently witnessed? It also recently came to light that a veterinarian performed amputation of the rostral part of the tongue of a dressage pony that was being penalised for tongue lolling. How can this conceivably be justified unless the tongue had been severely injured? I have heard anecdotal reports that this is not a unique case.

36.4 APPROPRIATE TRAINING TO DEAL WITH THE CHALLENGES

The undergraduate training of equine veterinarians is inadequate to prepare them for the challenges of investigation and diagnosis of performance-related problems in horses. Veterinarians are trained to recognise overt unilateral forelimb or hindlimb lameness that is evident when a horse is trotted in hand. They are taught how to perform basic diagnostic anaesthetic techniques but are rarely aware of the challenges of interpretation. Moreover, they are not trained to recognise ridden horse performance problems, some of which are specific to different sports disciplines. Veterinarians have been conditioned, like so many people in the equestrian world, that many ridden horse problems reflect a horse's behaviour or the way in which it has been trained rather than underlying musculoskeletal pain. This results in the horse being blamed and encourages more coercive training rather than identification of the underlying problems. Often gastroscopy is offered as the first diagnostic test, and if equine gastric ulcer syndrome is diagnosed, a cycle of treatment with omeprazole ± sucralfate or misoprostol and repeat gastroscopy ensues, despite the limited evidence that gastric ulcers are a primary cause of reduced performance and the increasing recognition that underlying stress, often the result of musculoskeletal pain, is a major predisposing factor.

Failure to recognise overt lameness encourages the use of expensive advanced imaging techniques as a 'fishing exercise'. For example, it may result in whole body skeletal scintigraphy, despite the evidence that in mature sports horses the investigation of poor performance by skeletal scintigraphy results in a high proportion of false negative or false positive results. If the latter are followed up by additional imaging (for example, radiography) and treatment, the owner may face a large invoice and no improvement in the horse's performance.

The veterinary profession needs to improve its diagnostic skills. Equine veterinarians must learn to recognise that failure to see horses ridden will result in the lack of appreciation of the underlying problems a rider may encounter during ridden exercise. Just because a veterinarian cannot recognise overt lameness does not mean that there is an absence of musculoskeletal pain. Veterinarians need to learn to listen carefully to riders and grooms and to understand their complaints. The failure of equine veterinarians to develop the prerequisite skills jeopardises equine welfare and endlessly frustrates owners and riders.

36.5 COMMUNICATION BETWEEN VETERINARIANS AND CLIENTS; THE CONFLICTS THAT FEE SCALES GENERATE AND MANAGING CLIENTS' EXPECTATIONS

Equine veterinarians face many economically driven challenges, both from clients and their own need to generate income, which are sometimes conflicting. While most professionally owned horses are not insured, many lower end sports horses are insured for veterinary fees. Consider what is morally appropriate to do from a diagnosis and management perspective versus what is affordable by the client or may be permissible under the limit of insurance fees. Insurance should not be a ticket to doing everything possible, unless that is genuinely in the best interests of the horse.

Once again there are potential conflicts between what a client may request or demand, and what may be morally correct, and the need for transparent communication. For example, the failure to describe all clinical findings on a pre-purchase examination certificate that could influence insurance cover and the failure to declare all findings on clinical assessment during a lameness investigation that could jeopardise future insurance cover are misleading and potentially fraudulent acts.

Clients often have a poor understanding of the wording of insurance policies or, more likely, have never read them. They frequently fail to understand the difference between elective euthanasia on humane grounds versus fulfilling insurance criteria for humane destruction. For example, consider a horse with navicular disease characterised by an erosion of the palmar compact bone and adhesions of the DDFT; the horse is chronically lame and likely to remain so. It does not fulfil insurance criteria for humane destruction, but it may be in the welfare interest of the horse that it undergoes euthanasia, particularly if the environment in which the horse can be kept is unsuitable for retirement.

A veterinarian has to deal with owners' emotions and financial situations which bring moral conflicts, especially as veterinarians have generally been educated on the basis of preserving life, although this may not always be in the best interests of either the owner or the horse. Some common examples include a client who has limited funds, but the horse has career-ending musculoskeletal problems. The horse could be retired and lead an adequately comfortable life, but the owner has no facilities or money to keep this horse. She wants a horse to ride; should a veterinarian stand in the way of a request for euthanasia? In contrast, there are owners who wish to continue to treat a horse with multiple musculoskeletal problems and to ride the horse, despite inadequate responses to treatment to maintain an adequate quality of life; the owner, is seemingly blind to the level of discomfort that the horse experiences during ridden exercise. This is abuse of the horse. The veterinarian should be the ultimate guardian of equine welfare, but this may not be easy to achieve. At the other extreme, consider a horse with a life-threatening condition, for example, a small intestinal obstruction that could be resolved by surgical management (assuming that it was treated early enough by a team with the requisite skills), but the horse is not insured, and the owner cannot afford surgery. Euthanasia may be the only option.

36.6 THE CONFLICTS GENERATED BY THE PRESSURES OF HORSE SPORTS

We then need to consider the use of horses in individual sports, many of which carry a risk of musculoskeletal injury. At the top end of most equine sports, there are huge sums of money involved in the prices of horses, prize money and sponsorship deals, in addition to income generated through public attendance at sporting events, television, and other news media coverage. There may be extreme owner pressure on riders. In some instances, there is a desire from a rider to compete and win at all costs. With children comes the added dimension of parental aspirations for their child, sometimes with complete ignorance of the equestrian world. In the middle of all this are the horses, and the horses being viewed by a largely ignorant general public, and the increasing public scrutiny and criticism of horse sports. This does not just come from outside the equine industry; there is a body of enthusiastic, vociferous equine people who are against the use of bits, horseshoes, individual stabling, or the use of horses in competitive sports.

Each individual sport brings its own problems which could involve the veterinary profession. We need to be educated if we are to offer a meaningful and helpful contribution, preserve horse sports, and optimise equine welfare. This means that as veterinarians we need to identify problems by the acquisition of data-based facts, to highlight what are the most serious problems, and to propose practical and palatable solutions that could mitigate each situation. There are many examples.

36.6.1 Steeplechasing

The number of horse falls in steeplechasing is unacceptably high, some resulting in career-ending injuries or death, highlighted by the Grand National, but not limited to this race. Could this be averted by reducing the number of runners, reducing the distance between the start and the first fence, superior pre-race checks, or reducing the frequency of racing? Could positron emission computed tomography (PET) scans identify individuals more at risk of injury, or would this just discredit the veterinary profession by increasing costs for the racing industry and withdrawing some horses unnecessarily? Do we really know why horses fall and how the risk could be reduced? Steeplechasing in Australia has already been banned in all states except Victoria; proactive action is needed if the sport is to remain elsewhere.

36.6.2 Flat Racing

Flat racing is a more lucrative sport than steeplechasing and there are more data available globally about injury risk and track design and surface, types of horseshoes, pre-race medication, and injury frequency after periods of lay-off. The issue of racing immature two-year-olds highly susceptible to stress-related bone injuries has long been debated in both the racing and veterinary industries. Career-ending injuries, often resulting in early euthanasia, are increasingly challenged by the lay public, given the high level of publicity which has surrounded recent multiple deaths at high-profile race meetings in the USA. The veterinary profession has been proactive in trying to provide fact-based commentaries on the day; more pre-race checks and stricter medication rules have unquestionably benefited the industry. However, the veterinary profession probably needs to take a lead to encourage racing practices to change, in recognition of the principle of 'friends, freedom, and forage'. It is no longer acceptable to the public to be told that horses are 'treated like kings', on an individual basis when most spend at least 22 hours per day confined in a stall. Provision of turnout and prospective evaluation of injury type and occurrence might improve understanding of what could be achieved to reduce injury risk, by provision of a more natural environment, with greater daily exercise. The British Horseracing Authority's (BHA) inconsistency in their ruling concerning use of the whip does not help public confidence (Elder 2023; PA Media 2023); the BHA has veterinary advisors – how can they condone the use of a whip given the evidence from Scandinavian countries in which the use of a whip has been banned? How can we morally justify the use of a tongue tie to restrict the movement of a horse's tongue?

The racing industry wants to be seen to be proactive in the rehoming of racehorses after the end of their racing careers and tries to imply that the majority can be successfully rehomed. This is despite the fact that many ex-flat racehorses have accumulated multiple injuries, have an inherent predisposition to impinging spinous processes often associated with thoracolumbar pain, and may be either physically or temperamentally unsuitable for rehabilitation as a sports horse or pleasure horse. The onus then falls on equine veterinarians to facilitate decision-making about a horse's future, with a possible financial conflict of interest, because there is little doubt that there is a potentially highly lucrative income from trying to manage these horses.

There are specific races globally that have become cultural events: for example, the Palio in Italy, the Ageuma Shinji in Japan, the Parbudice in the Czech Republic, and the Mongol Derby, all of which are under veterinary control. There is, justifiably, much concerned debate about the conditions the horses are subject to.

36.6.3 Eventing

In one- and three-day eventing, global effort has been made in recent years to collect and analyse horse and rider fall data, with the identification of risk factors related to dressage performance, fence type, frequency of competition, and previous competition record at the level of an event or at a lower level to achieve minimal eligibility requirements. The ground juries at international competitions have been empowered to be more proactive in issuing yellow cards to competitors openly abusing horses by excessive pressure on a fatigued horse. As a result, there has been a small but progressive decline in horse falls in the last 20 years. Falls are multifactorial: horse error, rider error, fatigue (which could relate to, among others, fitness, terrain, weather, and ground conditions), discomfort, excessive speed, approach speed too slow, and loss of confidence of horse and/or rider. Perhaps there could be more collaboration between owners, riders, veterinarians, and other paraprofessionals to promote regular health monitoring, to include ridden horse assessment, to recognise injuries early on and to educate riders and owners about the frequency of competition and the need for adequate recovery time after competitions for resolution of subclinical soft tissue injuries.

36.6.4 Dressage

The whole ethos of dressage is under increasing public scrutiny from the selection of the type of horse that is likely to be rewarded with high marks, the sometimes coercive training methods employed, including rollkur, the use of bits (including double bridles) and spurs, the tightness of nosebands, bit-associated lesions, and spur marks. Much of this criticism is justified, but why does showjumping escape similar close examination? In the warm-up arenas of international shows, similar coercive training methods, with the practice of hyperflexion facilitated by the use of draw reins, can be observed. What can and should the veterinary profession do – treat the injuries sustained or try to be more proactive in promoting change? Those that are knowledgeable about the sports could be more open in challenging the current training techniques. Although there is evidence that the very top dressage horses, by and large, have longevity of performance, competing successfully in their mid to late teens, what happens to the huge number of three- and four-year-old horses that fall by the wayside through injury early on in in their careers, because of their inherent athleticism and the way in which they are produced as young horses? The Helgstrand saga brought this to the headlines, but this is not an isolated problem (Anon 2023a, 2023b).

36.6.5 Showjumping

In showjumping in particular, equine sports horse veterinarians are faced with a potential problem, particularly at just below the top professional level. There are many talented showjumpers that can jump consistently and well, despite obvious lameness, particularly hindlimb lameness, and work reasonably comfortably in walk and canter. These horses will continue to be used whether or not a veterinarian can 'fix them'. To what extent should a veterinarian insist upon proper investigation and targeted treatment rather than a 'shotgun' approach to treatment through multifocal treatments? What are the moral considerations of actively facilitating the use of lame horses, which will be jumped anyway? Noseband tightness and bit use have been debated in the dressage world, but largely ignored in showjumping. The combination of bits, nosebands and hackamores in widespread use is truly remarkable. Why is this sport not under more scrutiny? Is there any awareness within the veterinary profession, and if so, do we just turn a blind eye, to avoid drawing attention to the sport? Is there any will within the profession to try to change the status quo?

36.6.6 Western Performance Horses

Reining and other western performance sports are huge and highly lucrative sports, especially in the USA. Large (tall and/or overweight) riders relative to horse body size, highly demanding athletic sports, with horses often competing at high frequency for very high prize money at two and three years of age, result in a high injury rate and a short career. Within some disciplines sedation during competition is legal. Tail blocking, or neurectomy, is illegal, but rule enforcement appears to be ignored. So, are the trainers or riders acquiring the drugs and administering them, or are veterinarians aiding and abetting these situations, which are unquestionably contrary to equine welfare?

36.6.7 Endurance

Endurance has received bad press, largely due to unscrupulous practices commonly carried out in the Middle East (Horse & Hound 2020). The adoption of mechanical nociceptive testing during competition has been a small step forwards, but it seems that even large fines and lengthy bans imposed by the Fédération Equestre Internationale on a small number of individuals have not been an adequate deterrent. In other geographical areas, where there is better respect for the rules, the sport of endurance is probably one of the most highly policed equine sports, with multiple veterinary checks before, during, and at the end of each competition. Like most other sports, musculoskeletal injury is the most common cause of days off training and competing, although generally upper-level horses have a remarkable tolerance of injury.

36.6.8 Bull Fighting and Rodeos

Bull fighting and rodeo, which each have their particular welfare concerns, are embedded in cultures that those of us outside find difficult to understand fully. They highlight whether sports which are dependent on audience support and essentially represent pure exploitation of the animals involved should be condoned by the veterinary profession.

36.6.9 Showing

Showing brings about two other major moral issues with which veterinarians have to engage, both as providers of advice to owners, and as experts making recommendations to horse shows and showing organisations and their judges. The problem of equine obesity and all its incumbent problems (equine metabolic syndrome, laminitis, altered enzymatic function predisposing to musculoskeletal injuries, overloading the limbs, having to work harder to 'carry' the weight) is not unique to showing, but it appears that fatness is at least indirectly rewarded by judges. It is a sad reflection on modern day society that excessive body condition score has become normalised. The only person that can address these problems from an evidence-based scientific point of view is an equine veterinarian. The problem of rider size is not restricted to bodyweight, but also includes height, the ratio of trunk length to limb length, and the rider's general morphology, all of which influence both magnitude and distribution of forces. The rider size problem is not unique to showing; in all disciplines both child and adult riders have become progressively larger over the last 40 years (Wang et al. 2017).

36.6.10 Polo

Polo places incredible demands on horses: speed, sudden accelerations and decelerations, frequent and abrupt changes of direction, tall riders, and the potential for direct trauma from a polo mallet or a collision with another horse. The prevalence of musculoskeletal injury is high. Matches are not under veterinary supervision. However, there is pressure from players on veterinarians to keep horses sound enough to play. Ironically, phenylbutazone and other non-steroidal anti-inflammatory analgesic drugs are permitted under many polo jurisdictions and have been shown to reduce the risk of equine gastric ulcer syndrome (Banse et al. 2018).

36.6.11 Lower-Level Sports and Leisure Horses

Among lower levels of competition in all disciplines and in the leisure horse industry, there is evidence that there is a higher prevalence of lameness, and more ignorance that equine behaviour during grooming, tacking-up, and ridden exercise may be a reflection of underlying musculoskeletal pain rather than just a reflection of a horse's challenging behaviour (Dyson et al. 2021, 2022; Dyson & Pollard 2022). Rider size, weight distribution, and saddle fit for horse and rider become a greater challenge, problems that equine veterinarians may be reluctant to address, but if they do not, who will?

36.7 CONCLUSIONS

The moral and ethical use of horses for sport and general leisure purposes requires that we identify the causes of trauma/injury and develop ways of minimising the risk of such trauma/injury occurring during training and competition. There are potential financial conflicts, conflicts of interest of data reporting versus client confidentiality, but without facts, decisions for change are unlikely to occur. The veterinary profession should consider trying to clarify conceptually and distinguish practically between optimal, excessive, and performance-enhancing treatment. It should also recognise the broader issues that veterinarians, as the ultimate guardians of the horse, have an obligation to address. These include training methods, rider size, equipment used, general management, and the recognition that there are reasons for so-called bad behaviour.

REFERENCES

Anon. Danish equestrian world in turmoil as ethics of national federation are questioned. *Eurodressage* [Internet]. 2023a Sept 29. Available from: https://www.eurodressage.com/2023/09/29/danish-equestrian-world-turmoil-ethics-national-federation-are-questioned.

Anon. Operation X documentary causes cascade of anger, indignation, disapproval. *Eurodressage* [Internet] 2023b Nov 23. Available from: https://www.eurodressage.com/2023/11/23/operation-x-documentary-causes-cascade-anger-indignation-disapproval.

Banse H, MacLeod H, Crosby C, et al. Prevalence of and risk factors for equine glandular and squamous gastric disease in polo horses. *Can Vet J*. 2018;59(8):880–884.

Dyson S. The ridden horse pain ethogram. *Equine Vet Educ*. 2022;34(7):372–380.

Dyson S, Bondi A, Routh J, et al. An investigation into the relationship between equine behaviour when tacked-up and mounted and epaxial muscle hypertonicity or pain, girth region hypersensitivity, saddle fit, rider position and balance and lameness. *Equine Vet Educ*. 2021;34(6):e258–e267.

Dyson S, Bondi A, Routh J, et al. Do owners recognise abnormal equine behaviour when tacking-up and mounting? A comparison between responses to a questionnaire and real-time observations. *Equine Vet Educ*. 2022;34(9):e375–e384.

Dyson S, Pollard D. Application of the ridden horse pain ethogram to horses competing in British eventing 90, 100 and novice one-day events and comparison with performance. *Animals (Basel)*. 2022;12(5):590.

Elder L. Last-minute changes to new whip rules for 2023. *Horse & Hound News* [Internet]. 2023 Jan 4 [cited 2023 Dec 27]. Available from: https://www.horseandhound.co.uk/news/last-minute-changes-british-racing-whip-rules-2023-813227.

Jones E. 'No improvement' seen at first Middle Eastern FEI endurance ride of 2020. *Horse & Hound News* [Internet]. 2020 Feb 11. Available from: https://www.horseandhound.co.uk/news/no-improvement-seen-at-first-middle-eastern-fei-endurance-ride-of-2020-hh-plus-706654.

PA Media. 'More palatable': BHA revises changes to whip rules after jockeys voice concerns. *The Guardian* [Internet]. 2023 Jan 4. Available from: https://www.theguardian.com/sport/2023/jan/04/bha-revises-changes-to-whip-rules-after-jockeys-voice-concerns-horse-racing.

Wang Y, McPherson K, Marsh T, et al. Health and economic burden of the projected obesity trends in the USA and UK. *Lancet*. 2017;378(9793):815–825.

FURTHER READING

Allen K, Anderson L, King M, et al. Competing interests at the heart of equine sports medicine ethics: a scoping review and thematic analysis. *Equine Vet J*. 2024;56(1):26–36.

37 Vets Speaking up for Animal Welfare

Sean Wensley

Some contemporary challenges are presented to promote ongoing reflection and engagement with veterinary and animal ethics and to encourage a confident profession-wide approach in helping animal-using industries transition away from harmful norms.

37.1 VETERINARY ANIMAL WELFARE RESPONSIBILITY

Enhancing, protecting, and securing the health and welfare of animals is the fundamental purpose of the veterinary profession (BVA & RCVS 2015; BVA 2021). In the UK, this primacy of animal welfare for veterinary surgeons is reflected in the declaration that each veterinarian makes upon admission to the Royal College of Veterinary Surgeons (RCVS 2012):

> *ABOVE ALL, my constant endeavour will be to ensure the health and welfare of animals committed to my care.*

While the RCVS declaration conveys the responsibility that veterinarians have to the welfare of animals *under their care*, the last decade or so has seen veterinary professional bodies clarifying the wider responsibility that the veterinary and veterinary nursing professions have, to provide animal welfare leadership at the societal level. Veterinary clinical work may optimise animal welfare within the status quo of currently accepted animal uses (e.g. animals used for food, sport, companionship and so on), but speaking up about the root causes of animal welfare harms is now also established as being central to the profession's overall welfare responsibility (BVA 2021; FVE 2021). This requires the profession to publicly highlight how animal-using activities give rise to welfare risks, as well as challenging whether these risks (and sometimes the underlying activity *per se*) are ethically justifiable.

Veterinary animal welfare policies and recommendations that result from this wider activity are valuable for practitioners, through their providing validation of welfare concerns that practitioners may be holding, as well as practical guidance on how to advance animal welfare beyond the provision of indicated remedial treatment. This chapter will describe how consensus on this wider veterinary animal welfare responsibility has been established, noting that it is a contested and evolving area, and describe some outstanding challenges.

37.2 VETERINARY ANIMAL WELFARE STRATEGIES

In the early 2010s there was growing international interest in veterinary animal welfare leadership, with professional statements being published such as this from the World Organisation for Animal Health (OIE, now WOAH 2012):

Veterinarians should be the leading advocates for the welfare of all animals [and] ... provide leadership to society on ethical considerations involved in the use and care of animals by humans.

Building on this growing imperative and responding to increasing member demands domestically, in the UK the strategic *Vet Futures* project, jointly powered by the British Veterinary Association (BVA) and the RCVS, identified leadership in animal health and welfare as one of its six key ambitions for the profession by 2030 (BVA & RCVS 2015). To help realise this ambition, BVA launched its first animal welfare strategy, *Vets Speaking Up for Animal Welfare*, in February 2016 (BVA 2016).

In approaching this strategy, BVA recognised that there is a plurality of views towards animal welfare within the veterinary profession, as in wider society. High-profile issues such as slaughter without pre-stunning for religious purposes and breeding animals with brachycephaly had led to accusations that the veterinary profession was complicit with animal harm if it did not use its voice to challenge harmful practices.

Reasons why the veterinary profession does not always approach animal welfare from a position of unification include the following:

- A minority of vets apparently denounce animal welfare. When I began my term as BVA president in 2015, I received a letter from a retired member of the profession who told me that *'Animal welfare is (more than it ever was) a label for unscientific, anthropomorphic, sentimental clap trap'*.
- Some vets might accept the premise of animal welfare, but may openly dismiss or misinterpret animal welfare science, concepts, and their implications.
- Some vets feel threatened by questions of animal ethics and what they might mean for their livelihoods.
- Some vets may feel an allegiance to an industry, born of long-standing, sometimes lifelong, involvement and identity.

To structure its approach, BVA considered opportunities for the profession to advocate animal welfare at three levels:

1. Through individual veterinary professionals to animal keepers and owners
2. Through veterinary practices to the surrounding community
3. Through national veterinary associations to create political impact and challenge societal norms

The association undertook a stakeholder survey to map perceptions and expectations of BVA's role in promoting animal welfare and on what stakeholders felt was being done well, and could be done better, at each of the three levels.

The resulting strategy, containing 30 actions, was structured around six emergent themes, presented as 'priority areas':

1. Animal welfare assessment
2. Ethics
3. Legislation
4. Advocacy
5. Education
6. International

It was BVA Council's view, across these six areas, that a progressive, fit-for-purpose veterinary profession would, for example:

1. Promote positive welfare, utilise contemporary animal welfare frameworks, and disseminate animal welfare research findings to members.
2. Assist members with ethical decision-making and apply ethical frameworks to policy development.
3. Provide guidance on animal welfare legislation, including on reporting suspected non-accidental injury.
4. Work collaboratively, particularly with species-specialist associations, to develop a list of specific animal welfare problems on which they would develop positions and proactively campaign.
5. Deliver high-quality teaching in animal welfare science, ethics, and law to undergraduates and through continuing education.
6. Have a position on humane, sustainable animal agriculture and advance work, with international partners, at the intersection of animal welfare, climate change, biodiversity loss, food safety and security, antimicrobial resistance, and other pressing global challenges.

From this vision, and subsequent policies, the following fundamental points and principles were agreed:

1. The profession has a dual duty: to advocate the best interests of animals under the care of individual veterinary surgeons – as required by its UK oath and similar international veterinary oaths – as well as to advocate for changes and solutions to address the root causes of animal welfare problems, beyond the bounds of animals under its direct care.
2. The veterinary profession should provide strong and visible leadership on animal welfare at individual, community, national, and international levels.
3. Vets are rightfully animal-welfare-focused, as opposed to client- or industry-focused, or business-focused. They must have positive, empathic

relations with clients and they must charge appropriately and unashamedly to remain commercially viable, but these are enablers for achieving their overriding, motivating objective of improving animal welfare. This does not mean pursuing animal welfare at all costs, it is about animal welfare being the primary aim, at each of the levels.
4. Attaining good physical health is necessary but not sufficient for attaining good welfare. Mental wellbeing and quality of life, particularly arising from the expression of species-typical behaviours, are also essential.
5. Recognition of the shift in societal and legal focus, away from simply sparing animals the worst of being under human stewardship, towards actively promoting positive welfare states and the animals experiencing a good life.
6. The profession may sometimes adopt an abolitionist stance; that *'there is a limit to acceptable animal welfare compromises associated with each area of animal use. If these limits are reached and cannot be adequately addressed, the veterinary profession will oppose that use or practice'* (BVA 2021). BVA and the Federation of Veterinarians of Europe (FVE)'s opposition to the use of performing wild animals in travelling circuses gives an example of this.

FVE, on behalf of the profession across Europe, also adopted these principles, stating, for example, in their 2020 revised policy position on animal welfare with the American and Canadian Veterinary Medical Associations that kept animals should experience a Good Life and a humane death (FVE 2020), and in their first animal welfare strategy, that the profession's overall primary aim is to *'help make the world a better place for animals'* (FVE 2021).

37.3 VETERINARY ANIMAL WELFARE ADVOCACY

Both BVA and FVE's strategies committed the associations to developing the policy positions that would underpin advocacy in collaboration with species-specialist colleagues and associations.

A first step was to agree the welfare problems on which it was felt the associations should take a leadership role in highlighting and addressing, and the FVE General Assembly, with the specialist associations' full input, agreed a long list of 152 such problems across Europe. These are 152 hurdles to fulfilling the ethical prescription of a good life and a humane death for kept animals and represent 152 welfare risks to the ongoing granting of social licence to use animals for human benefit.

- **Farmed animals**

Some of the first policy positions produced off the back of the strategies focused on mutilations in farmed animals. For instance, castrating lambs using a tight rubber ring to restrict the flow of blood to the scrotum is permitted in the UK without an anaesthetic if the device is applied during the first week of life. This causes pain that typically lasts for around two hours, then is followed by further inflammation and pain which can persist for more than two days. What does the veterinary profession think about the fact that several million lambs are castrated without pain relief each year in the UK and many more are tail docked?

A policy position published by BVA with the Sheep Veterinary Society in 2019 presses for a 3Rs approach to castration and tail docking – replacing the need to perform these procedures through alternative management approaches, reducing the numbers of animals to the minimum necessary, and refining the procedures through lobbying government and industry to develop and authorise a local anaesthetic and analgesic protocol for use in field conditions.

That position followed BVA's 2017 policy position with the British Cattle Veterinary Association, which also advocated a 3Rs approach to castration and disbudding of calves, and emphasised the importance of using both a local anaesthetic and a non-steroidal anti-inflammatory drug (NSAID) to manage pain once the effect of the local anaesthetic has subsided.

In 2019 BVA published a comprehensive and visionary position on UK sustainable animal agriculture, in which, amongst 13 recommendations, it presented the imperative for an evolved agricultural system that does not depend on routine use of mutilations, offers stimulating living environments to allow for the performance of highly motivated behaviours, and sees animals bred in an ethically responsible way to improve animal health and welfare. The veterinary profession is sometimes asked what it thinks about 'intensive' or 'factory' farming. These terms can be divisive, but if we look beyond the terms, the profession is unified with the broader animal protection movement in its opposition to some of the agro-industry's worst animal welfare practices.

- **Companion animals**

In recent years, BVA has published policy positions with the British Veterinary Nursing Association, the British Small Animal Veterinary Association, and the British Veterinary Zoological Society on topics including obesity, the importance of housing pet rabbits in compatible pairs or groups, breeding for extreme conformation and the welfare of non-traditional companion animals (exotic pets).

Advocacy on health harms linked to selective breeding has been delivered through BVA's *Breed to Breathe* and *Health Over Looks* campaigns, and similar veterinary campaigns elsewhere, such as the Australian Veterinary Association and RSPCA Australia's joint *Love Is Blind* campaign.

The companion animal sector has also given examples of the need for the profession to remain responsive to emergent welfare challenges. There has been a concerning rise in ear-cropped dogs in the UK – a painful mutilation of dogs' ears undertaken for purely cosmetic reasons, which is illegal but increasingly seen in dogs who have been imported. BVA's *Cut the Crop* campaign, working alongside NGOs, has resulted in the UK government committing to addressing this problem.

Individual practitioners have been effective advocates, promoting the campaign's messages in the media and elsewhere.

- **Equids**

The BVA welfare prioritisation exercise, with input from the British Equine Veterinary Association, listed 12 priority welfare problems affecting horses, including inappropriate stabling and turnout, obesity, unresolved stress and pain behaviour, training methods, and tack fit including nosebands, bits, and saddles. There is now considerable evidence for the welfare implications of these issues for horses, as well as significantly heightened focus on the equine industry's social licence to operate. A multi-stakeholder workshop organised by the Animal Welfare Research Network in 2021 asked, '*How happy are equine athletes?*' Equine physical health is vital for competitive success, but, as in other areas of animal use, there has historically been less consideration of equine mental well-being. The workshop reported that in the view of its participants, it is questionable whether any horse would choose to take part in equestrian sport if given such a choice. A year later, the International Federation for Equestrian Sports, the FEI's Equine Ethics and Wellbeing Commission, reported that the majority of the public, 67%, in 14 countries do not believe that horses enjoy being involved in sport or only enjoy it sometimes. Their survey of equestrian stakeholders found that the majority, 78%, believed that equine welfare standards need improving (FEI 2022). Visible issues, such as use of the whip and racecourse fatalities rightfully generate public concern and debate, but a necessary spotlight is now being shone on quality of life in the less visible areas of horse management and training. The charity World Horse Welfare and others are promoting the 3Fs of horse welfare: freedom, friendship, and forage, which are championing cultural change to ensure regular turn-out to pasture, opportunities for social contact and constant access to high fibre food.

37.4 ONGOING CHALLENGES

With these veterinary welfare strategies in the world, and a refreshed BVA welfare strategy published in 2025, where are we now? While we can be encouraged and energised by successes to date, we must be honest about ongoing challenges. I will share some recent observations and pose some questions, from across the priority areas.

- **Animal welfare assessment**

BVA is promoting the Five Domains model and recommending it as the basis for revised UK animal welfare legislation (BVA 2021). I recently chaired a working group on the welfare of non-traditional companion animals (exotic pets), where some external contributing veterinarians characterised welfare in the narrow and outdated way of mortality rates and disease prevalence. Other veterinarians have recently and publicly claimed that racehorses love racing and therefore, when there are sadly fatalities, the horses 'die doing what they love' – can that claim be substantiated and is it part of a holistic welfare assessment, incorporating harms arising from management and training, as well as competition? Ongoing work is needed to embed welfare science and contemporary assessment approaches within the profession.

- **Education**

De Briyne and colleagues (de Briyne et al. 2020) gave a good insight into the veterinary teaching of Animal Welfare Science, Ethics and Law based on survey responses from 57 veterinary schools from 25 European countries. They reported, for example, a nearly 40 percentage point increase in the number of schools that were teaching the importance of positive animal welfare, up from 59% to 98%, while they commented that the teaching of ethics fares worse than animal welfare science and law: 37% of schools did not meet or only partially met the agreed day 1 competencies.

In her illuminating book *Learning Animals* (Dolby 2022), Nadine Dolby, Professor of Curriculum Studies at Purdue University, examines how veterinary education shapes the ways veterinary students experience animals and construct professional identities, based on in-depth personal narratives collected over five years. She describes moral stress, burnout, and the feeling of being engulfed in the 'mechanic' model (Rollin 2006) of veterinary education, without concentrated attention on the central, ever-present ethical issues, including those arising from society's increasing questions and unease about our relationships with animals.

In the wake of high-profile protests at the 2023 Grand National and other UK horse-racing events, a hot topics session at the BVA Live event the same year debated the social licence of animal sport. Some contributing vets, still today, openly questioned whether vets know enough about animal welfare to make ethical judgements. Is this acceptable in the present day? While all professionals must be honest about their knowledge limits, would we accept similar responses from veterinarians about basic aspects of veterinary pathology or pharmacology?

- **Advocacy**

While some 20 comprehensive policy positions on animal welfare topics have been published by BVA since 2016, transforming the nature of veterinary engagement with animal welfare, that is still less than a fifth of the welfare problems that were originally identified as requiring a position. There are practical and other reasons for this. Practically, representative veterinary bodies are overwhelmed with topics on which their members need support. Other factors can include a reticence by some Veterinarians and Veterinary Associations to proactively engage.

When, in 2022, three leading animal welfare charities called for the abolition of greyhound racing in the UK, the Society of Greyhound Veterinarians, while voicing concerns about a ban, said that the Society 'does not take an ethical view of the sport'. Does this reflect indifference and a lack of moral courage, or a justifiable agnosticism?

- **Ethics**

We continue to see examples of apparent industry-focused rather than animal-welfare-focused veterinary approaches to some ethical issues. During the BVA exotic pets' policy development, some fish veterinarians argued for the ongoing wild capture of marine fish to be kept as pets because of the economic returns for exporting countries.

I have mentioned BVA's support in principle for seeking abolition of certain animal-use practices on animal welfare grounds, and the possibility of a veterinary body being agnostic about animal use practices but should a veterinary organisation ever actively promote animal use?

Some UK farm veterinary practices support the National Farmers' Union's *Back British Farming* campaign through their social media posts. Is there a clear ethical basis for doing so, when British farming, despite its relatively high standards, includes harmful practices such as confining sows in farrowing crates and breeding fast-growing broilers, about which the UK veterinary profession currently has no published position? What is the ethical basis on which an animal-welfare-focused profession might actively promote an area of animal use? If resources are too stretched for veterinary bodies to advocate animal welfare improvements in high priority areas, is it ever justifiable to divert those limited resources to promoting animal use? Perhaps veterinary advocacy should be reserved for addressing pervasive animal health and welfare problems, then consider promoting an activity writ large once, and if, that is achieved?

In a letter to the Vet Record, '*The profession has a duty to support its farmers*', the author says, '*In the 21st century, those of us working in the farm sector still pride ourselves on the strength of the relationships we develop with our farm clients. Many clients, who we work alongside daily, become lifelong friends and mutual confidants . . . We must continue to work alongside farmers, as we always have done, promoting British produce and showing our undivided support*' (Parrish 2020). Would similar imploring sit uneasily beneath a headline '*The profession has a duty to support its breeders of dogs with brachycephaly*', and if so, why?

In an example from New Zealand, veterinary advocacy of the pork industry has been coupled with a bid to reframe farrowing crates as 'maternity hospital beds', to secure public sympathy and support for the controversial practice (Hill 2020). Is this ethically justifiable?

37.5 A TWO-TIER VETERINARY PROFESSION?

Associations like BVA and FVE are trying to navigate these ethical questions on behalf of their members, but for some veterinarians, they are not going fast or far enough. Consequently, we have seen the formation of additional veterinary associations who are aiming to provide clearer animal welfare leadership; these include the Caring Vets in the Netherlands, the Humane Society Veterinary Medical Association in the US, and the Progressive Veterinary Association launched in 2022 in the UK. These associations pursue important issues. If their objective is to put scrutiny and pressure on the national associations, then that seems valuable; if not, do they risk legitimising a two-tier veterinary profession: those who advocate animal welfare at the societal level and those who take a more passive or traditional stance?

These potential fault lines are drawing media attention. In the US, Vox, with its 10 million YouTube subscribers, recently probed the American Veterinary Medical Association (AVMA)'s stance on animal ethics, following the public defence of sow stalls by US pig veterinarians and the AVMA's support for the emergency killing of millions of farmed animals using heatstroke (Bolotnikova 2023).

Peter Singer's recently published *Animal Liberation Now* – updating his foundational text – takes aim at the veterinary profession, saying on its jacket that the '*complicity of the American Veterinary Medical Association in some of the most horrific practices*' is '*most shocking*' in the present-day context (Singer 2023).

The business and veterinary ethics of small-animal practice continue to be challenged in the media and, in the UK (at the time of writing), are the subject of a Competition and Markets Authority (CMA) review. While I do not think that particular challenge will simply dissipate in response to the profession's broader animal welfare advocacy, it is nevertheless likely to be essential that the profession's perpetual public positioning should unequivocally demonstrate its focus on protecting and advancing animal welfare.

The espoused veterinary vision of a good life and a humane death for animals kept and impacted by humans is a radical one, despite its apparent simplicity. Achieving it would require a global transformation in how we manage and use animals, and for many the rate of change is unacceptably slow. Animal rights are being invoked by some veterinary advocates. The recently formed US-based veterinary advocacy association, Our Honor, for example, promote animal rights through their communications, while in the UK, veterinarian Steven McCulloch has promoted animals having a 'right to wellbeing' (McCulloch 2023).

- **International**

We are seeing both potential risk and reward for animal welfare as the veterinary profession becomes more involved with sustainability. On the one hand, veterinary advocacy should be invaluable in helping ensure the interests of sentient animals are increasingly accounted for within the currently anthropocentric sustainable development agenda. On the other, we should be aware of colleagues who are willing to de-prioritise animal welfare in their rush to embrace environmental sustainability. In a recent example, a veterinarian who leads an agricultural trade association challenged the promotion of slower-growing broilers, who can have improved welfare, stating that carbon emissions and feed and water use would each rise and raising doubts about the ability to balance these sustainability objectives. She should have advocated animal welfare and could have proposed solutions such as 'less and better' consumption (as recommended by BVA and others) – which in this case was instead proposed by a senior European food policy officer who was not a veterinarian.

37.6 A THREE-STAGE EVOLUTION

On the basis of these reflections, I see something of a three-stage process in the evolution of veterinary animal welfare advocacy:

1. In the first stage, the veterinary profession identifies as standing shoulder-to-shoulder with animal-using industries, there to assist them with deriving human benefits from animals through the protection and restoration of physical health.
2. As societal awareness of animal sentience grows, together with concern for humane animal treatment, the profession functions as a canary in the mine: detecting and sympathising with this rising public demand for ethical treatment and, in stage 2, identifying as advocates of animal health and wellbeing in order to help future-proof industries and assist them in retaining their social licence to operate.
3. In the third stage, the veterinary profession comprises a workforce that is taught and motivated to proactively challenge the status quo of animal use and shape public opinion to do the same. It identifies as a leader in protecting animals' interests, with little reverence for the status quo – advocating either the purposeful reform of traditional industry practices or making organised calls for an irredeemable animal-using activity to be abolished.

While none of the ethical issues inherent in this landscape are new, as the global profession publishes policy positions on the roles of veterinarians in animal welfare, based on consultation and consensus, so the number and range of justifiable ethical stances reduces and the risk of claims of complicity with institutionalised animal harm being substantiated increases. As Nadine Dolby writes in *Learning Animals*, *'historically, veterinary medicine . . . has tacitly and quietly accepted that animal suffering and human violence towards animals is necessary. However, more recently, societal pressure on these norms and practices has required the profession to rethink its response to how it both represents and participates in these acts'*.

Making comparisons between veterinary work and the role of physicians and surgeons in the trans-Atlantic slave trade can be unhelpful and distracting, but

I raised it in 2023 when speaking in the impressive Liverpool Town Hall, which was infamously built on the proceeds of slavery. Doctors worked on slave ships and plantations, ostensibly to safeguard the health of those who were enslaved. But, as we now know, aside from the morally indefensible enslavement itself, there was no prospect of the slaves' conditions being compatible with good health and wellbeing. While most doctors who witnessed those conditions would have accepted that, at least two, Alexander Falconbridge and James Arnold, wrote about their first-hand experiences, so that they could be used as powerful evidence against the trade. Our similarly compelling veterinary testimony, about how animals typically fare while being used by humans, should also be a powerful driver of social change, albeit that we are currently typically seeking improved conditions rather than abolition. The need for veterinary ethics to help navigate these contentious waters has never been greater.

REFERENCES

Bolotnikova M. The bitter civil war dividing American veterinarians. *Vox* [Internet]. 2023 Jan 4. Available from: https://www.vox.com/future-perfect/23516639/veterinarians-avma-factory-farming-ventilation-shutdown.

British Veterinary Association (BVA). Vets speaking up for animal welfare: BVA animal welfare strategy. *BVA Media* [Internet]. 2016 [cited 2024 Jun 28]. Available from: https://www.bva.co.uk/media/3124/bva-animal-welfare-strategy-final-version.pdf.

British Veterinary Association (BVA). BVA position on animal welfare. *BVA Media* [Internet]. 2021 Jul. Available from: https://www.bva.co.uk/media/4273/full-bva-position-on-animal-welfare.pdf.

British Veterinary Association (BVA) and Royal College of Veterinary Surgeons (RCVS). VetFutures: taking charge of our future: a vision for the veterinary profession for 2030. *VetFutures Resources* [Internet]. 2015 Nov 20. Available from: https://vetfutures.org.uk/resource/vet-futures-report/.

De Briyne N, Vidović J, Morton DB, et al. Evolution of the teaching of animal welfare science, ethics and law in European veterinary schools (2012–2019). *Animals (Basel)*. 2020;10(7):1238.

Dolby N. *Learning animals: curriculum, pedagogy and becoming a veterinarian*. 1st ed. London: Routledge; 2022.

Fédération Equestre Internationale (FEI). Public attitudes on the use of horses in sport: survey report. *Equine Wellbeing FEI Assets* [Internet]. 2022 Nov. Available from: https://equinewellbeing.fei.org/assets/documents/Results%20of%20General%20Public%20Survey%20-%20%20Equine%20Ethics%20and%20Wellbeing%20Commission%20Report%202022.pdf.

Federation of Veterinarians of Europe (FVE) [Internet]. AVMA-FVE-CVMA joint statement on the roles of veterinarians in promoting animal welfare (2020 Apr). *FVE Publications* [Internet]. 2020 Apr 30. Available from: https://fve.org/publications/avma-fve-cvma-joint-statement-on-the-roles-of-veterinarians-in-promoting-animal-welfare-april-2020/.

Federation of Veterinarians of Europe (FVE). Animal welfare strategy: the veterinary voice for Europe's animals. *FVE Publications* [Internet]. 2021 Nov 18. Available from: https://fve.org/publications/fve-animal-welfare-strategy-the-veterinary-voice-for-europes-animals/.

Hill D. Vet says kiwi farmers rate well on pig welfare. *New Zealand Herald* [Internet]. 2020 Aug 16. Available from: https://www.nzherald.co.nz/the-country/news/vet-says-kiwi-farmers-rate-well-on-pig-welfare/3QCT2R2TVXOQU3MXQF3OT3ZWYE/.

McCulloch S. Vets must be strong advocates for animal rights. *Vet Rec*. 2023;192(12):491.

Office International des Epizooties (OIE). OIE recommendations on the competencies of graduating veterinarians ('day 1 graduates') to assure national veterinary services of quality. *WOAH Uploads* [Internet]. 2012 May. Available from: https://www.woah.org/app/uploads/2021/03/dayone-b-ang-vc.pdf.

Parrish K. The profession has a duty to support its farmers. *Vet Rec*. 2020;186(6):192.

Rollin BE. *An introduction to veterinary medical ethics: theory and cases*. 2nd ed. Oxford: Blackwell Publishing; 2006.

Royal College of Veterinary Surgeons (RCVS). Code of professional conduct for veterinary surgeons. *RCVS Advice & Guidance* [Internet]. Undated [cited 2024 Jun 28]. Available from: https://www.rcvs.org.uk/news-and-views/news/new-codes-of-professional-conduct-launched/.

Singer P. *Animal liberation now: the definitive classic renewed*. 3rd ed. New York: Harper Perennial; 2023.

38 An Approach to Ethical Conflicts in Clinical Practice

Brennen McKenzie

Veterinarians have legal and ethical duties to both our patients and our clients. Often, the interests of these parties align, but when they do not, the clinician can face challenging ethical dilemmas.

There are no universal rules for solving these, and we must all use our own beliefs and values as foundations for our ethical judgements. However, we need not do so in a vacuum. The disciplines of ethics and psychology and the history of science and medicine offer us useful insight and instruction. Veterinary students should be given the opportunity to study and critically evaluate the lessons available from these domains.

We also can benefit from an explicit, systematic approach to balancing the interests of our patients and clients within the financial, legal, and logistical context of clinical practice. In this chapter, I suggest one such method for approaching ethical dilemmas based on my own experiences in clinical practice.

I believe we owe our clients kindness and compassion, but our primary responsibility is to promote and advocate for the best interests of our patients. We must use our experience and expertise to identify what patients need and our skills as communicators and doctors to meet those needs as best we can within the constraints imposed by each unique situation.

38.1 INTRODUCTION

Ethics can be an unsatisfying subject. Enormous quantities of ink have been passionately spilled over it for ages, and yet humans have never come to an enduring consensus on universal ethical principles. Such agreement as we do achieve is tenuous and transient, and disagreements about ethical precepts seem to cause more conflict than the lack of such precepts.

The general societal values and beliefs that underlie ethical reasoning also change significantly over time, altering the context which defines specific societal and economic roles, such as that of veterinarian. Veterinary medicine exemplifies this, having changed dramatically in response to shifts in cultural beliefs about animals.

An Approach to Ethical Conflicts in Clinical Practice

The concepts of animals as soulless mechanisms designed to serve specific utilitarian purposes in support of human needs, which is often how the historical view is characterised, may never have been absolute or universal, but such concepts were certainly more widespread than they are today. A society that relies on dogs for hunting and livestock guarding, or that depends on a few animal species for the majority of its food, or one that venerates the horse as an instrument of war, may well support some medical treatment for animals to preserve their ability to perform these roles. However, debates about the merits of chemotherapy or heart valve transplants for ageing dogs and cats are not going to happen in such societies.

Many of the ethical issues now discussed in our profession exist only because of a growing acceptance of a very different view of animals and their relationship to human society. While some species continue to be seen, or at least treated, as utilitarian objects producing food and raw materials, others are widely understood as sentient beings with interests and preferences that deserve to be respected. Healthcare for animals fulfilling a role as companions, or even children in some sense, is going to look very different and face different ethical issues from the care given to animals seen as sources of food, clothing, or labour.

As a general practice vet, I am nothing if not a pragmatist. My goal is to achieve the best medical outcome and the best quality of life possible for my patients while respecting the needs and interests of my clients and my colleagues. We are not all likely to interpret the interests of clients and patients in exactly the same way or even to agree on a complete set of foundational ethical principles, but I don't believe this is necessary for consideration of these subjects to be useful and productive. Discussion in itself can have some value in stimulating, and perhaps aligning, our thoughts and producing more intentional and systematic practices.

So I will wade a short way into the quagmire of veterinary medical ethics. Specifically, I want to talk about the dilemmas and conflicts that arise when vets and their clients have different perspectives on what is best for the animals in our care. An owner may reject treatment that the vet sees as vital to maintaining an acceptable quality of life for the pet. Or conversely, the owner may seek aggressive care that the vet sees as futile or doing more harm than good for the patient. Though the actions we take will depend on the specifics of each situation and must align with our personal ethical principles, I believe a systematic and informed method of thinking about such dilemmas can make these decisions less stressful and better serve the interests of all involved.

My hope is not to lay out a set of rules for every situation or to create a universal framework for ethical reasoning (if Kant couldn't do it, what chance do I have!). I aim only to familiarise veterinarians with some of the ways such issues have been framed in the more expansive domain of human medical ethics and share my thoughts and observations from 25 years of practice on one effective way to approach common ethical dilemmas.

38.2 GENERAL PRINCIPLES OF MEDICAL ETHICS

Veterinary medical ethics are often adapted from the approach dominant in human medicine at any given time. The most common broad principles cited as the basis for current human medical ethics are as follows (Beauchamp & Childress 2013):

- Autonomy – patients have the right to informed consent and to accept or reject treatment.
- Beneficence – doctors should act in the best interests and for the benefit of patients.
- Non-maleficence – doctors should endeavour not to cause harm or at least ensure treatments do more good than harm.
- Justice – all people should be treated equitably and fairly.

These principles are then elaborated into codes of ethics, such as those published by medical associations. Legal rules and government regulations constraining medical practice incorporate some of the concepts underlying medical ethics, though they also encode general societal moral and ethical standards, which can sometimes lead to conflict between professional ethical guidelines and the law. A prominent current example is the restriction of reproductive healthcare in the US, where the religious views of influential segments of society are encoded in laws that override the principles of patient autonomy and equal medical treatment for patients.

There are, of course, challenges in adapting human medical ethics to veterinary medicine. Even in the current cultural environment, in which pets are often felt to be family members with wants and needs that should be respected, the legal and economic context still identifies them firmly as property with no right to true autonomy.

Furthermore, animals are generally thought to lack the capacity to understand their own health and healthcare, and so they are not able to consent to nor allowed to reject medical treatment. Legally and cognitively, they cannot be granted autonomy in making healthcare decisions for themselves. Pets are very much still treated under the paternalistic model of medicine, where the authority of the caregiver outweighs the autonomy of the patient. This authority is legally and practically in the hands of the owner, rather than the veterinarian, which can set us at odds with our clients even when both parties want what is best for the patient.

Despite the status of our patients as property, most codes of ethics in veterinary medicine attempt to incorporate the principle of beneficence, making at least some reference to the primacy of the patient's best interests, though usually still identifying potentially competing interests as well:

- Australian Veterinary Association (2024):
  - '[Vets should] hold as a key concern, the health, welfare and respectful treatment of animals'.

- '[Vets should] ensure veterinary recommendations and decisions are based upon the health and welfare of the animal, the safety of the public, the needs of the client and the need to uphold the public trust vested in the veterinary profession'.
- American Veterinary Medical Association (AVMA) (2024):
  - 'A veterinarian shall be influenced only by the welfare of the patient, the needs of the client, the safety of the public, and the need to uphold the public trust vested in the veterinary profession'.
- Royal College of Veterinary Surgeons (RCVS) (2024):
  - 'Veterinary surgeons must make animal health and welfare their first consideration when attending to animals'.
  - 'Veterinary surgeons must be open and honest with clients and respect their needs and requirements'.

So we are supposed to centre the welfare of the patient while still respecting the needs of the client and society as a whole in a context in which the patient is the property of the client, who has the legal and economic control over all healthcare decisions. How hard could that be?

In practice, most vets and animal owners share the goal of doing what is in the best interests of the patient. Unfortunately, sometimes they can have very different understandings of what that entails. Owners may wish to employ treatments that clearly have no real value (e.g. homeopathy, energy medicine) or have only unproven safety and efficacy (e.g. most supplements and herbal remedies, acupuncture) (McKenzie 2019). Or they may wish to pursue aggressive medical treatment that is likely futile or has adverse effects that appear, from the clinician's perspective, to clearly outweigh the benefits (e.g. tertiary chemotherapy protocols in patients with advanced metastatic disease).

In some cases, intensive and invasive treatments commonly employed in human medicine but rarely used in veterinary patients may be sought (e.g. kidney or bone marrow transplantation, heart valve replacement), and this certainly presents challenges to all of the standard ethical principles – would the patients choose these treatments (autonomy), do they really provide meaningful benefit (beneficence), are the high risks and significant suffering involved justified (non-maleficence), and is this an appropriate way to utilise the very limited resources available for animal healthcare (justice)?

Often, these conflicts look quite different from the perspectives of the pet owner and the veterinary professional. Owners may strongly advocate for treatment and feel their vet has 'given up' when they suggest less aggressive intervention or even euthanasia. Or conversely, they may feel the vet doesn't appreciate the emotional, financial, and practical burden of a recommended treatment that seems to the owner unlikely to have a guaranteed or lasting benefit.

As an example, some of my clients have been surprised, even horrified, at my suggestion to treat cancer in their pets with chemotherapy despite the evidence that this can extend life and preserve wellbeing significantly in some cases. While some of this response may stem from misleading comparisons to the experience of human cancer patients, there are genuine and fair ethical questions about the use of chemotherapy in animals (Stephens 2019). On the other hand, other clients have demanded continued chemotherapy, or the use of implausible or experimental cancer treatments when it seemed clear to me that such therapy was futile and could only inflict and prolong the suffering of the patient.

Sometimes we forget that our perspective on medical treatment of patients is dramatically different from the perspective of our clients, whom we asked to authorise, fund, and participate in uncomfortable treatments for their pets that they may not fully understand. Yet we have an ethical responsibility to balance the needs of our patients and the goals and values of our clients, in the context of the scientific evidence and available interventions, as best we can despite such disparate perspectives.

38.2.1 Preserving Life Versus Relieving Suffering

Another guiding principle in human medicine is that the physician has a duty to preserve life. While relieving suffering is also part of the doctor's job, physicians often aren't given the option to prioritise relief of suffering over sustaining life. In many countries, despite the principle of autonomy, even patients are not permitted to choose the relief of suffering by active euthanasia, though sometimes they may be able to choose the withdrawal of life-sustaining treatment and the use of palliative care only.

In contrast, the option of euthanasia is routinely available in veterinary medicine. This is widely seen as serving the best interests of our patients, even though the availability of this option is a consequence of the status of our patients as property and a legacy of the religious distinction between humans as beings with souls and animals as inanimate.

This sets up another very familiar potential for conflict, between the interests and desires of the patient as perceived and expressed by the patient, the owner, and the veterinarian. What do we do if our client wants to euthanise a pet with a problem that we can effectively treat? Does it matter if their choice is based on financial constraints or on their personal beliefs, religious convictions, or simply a lack of interest in dealing with the issue? And how do we approach the client who refuses euthanasia even when there seems to us little comfort or joy left in life for the pet? Again, do their motivations matter?

While the specific choices we make in such situations depend on the unique circumstances of each case, and on our own beliefs and feelings, we should strive for at least a rational and consistent approach to these dilemmas.

38.3 AN APPROACH TO CLINICAL ETHICS?

Veterinarians have a range of views and perspectives based on their cultural and personal beliefs. They are also inevitably constrained by the legal and regulatory environment, the economic context in which they practise, and the beliefs of individual clients. In my view, a universal set of strong and specific ethical rules is no more achievable in veterinary medicine than it has proven to be in society at large.

What I believe we should strive for instead is to prepare individual vets to make ethical decisions in a thoughtful and informed way, and to encourage ongoing and effective communication about ethical issues within the profession and between veterinarians and the public. All prospective veterinarians should be taught about the history and evolution of human and veterinary medical ethics and required to discuss, debate, and critically evaluate the existing guidelines and laws applicable to veterinary practice.

Such subjects are currently given quite superficial treatment in most veterinary training programs, likely because of their controversial nature or because such material is seen as less important than didactic content directly related to the diagnosis and treatment of disease. However, just as the veterinary curriculum has changed in response to a recognition that vets must learn communication skills to do their job effectively, so it needs to change to support the core activity of primary care practice – making and communicating decisions in the complex context of the VCPR and the larger cultural and economic environment in which we must operate. Learning about ethics, cognitive psychology, and interpersonal communication is not a luxury but a necessary element of preparing us for our role as clinicians.

The burden of day-to-day ethical decision-making is inevitably on the individual vet, so our emphasis should be on preparation and practise for this. Guidelines are useful, but they can only provide a vague sense of what the professional community thinks about broad ethical principles, and often organisational guidelines may seem driven by legal or political considerations as much as by a desire to help clinicians in their daily practice.

This approach requires individual vets to intentionally and conscientiously integrate critical thinking about ethics into their work. Sadly, not every vet will do this. But without the expectation that this is a core part of our work, and without appropriate training and experience, vets are not going to be able to move from a reflexive, *ad hoc* approach to ethical issues to a more thoughtful and structured approach.

Evidence-based medicine is similar, in some ways, to this approach to clinical ethics. A common misconception about EBVM is that it is intended to be a rigid set of rules derived from population research and dictated to clinicians for how to manage patients. The reality is that EBVM is a method or a set of concepts and techniques that is meant to support more effective patient care by preparing individual clinicals to conscientiously and judiciously integrate scientific evidence with their own expertise and the goals and values of clients (Sackett et al. 1996). My view of clinical ethics is that it, too, should be a set of methods and principles that support thoughtful, explicit ethical reasoning and clear communication about ethical issues.

What follows, if I haven't already emphasised it sufficiently, is just my opinion. It is based on extensive study and two decades of experience as a clinician, but it is also rooted in my personal ethical beliefs. These reflect my inherent temperament and the culture I grew up and live in. You will very likely agree with some of what I say and disagree with some. My hope is that these ideas will be useful to you even, or perhaps especially, if you don't agree with them.

Regardless of what conclusion you finally reach in specific situations, the process can be more efficient, more thoughtful, and less painful if you have a method to work through such challenges.

My personal method involves these general steps, which I will elaborate here:

- What is best for the patient?
- What does the owner want, need, and believe about their pet's needs?
- What limitations are imposed by the context?
- What is the best approach to meet the needs of the patient within the limits set by the owner and general context?
- How will I know if this approach is 'good enough' now and in the future?
- What will I do if the patient's needs are not being adequately met?

38.3.1 What is Best for the Patient?

Today, most people accept that animals have sentience – a general awareness of their circumstances and the capacity to experience both positive feelings and suffering. Most would also agree that even the most intelligent species lack the cognitive capacity to understand their health and make decisions about their own care in the way most competent adult humans can. Many of the ethical dilemmas veterinarians face arise because we operate in the grey area between the extremes of treating animals as inanimate machines and seeing them as equivalent to human beings. We must decide for them what their interests are and what obligation we have to accommodate these.

The degree of moral obligation we impose on ourselves is often determined by the role particular animals play in human life. We may make some accommodations to reduce the suffering of production animals, but this is pretty minimal compared with the obligation most pet owners and companion animal vets feel to support the wellbeing or dogs and cats. The degree to which such differences are justifiable based on the different characteristics of these species is a subject for another day. As I am a companion animal vet, I will focus on issues that pertain to that category.

In deciding what is best for my patients, I assume that their interests include the following:

- Continued life
- Continued participation in experiences that are pleasurable
- Minimisation of physical and psychological suffering

'Psychological' may be a controversial word for some, but in my pre-veterinary career as a behavioural biologist working with primates, I became convinced that other mammals experience homologues of most of the primary emotions that humans experience – fear, joy, sadness, anger, anxiety, etc. The evidence of decades of behavioural science is pretty compelling that animals have desires and aversions, and it is difficult to argue that their wellbeing is not influenced as much by these as by physical discomfort and pleasure (Bekoff 2000).

Determining what is best for a particular patient, then, involves identifying the components of wellbeing for that individual. This may involve relatively objective measures, such as using validated clinical metrology instruments to assess pain, function, and quality of life (Fulmer et al. 2022; Schmutz et al. 2022; McKenzie & Chen 2022). The creation and improvement of more such instruments should be a priority in order to make clinical management more objective and effective. One responsibility I believe we do have is to make use of the most accurate and effective tools for assessing our patients' welfare, and I think clinicians should make a greater effort to consistently employ such instruments rather than relying solely on subjective owner perceptions and our brief interactions with patients to assess their wellbeing.

Subjective assessment, on the part of both the owner and the clinician, of course, is also a part of determining what is best for a particular patient. Owners are especially helpful in identifying the activities and experiences a specific patient most enjoys and in assessing the extent to which changes in these caused by health problems or medical treatments may be compromising quality of life.

What is best for patients is also informed by EBVM. Scientific evidence is the most effective way to assess the effectiveness and the risks of medical treatments, and this must be explicitly incorporated in the assessment of whether treatment truly serves the needs of the patient. Ineffective therapies can never serve the interests of patients, and they can diminish wellbeing, either directly through adverse effects or indirectly by fooling humans into believing they are working and interfering with the use of truly effective treatment.

Perhaps the most common ethical dilemma vets face is the tension between the interest in continued living and the interest in a favourable balance between positive and negative physical and psychological experiences, which we often call 'quality of life'.

Some owners are unable to truly see the extent to which their pets may be suffering, and they may refuse needed palliative care for this or other reasons. I once treated a dog with humeral osteosarcoma whose owner was firmly opposed to conventional, science-based medicine. Despite the herbal and homeopathic remedies she was using, it was clear to me that the patient was in significant pain. Yet the owner was shocked and offended at the suggestion that more pain control was needed because she truly believed her dog was not in pain. Her ideological commitment to a certain approach blinded her to the extent of her dog's suffering.

In a situation such as this, I believe we have a strong responsibility to advocate for the welfare of the patient, even if it means coming into conflict with the owner's views. Of course, to do so successfully means not alienating owners, and communications strategies have to be employed which are most likely to be effective at changing behaviour. However, the abdication of responsibility to engage, either because the dog is ultimately the owner's property or because we believe an attempt to change their views will be futile, does not seem an ethically sound approach.

Perhaps even more often, I have encountered owners who were cognisant of their pets' suffering but simply too emotionally invested to be able to abandon futile therapy, or perhaps opposed in principle to euthanasia. While I am a great admirer of the animal hospice and palliative care movement, one area in which I disagree with the consensus in that domain is the principle that vets must respect such decisions to the extent of not trying to influence owners to pursue euthanasia. While we may not be successful in such efforts, and we should always treat clients with kindness and respect, our role includes a perspective informed by knowledge and experience not directly available to our clients. We have a responsibility to share that perspective with them whether it readily aligns with their own or not.

Doing this effectively, and influencing clients in a way that supports the best interests of our patients, of course, begins with understanding and even empathising with the perspective of our clients, even if we may have a different view and even wish to shift their perspective closer to ours.

38.3.2 What does the Owner want, Need, and Believe about Their pet's Needs?

Understanding the owner's perspective on their pet's healthcare is important for two reasons: (1) the owner has their own interests, and vets have some ethical, legal, and fiduciary obligation to serve these as well as those of our patients, and (2) the owner is the ultimate decision-maker, and both understanding and responding to their perspective is necessary to achieve our goal of serving the interests of the patient.

There is debate in our profession about the extent of our obligations to owners. Some would argue that their interests are paramount, even above those of patients, because they legally own the patient and they pay the bill for veterinary care. The other extreme is that our obligation is only to meet the needs of the patient and that owners are, at best, a means to this end or, at worst, and impediment to it. My own perspective lies somewhere between these poles.

I do, of course, feel a general obligation as a human being to be kind to others and behave compassionately as far as I am able. And our clients often come to us at particularly trying moments in their lives, faced with the suffering of a family member they love. We are also often unaware of the larger context of our clients' lives, and many of them are experiencing the challenges of having a sick pet added to other sources of pain and stress in their lives. Acknowledging and accommodating the needs of clients is both ethically appropriate and pragmatically necessary.

However, I believe the primary responsibility of veterinarians is to the wellbeing of our patients. If we cannot effectively meet their needs, I don't believe we are fulfilling the purpose of our role. While we have ethical duties to our clients, our greater responsibility is to advocate for and promote the interests of the patient rather than the clients, both as a feature of our role and because our patients cannot advocate for their own interests. When the interests of patients and clients conflict, we must do what we can to promote what is best for our patients, and while we should be kind, we should also be clear and direct with clients and try to be as effective an advocate as possible for what our patients need.

I also believe that while owners provide critical information and insight necessary for understanding the interests of the patient, they lack the knowledge and experience that veterinarians have. Part of our responsibility is to make this knowledge and expertise available to owners, and this includes trying to correct mistaken beliefs and inaccurate understanding.

Some have argued that it is paternalistic to assume we can determine what is best for a patient better than their owner can, but I think this ignores the significance of our specialised training and knowledge. We should not be shy about telling owners what we believe to be true about the welfare of their pets and correcting misapprehensions they may have. That is, to a significant extent, why they come to us!

Effective communication is a key element in managing the tensions that can arise between our duty to our patients and the needs and views of their owners. The best way to understand the perspective of our clients and incorporate it into developing diagnostic and treatment plans is to ask! While the limited time available for most primary care consultations is a barrier, we cannot effectively meet a patient's needs without making the time and effort to understand how the owner perceives these and what constraints they may have on pursuing testing and treatment.

Direct discussion is the core of this effort, but there are also a few other tools available to us. The concept of caregiver burden is a key component of managing chronically ill human patients, and there is evidence that owners of seriously ill pets face financial, practical, and psychological burdens similar to those experienced by the caregivers of humans with chronic illness (Britton et al. 2018; Christiansen et al. 2013). A couple of clinical metrology instruments have been developed to assess this caregiver burden, and hopefully more will be available in the future (Spitznagel et al. 2019). These can aid us in assessing the capacity of our clients to accommodate various types of treatment we may wish to offer for their pets.

38.3.3 What Limitations are Imposed by the Context?

We do not live in a perfect world where the capacity and resources available to us, and our clients are infinite. The ideal medical treatment is of no use if it is unavailable, unaffordable, or impossible for the veterinarian or the client to employ.

I give a few examples here: Giving multiple doses of antivenin is a standard and critical component of treatment for rattlesnake envenomation, yet many of my clients cannot afford even a single vial, and often the local hospitals won't sell me one anyway. Chemotherapy is a very successful treatment for diffuse B-cell lymphoma in dogs, yet I can no longer offer it because changes in regulatory requirements have made it impossible for me to store and deliver the drugs in my hospital.

Intensive palliative care may ease suffering and improve quality of life for veterinary patients with terminal illnesses, yet the time and effort needed to do this effectively is beyond many clients and clinicians.

The list of situations in which a preferred treatment exists but cannot be used for a particular patient due to contextual limitations is nearly endless. Part of our ethical responsibility is to understand such limitations and to optimise the wellbeing of patients as best we can within them.

This may sometimes involve compromises in what we believe or have been taught is gold standard care. I have argued elsewhere in this book that there are situations in which general practitioners may be better able to provide better care for some patients than specialists. Certainly, the care provided by a GP is better than no care at all, which may be the alternative if referral is unavailable or unaffordable.

The concept of a spectrum of care is the centre of growing discussion, and it is a useful articulation of the need for veterinarians to adapt our treatment plans to the limitations imposed by context (Stull et al. 2018). An explicit, thoughtful, and evidence-based choice among available options for diagnosis and treatment is ethically superior to a rigid insistence on an unachievable, mythic gold standard. Rather than being made to feel bad about 'compromising' patient care, veterinarians should be trained to think about the spectrum of available and realistic care options in a systematic and evidence-informed way and to communicate this process and these options effectively to clients.

Making such decisions involves being informed and aware of evidence-based treatment options for conditions we commonly seen, as well as understanding limitations to the availability and accessibility of these treatments. These limitations may be related to the client, or they may stem from other elements of the overall context in which a specific case is managed. Being prepared to identify and discuss with our clients alternatives to any treatment that is not acceptable or appropriate, for whatever reason, is part of our responsibility. This preparation includes thinking about the ethical dimensions of various management approaches and any 'red lines' we may have about therapies that we feel are not appropriate to employ.

Once again, communication is critical to identifying and managing ethical decisions around the spectrum of care, particularly in understanding what limitations the client's circumstances or perspective may place on management options. There is a large space between automatic acquiescence to whatever the client initially demands or rejects and a rigid 'my way or the highway' approach to insisting on a perceived gold standard approach as the only option. The most ethically appropriate strategy will often lie between these poles.

38.3.4 What is the Best Approach to Meet the Needs of the Patient Within the Limits Set by the Owner and General Context?

This is the real heart of ethical decision-making in clinical practice. Integrating our medical understanding of the patient's condition, our professional and personal assessment of their needs, our understanding of the client's perspective, and

An Approach to Ethical Conflicts in Clinical Practice

our awareness of the contextual limitations on our treatment options into a plan that effectively meets the needs of the patient. The details of the process and the final plan will, of course, be unique to each patient. However, the tools we have already discussed, such as the methods of evidence-based medicine, effective client communication, and the concept of a spectrum of care, will be useful in all cases to support the best plan for each patient.

I can't tell you what the 'right' answer is for any given patient. However, you will be much better prepared to choose it if you have put in the work to think deeply about these issues, to develop a consistent approach, and to gain the necessary knowledge base and communication skills. Hopefully, you will also find the process of making such choices less stressful and unsatisfying.

38.3.5 It's a Circle, not a Point

Like many aspects of medicine, ethical clinical decision-making is an iterative process, not a single event (Figure 38.1). The needs of the patient, the capacity of the owner, the available treatments, and the contextual constraints all change over time, and we must be committed to regular, systematic re-evaluation of all of these elements. During each recapitulation of this process, we must apply the general

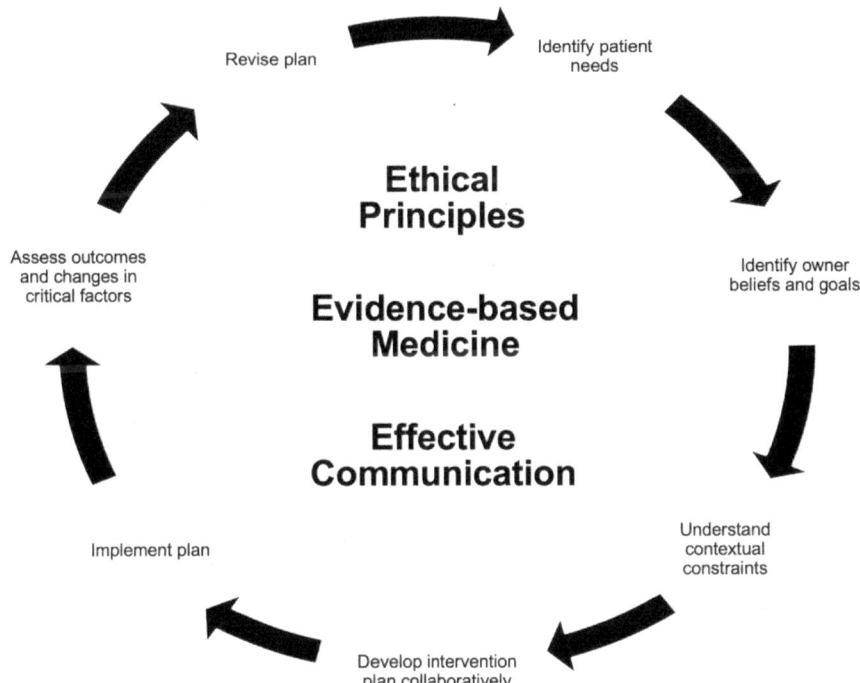

FIGURE 38.1 Process and key elements of ethical clinical decision-making.

principles that inform our individual ethical perspective and the techniques of evidence-based medicine and effective communication to ensure that we optimise the care for the patient as far as possible for that case.

In terms of patient needs, regular and explicit reassessment will involve ongoing communication with the owners, regular examinations, and re-evaluation as appropriate for the particular case, and ideally use of objective clinical metrology instruments to assess pain, quality of life, and other key aspects of wellbeing.

Similarly, regular communication with clients should include not only assessment of the patient but of the capacity and perspective of the owner. The failure of theoretically effective treatments often results from the inability of clients to effectively employ these treatments or a change in the owners' view of what they can or should be doing. If a treatment is unsustainable for the owner – financially, logistically, or psychologically – then it is no longer the best treatment for the patient, and alternatives on the spectrum of care should be evaluated.

With chronic or incurable conditions, the question 'Is this good enough?' should be asked early and often. Explicit discussion of quality of life and alternative approaches, including hospice or euthanasia, should be a regular part of patient assessment. Perhaps the most common source of ethical dilemmas for veterinarians is when the clinician and the owner have different answers to this question.

38.4 MANAGING CONFLICT AND DISAGREEMENTS ABOUT PATIENT CARE

There are many possible reasons for divergent perspectives on patient wellbeing and the merits of specific treatments. Veterinarians have a perspective on patients that is informed by extensive science-based knowledge and often by individual experience with prior patients. It is also a perspective that is less personal and laden with our own needs and emotions. This is an advantage in some ways. We are less likely than our clients, for example, to refuse to acknowledge the futility of medical treatment because of the personal need to maintain our relationship with a beloved family member. However, the personal relationship between an owner and their pet is also a critical element of the context in which we must make medical decisions, and we should acknowledge its importance even as we may try to shift the owner's view of the situation.

The relevance of our scientific knowledge to decisions about the best interests of patients cannot be overstated. While issues of ethics and values may be relative and contingent on each person's unique perspective, facts about the natural world have their own reality independent of what we believe or feel. And the scientific evidence concerning such facts is by far the most reliable guide to knowing them. A huge part of our value to clients is knowing things they do not know and having an approach to developing reliable knowledge founded in the long, successful history of science. For this reason, it is not only acceptable but ethically incumbent upon us to correct misconceptions or misperceptions owners have about their pets' health.

It is not inappropriate or disrespectful to help a client change a mistaken belief about the cause of their pets' medical problems or about the safety and efficacy of various medical treatments. It is not patronising or paternalistic to try and change a client's mind when such misconceptions lead them to make choices that do not truly support the wellbeing of their pets.

As I sometimes say to my own clients, 'You are not obligated to agree with my opinion or following my recommendation, but since you are paying me for them, I am obligated to give them to you whether you want them or not'. This is generally delivered with humour, and it centres the owner in a position of power, which makes unwelcome advice more palatable. Of course, the primary obligation to challenge owner misperceptions is not our financial dependence on the client; it is our duty to the welfare of the patient.

We may often be tempted to avoid conflict with clients, and it can be exhausting to feel like we are always having to battle against beliefs or practices which interfere with effective patient care and which often don't seem to change despite our best efforts. But the effort involved and the degree to which we succeed or fail do not seem to be all that relevant to whether or not we are obligated to try. If we have a clear understanding of what is best for the patient, we have a responsibility to promote that. The best response to the challenges we face in doing so is to try and get better at it!

Clinical practice is a wonderful place to grow and improve personally and professionally. Learning to listen better and to communicate more effectively, learning to adapt our style, and providing recommendations to best suit the context and the needs of patients and owners are as important as learning new surgical techniques or keeping up with the latest therapeutic options. It may not be as enjoyable or suited to our temperament for all of us as direct patient care, but helping our patients is our responsibility, and doing this effectively requires as much interpersonal skill as it does medical knowledge or surgical acumen.

My hope is that some of the tools and techniques I have discussed will make it a little bit easier for you to navigate some of the ethical challenges you encounter and successfully support the needs of your own patients and their human family.

REFERENCES

American Veterinary Medical Association (AVMA). Principles of veterinary medical ethics. *AVMA Policies* [Internet]. 2024[cited 2024 May 19]. Available from: https://www.avma.org/resources-tools/avma-policies/principles-veterinary-medical-ethics-avma.

Australian Veterinary Association (AVA). Members code of professional conduct. *AVA About* [Internet]. 2024 [cited 2024 May 19]. Available from: https://www.ava.com.au/about-us/code-of-professional-conduct/.

Beauchamp TL, Childress JF. *Principles of biomedical ethics*. 7th ed. Oxford: Oxford University Press; 2013.

Bekoff M. Animal emotions: exploring passionate natures: current interdisciplinary research provides compelling evidence that many animals experience such emotions as joy, fear, love, despair, and grief – we are not alone. *BioScience*. 2000;50(10):861–870.

Britton K, Galioto R, Tremont G, et al. Caregiving for a companion animal compared to a family member: burden and positive experiences in caregivers. *Front Vet Sci.* 2018;5:325.

Christiansen SB, Kristensen AT, Sandøe P, et al. Looking after chronically ill dogs: impacts on the caregiver's life. *Anthrozoös.* 2013;26(4):519–533.

Fulmer AE, Laven LJ, Hill KE. Quality of life measurement in dogs and cats: a scoping review of generic tools. *Animals (Basel).* 2022;12(3):400.

McKenzie BA. *Placebos for pets? The truth about alternative medicine in animals.* London: Ockham Publishing; 2019.

McKenzie BA, Chen FL. Assessment and management of declining physical function in aging dogs. *Top Companion Anim Med.* 2022;21(51):100732.

Royal College of Veterinary Surgeons (RCVS). Code of professional conduct. *RCVS Advice & Guidance* [Internet]. 2024 [cited 2024 May 19]. Available from: https://www.rcvs.org.uk/setting-standards/advice-and-guidance/code-of-professional-conduct-for-veterinary-surgeons/#:~:text=%22%20I%20PROMISE%20AND%20SOLEMNLY%20DECLARE,welfare%20of%20animals%20committed%20to.

Sackett DL, Rosenberg WM, Gray JA, et al. Evidence based medicine: what it is and what it isn't. *BMJ.* 1996;312(7023):71–72.

Schmutz A, Spofford N, Burghardt W, et al. Development and initial validation of a dog quality of life instrument. *Sci Rep.* 2022;12(1):12225.

Spitznagel MB, Mueller MK, Fraychak T, et al. Validation of an abbreviated instrument to assess veterinary client caregiver burden. *J Vet Intern Med.* 2019;33(3):1251–1259.

Stephens T. The use of chemotherapy to prolong the life of dogs suffering from cancer: the ethical dilemma. *Animals (Basel).* 2019;9(7):441.

Stull JW, Shelby JA, Bonnett BN, et al. Barriers and next steps to providing a spectrum of effective health care to companion animals. *J Am Vet Med Assoc.* 2018;253(11):1386–1389.

Index

A

acupuncture, 127
   and caregiver placebo, 40
   current evidence, 131–134, 143, 196–197
   definition, 139
   veterinary guidelines, 134, 140, 252
ageing, 29, 34, 69, 192–197, 199–200, 265
   dog ageing project, 100, 197–198
   geriatric zoo animals, 165
   process, 192–193, 198
   and rehabilitation, 196–197
alternative medicine, *see* complementary and alternative veterinary medicine
amphibians, 156, 165
amputation, 91, 208, 224, 261, 347
anaesthesia, 16, 47
   advancement of, 271
   local, 211, 277, 360
   in undergraduate education, 222
   zoo animals, 163
analgesia, 113, 195–196, 271, 273
animal
   behaviour, 317, 319–320
   rights, 31, 73, 189, 265, 319, 364
   sentience, 11, 22–23, 365
animal welfare
   assessment, 73, 162, 207, 361
   science, 22–23, 81, 358–362
anthropocentrism, 24, 266, 316, 320–322
anthropomorphism, 72, 266–267, 275, 315–325
anticipatory grief, 75, 207
arthritis, *see* osteoarthritis
autonomy
   beneficence, 262
   client, 71–75, 142–143, 257
   financial, 257, 260
   medical ethics, 26, 267, 370–372
   principle, 32–35, 76, 274, 324, 372
   veterinary ethics, 290

B

bedside manner, 215, 244
beneficence, 4, 32–35, 262–263, 370–371
best interests
   patient, 20, 27, 79–86, 260, 370, 380
best practice, 216, 248, 312
bias, 61, 241, 253
   clinical trials, 226
   cognitive, 38, 57, 135, 243–244, 253–254
   commission, 61, 252–253
   conflict of interest, 103
   publication, 39, 149
birds, 15, 162, 168, 336
blood tests, 61–62, 163
   cost of, 204
   preanaesthetic, 61–62, 64–65, 204–205
brachycephalic obstructive airway syndrome (BOAS), 187–191, 305
breeding, 207, 240, 360, 363
   laboratory mice, 173–174
   pedigree, 160, 183–190, 360
   zoos, 156–159, 163
burnout, 74, 236–243, 362

C

caregiver
   burden, 56, 75, 192, 241, 268–269, 322, 377
   placebo effect, 40, 72, 90, 149
chemotherapy, *see* oncology chemotherapy
chronic kidney disease, 56, 193, 329
climate change, 134, 340, 358, *see also* sustainability
clinical trials, 6, 90–95, 116, 121–122, 198, 225–227
Code of Professional Conduct, 104, 205, 288, 293
compassion fatigue, 242–243
complementary and alternative veterinary medicine, 127–145, 252, 382
   cannabidiol, 146, 150–151, 195
   chiropractic, 128–132, 138, 142
   herbal remedies, 132, 371
   homeopathy, 37, 127–132, 137–139, 145, 371
   supplements, 133–134, 146–148, 150–151
conflict of interest
   clinical research, 226–228
   ethical review, 103–105, 113
   overtreatment, 240, 244, 295
   pet food, 338
   pet insurance, 327, 349
   routine veterinary practice, 115
conservation, 32, 98, 100, 156–158, 167
contextualised care, 189, 247–257, 260, 262, 271–272

corporatisation, 24, 41, 60, 241, 294, 297, 304
costs of veterinary services, *see* financial costs
cranial cruciate ligament rupture, 92, 96, 234
crowdfunding, 5, 120, 268, 328
cruciate ligament repair
    cora-based levelling osteotomy (cblo), 89
    tibial plateau levelling osteotomy (TPLO), 50, 89, 92, 305
culture
    workplace, 243

D

Declaration of Helsinki (DoH), 92, 95
dental procedures, 56, 307–308
deontology, 32
depression, 30, 75, 248, 320
disease control, 12–13, 135
duty of care, 29, 172, 288, 293

E

emotional labour, 276
end-of-life care, *see* hospice care
ethical review
    AWERB (animal welfare and ethical review body), 105, 112–118, 124, 176, 226
    CERC (clinical ethical review committee), 227–228
    retrospective, 102
    VERC (veterinary ethical review committee), 226–228
ethology, 317–318
euthanasia, 10, 34, 120, 214, 227, 331, 372
    contextualised care, 260, 330
    fear of death, 267, 273
    methods, 14–16, 169
    withholding, 267, 271
evidence-based medicine
    definition of, 251, 271

F

fake news
    post-truth world, 36, 43
farming
    intensive, 101, 281
FDA, *see* Food and Drug Administration
financial
    burden, 73, 94
    incentives, 207, 296
    pressures, 83, 310
Five Freedoms, 22–23, 33, 162
Food and Drug Administration, 93, 150–151, 198
food
    production animals for, 98, 101

G

geriatric, *see* ageing
gold standard care, 13, 82–84, 225, 251, 271–272, 328–329

H

harm benefit analysis
    ethical review, 98, 110, 114, 176, 226, 228
    overtreatment, 80–81
hospice care, 208, 254, 267–268, 295, 331, 380, *see also* palliative care
    definition, 72
    oncology, 69–70
human medical ethics, 121, 369–370
human-animal conflicts, 319–320
humane endpoints, 5, 110–122, 176–177, 226, 267
humanisation
    of pets, 72, 131

I

informed consent, 64, 120, 214–216, 244, 370
    complementary and alternative medicine, 142–143
    discussions, 259–263
    gold standard care, 225
    for research, 94, 99, 198
insurance, 257, 294, 327–328, 349
intensive care, 77–82, 228, 240

K

killing humane, *see* euthanasia

L

lameness
    equine, 347–355

M

media, 23, 75, 208, 328, *see also* social media
moral
    distress, 10–17, 279
    obligations, 258, 266, 374
    reasoning, 289

Index

N

non-disclosure agreements (NDAs), 242
nurses
    veterinary, 228, 263, 270, 297

O

oath, 10, 21, 358
oncology, 69–75, 223–228
    chemotherapy, 69–73, 75–76, 377
osteoarthritis, 139, 149, 195
overdiagnosis, 6, 50–57, 225, 248, 295
    blood testing, 60–66
    reduction of, 51–52, 58, 230, 254
overtreatment, 5, 223–224, 257, 328
    clinical ethical review, 227–228
    definition, 273n2
    intensive care, 77, 80, 82–86
    reduction of, 58

P

pain, 4, 109, 118–119, 195, 259
    3Ps test, 268
    cancer, 71, 74
    farm animals, 360
    sentience, 30
palliative care, 72, 267–268, 326, 330–331, 375–376
    definition, 73
pedigree breeding, *see* breeding
pet food, 134, 146, 299, 337–339
pigs, 277–281, 363
placebo effects, 128, 131, 136, 144–145, 149, 382
population control
    zoo animals, 163
pre-anaesthetic testing, *see* blood tests pre-anaesthetic
predatory journals, 36–40

Q

quality of life assessment, 122, 194, 267

R

racing industry, 350–351
rats, 173–175, 239
refinement, 111–112, 176, 252, 321
regulatory oversight, 6, 189, 207
research
    biomedical, 25, 81, 166, 174, 178, 226
    clinical medical, 15, 78, 90, 167
    clinical veterinary (CVR), 92–95, 116, 122
    wildlife, 98, 100

risk-benefit analysis, *see* harm benefit analysis
routine veterinary practice (RVP), 26, 92–94, 104–105, 114–116, 268, 274

S

sentience, 10, 16–17, 21–26, 29–31, 168, 219
shareholders, 4, 27, 48, 83, 241, 297–299
slaughter, 11–16, 337, 357
social media, 48, 94, 120, 187, 208
    crowdfunding, 328
    public trust, 41
specialisation, 69–76, 78, 206, 223–224, 236
    credentials, 272
    human medicine, 234, 297
    palliative care, 331
    veterinary general practitioners, 231–235
spectrum of care
    definition of, 247, 251
suicide
    risk of for vets, 56, 59, 209, 249, 273–275
supervets, 3–9, 209, 266, 327
sustainability
    environmental, 339–340, 365

T

therapeutic misconception, 241

U

undergraduate education, 204, 222
utilitarianism, 25–33, 73, 98, 161

V

vaccinations, 306–307
    equine, 347
    Pet Club schemes, 311
veganism, 336
Veterinary Medicines Directorate (VMD), 93, 146

W

wild
    animals, 100, 132, 156, 359
    birds, 159, 163
World Health Organization, 37, 194

Z

zoo animals, 155